Clinical Manual of Sexual Disorders

T0176410

Clinical Manual of Sexual Disorders

Edited by

Richard Balon, M.D.

Professor, Department of Psychiatry and
Behavioral Neurosciences,
Wayne State University,
Detroit, Michigan

Robert Taylor Segraves, M.D., Ph.D.

Chair, Department of Psychiatry,
MetroHealth Medical Center; and
Case Western Reserve University,
Cleveland, Ohio

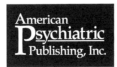

Washington, DC
London, England

If you would like to buy between 25 and 99 copies of this or any other APPI title, you are eligible for a 20% discount; please contact APPI Customer Service at appi@psych.org or 800-368-5777. If you wish to buy 100 or more copies of the same title, please e-mail us at bulksales@psych.org for a price quote.

Copyright © 2009 American Psychiatric Publishing, Inc.
ALL RIGHTS RESERVED

Printed in Canada on acid-free paper
13   12   11   10   09   5   4   3   2   1
First Edition

Typeset in Adobe's Formata and AGaramond.

American Psychiatric Publishing, Inc.
1000 Wilson Boulevard
Arlington, VA 22209-3901
www.appi.org

FSC
Mixed Sources
Product group from well-managed
forests and other controlled sources
Cert no. SW-COC-002358
www.fsc.org
© 1996 Forest Stewardship Council

Library of Congress Cataloging-in-Publication Data
Clinical manual of sexual disorders / edited by Richard Balon, Robert Taylor Segraves. — 1st ed.
    p. ; cm.
  Includes bibliographical references and index.
  ISBN 978-1-58562-338-9 (alk. paper)
  1. Psychosexual disorders—Handbooks, manuals, etc. 2. Sexual disorders—Handbooks, manuals, etc. 3. Psychotherapy patients—Sexual behavior—Handbooks, manuals, etc. I. Balon, Richard. II. Segraves, R. Taylor, 1941–
  [DNLM: 1. Sexual Dysfunctions, Psychological. 2. Sexual Dysfunction, Physiological. WM 611 C6409 2009]
  RC556.C575 2009
  616.85'83—dc22
                                     2009020934

British Library Cataloguing in Publication Data
A CIP record is available from the British Library.

I would like to thank my coeditor for all the wisdom, knowledge, patience, and encouragement he has provided to me and to the entire field over the years.

Richard Balon, M.D.

Contents

PART I

Assessment, Comorbidity, and Medication Effects

Melissa A. Farmer, B.A.
Alina Kao, B.A.
Yitzchak M. Binik, Ph.D.

Jeanne M. Lackamp, M.D.
Cynthia Osborne, M.S.W.
Thomas N. Wise, M.D.

PART III

Age-Related Sexual Issues

List of Tables

List of Figures

Contributors

Marc E. Agronin, M.D.
Associate Professor of Psychiatry, University of Miami Miller School of Medicine; Medical Director for Mental Health and Clinical Research, Miami Jewish Home and Hospital for the Aged, Miami, Florida

Richard Balon, M.D.
Professor, Department of Psychiatry and Behavioral Neurosciences, Wayne State University, Detroit, Michigan

Rosemary Basson, M.D., FRCP
Clinical Professor, Department of Psychiatry, and Associate Member, Department of Obstetrics and Gynaecology, University of British Columbia, Vancouver, British Columbia, Canada

Yitzchak M. Binik, Ph.D.
Professor, Department of Psychology, McGill University; Director, Sex and Couple Therapy Service, McGill University Health Centre, Montreal, Quebec, Canada

Miriam Boraz, Ph.D.
Staff Psychologist, Center for Marital and Sexual Health, Beachwood, Ohio

Lori A. Brotto, Ph.D.
Assistant Professor, Department of Obstetrics and Gynaecology, University of British Columbia, Vancouver, British Columbia, Canada

Anita H. Clayton, M.D.
David C. Wilson Professor of Psychiatry and Neurobehavioral Sciences, Professor of Clinical Obstetrics and Gynecology, University of Virginia, Charlottesville, Virginia

Leonard R. Derogatis, Ph.D.
Director, Center for Sexual Medicine at Sheppard Pratt; Associate Professor, Department of Psychiatry, School of Medicine, Johns Hopkins University, Baltimore, Maryland

Stacy Elliott, M.D.
Medical Director, BC Center for Sexual Medicine, Vancouver Coastal Health Authority; Clinical Professor, Departments of Psychiatry and Urological Sciences, Faculty of Medicine, University of British Columbia, Vancouver, Canada; International Collaboration On Repair Discoveries (ICORD), University of British Columbia, Vancouver, Canada

Melissa A. Farmer, B.A.
Doctoral Candidate, Department of Psychology, McGill University, Montreal, Quebec, Canada

David V. Hamilton, M.D., M.A.
Resident Physician, Department of Psychiatry and Neurobehavioral Sciences, University of Virginia, Charlottesville, Virginia

Samia Hasan, M.D.
Staff Psychiatrist, Center for Marital and Sexual Health, Beachwood, Ohio

Alina Kao, B.A.
Doctoral Candidate, Department of Psychology, McGill University, Montreal, Quebec, Canada

Jeanne M. Lackamp, M.D.
Assistant Professor, Department of Psychiatry, University Hospitals/Case Western Reserve University School of Medicine, Cleveland, Ohio

Stephen B. Levine, M.D.
Clinical Professor of Psychiatry, Case Western Reserve University School of Medicine, Cleveland, Ohio; Co-director, Center for Marital and Sexual Health, Beachwood, Ohio

Cynthia Osborne, M.S.W.
Department of Psychiatry and Behavioral Sciences, The Johns Hopkins University School of Medicine, Baltimore, Maryland

Derek C. Polonsky, M.D.
Clinical Instructor in Psychiatry, Harvard Medical School; Assistant Professor in Psychiatry, Tufts Medical School, Boston, Massachusetts; Private Practice, Brookline, Massachusetts

Alan Riley, M.Sc., M.B., B.S., MRCS, FFPM
Professor of Sexual Medicine, University of Central Lancashire, Preston, Lancashire, United Kingdom (retired); Consultant in Sexual Medicine, Lampeter, Wales, United Kingdom

Elizabeth Riley, B.Sc. (Hons)
Research Sex Therapist, Lampeter, Wales, United Kingdom

Robert Taylor Segraves, M.D., Ph.D.
Chair, Department of Psychiatry, MetroHealth Medical Center and Case Western Reserve University, Cleveland, Ohio

Rajeet Shrestha, M.D.
Resident, Department of Psychiatry, MetroHealth Medical Center, Cleveland, Ohio

Ronald Stevenson, M.D., FRCPC
Consultant Psychiatrist, BC Center for Sexual Medicine, Vancouver Coastal Health Authority; Associate Clinical Professor, Department of Psychiatry, Faculty of Medicine, University of British Columbia, Vancouver, Canada

Marcel D. Waldinger, M.D., Ph.D.
Neuropsychiatrist and Professor in Sexual Psychopharmacology, Department of Psychiatry and Neurosexology, Haga Hospital Leyenburg, The Hague, The Netherlands; and Section Psychopharmacology, Utrecht Institute of Pharmaceutical Sciences, Faculty of Beta Sciences, University of Utrecht, Utrecht, The Netherlands

Thomas N. Wise, M.D.

Professor, Department of Psychiatry and Behavioral Sciences, The Johns Hopkins University School of Medicine, Baltimore, Maryland; Chair, Department of Psychiatry, Inova Fairfax Hospital, Fairfax, Virginia

Jane S.T. Woo, M.A.

Doctoral Candidate, Department of Psychology, University of British Columbia, Vancouver, British Columbia, Canada

The following contributors to this book have indicated a financial interest in or other affiliation with a commercial supporter, a manufacturer of a commercial product, a provider of a commercial service, a nongovernmental organization, and/or a government agency, as listed below:

Marc E. Agronin, M.D. —*Speaker's bureau:* Forest (Namenda, Lexapro), Novartis (Exelon), Janssen (Risperdal Consta, Invega), Astra-Zeneca (Seroquel); *Research studies:* Forest, Elan, Eli Lilly, Lundbeck, Medivation, Merck, Teikoku, Wyeth.

Yitzchak M. Binik, Ph.D.—*Grant/Research support:* Canadian Institutes for Health Research and Pfizer Canada.

Anita H. Clayton, M.D.—*Grant support:* BioSante, Boehringer-Ingelheim, Bristol-Myers Squibb, Eli Lilly, GlaxoSmithKline, Novartis, Pfizer, Sanofi-Aventis, Wyeth; *Consultant/Advisory board:* Boehringer-Ingelheim, Bristol-Myers Squibb, Concert, Eli Lilly, Fabre-Kramer, GlaxoSmithKline, Novartis, Pfizer, PGxHealth, Sanofi-Aventis, Wyeth; *Speaker's bureau/Honorarium:* Eli Lilly, Pfizer, Wyeth; *Royalties/Copyright:* Ballantine Books/Random House, Guilford Publications, Healthcare Technology Systems.

Melissa A. Farmer, B.A.—*Grant support:* National Vulvodynia Association (nonprofit).

Stephen B. Levine, M.D.—*Grant support:* Palatur Technologies (investigator for study of bremalanotide for female sexual arousal disorder), Boehringer-Ingelheim (investigator for study of flibanserin for female HSSD), Johnson & Johnson (investigator for study of KJ lubricant for female sexual enhancement), and Procter & Gamble (investigator for study of safety testosterone patch for women).

Robert Taylor Segraves, M.D., Ph.D.—*Consultant:* Boehringer-Ingelheim, Eli Lilly.

Ronald Stevenson, M.D., FRCPC—*Research support:* Eli Lilly (member of panel developing physician CME on sexual disorders), *Speaker's bureau/Advisory board:* Bayer, Lilly, Pfizer, Paladin, Solvay.

The following authors have no competing interests to report:

Richard Balon, M.D.
Rosemary Basson, M.D., FRCP
Lori A. Brotto, Ph.D.
Leonard R. Derogatis, Ph.D.
David V. Hamilton, M.D., M.A.
Alina Kao, B.A.

Jeanne M. Lackamp, M.D.
Derek C. Polonsky, M.D.
Alan Riley, M.Sc., M.B., B.S., MRCS, FFPM
Rajeet Shrestha, M.D.
Marcel D. Waldinger, M.D., Ph.D.

Introduction

Robert Taylor Segraves, M.D., Ph.D.

Richard Balon, M.D.

Knowledge about the management of sexual disorders is important to the general psychiatrist for numerous reasons. Sexuality is an integral and important part of people's lives both in the general population and in psychiatric patients. Sexual health is important for one's well-being, and sexual enjoyment adds to quality of life at any age. Sexual expression can help define one's sense of personal competence, well-being, and masculinity or femininity, and it serves a large role in the expression of intimacy in interpersonal relationships. Conversely, sexual dysfunction can have adverse effects on one's sense of competence and well-being and on interpersonal bonding. Many people believe that an unhappy sex life can lead to numerous problems, including depression and marital breakup.

Only a minority of general psychiatrists in the United States specialize in the treatment of sexual disorders. In the remote and recent past, psychiatry as a field had a greater interest in human sexuality. Sexuality was a major focus in psychoanalytic psychotherapy. Sigmund Freud postulated that libido was one of the basic instincts. His work, including *Three Essays on the Theory of Sexuality* (Freud 1905/1953), was one of the triggers of psychiatry's interest in human sexuality and its importance for human development. Work of other pioneers, such as Havelock Ellis and Alfred Kinsey, brought a lot of attention and interest to the field, from both psychiatrists and the general public. Many psychiatrists became interested in the treatment of sexual disorders after publication of Masters and Johnson's *Human Sexual Response* (1966) and *Human Sexual Inadequacy* (1970). However, during the last several decades, various factors have led to a decreasing number of psychiatrists focusing on the treatment of sexual dysfunction:

- Many health insurance plans did not reimburse for the treatment of sexual disorders.
- The advent of managed care made the treatment of sexual disorders even less attractive financially.
- The field of psychiatry as a whole shifted away from the treatment of "problems in living" to the treatment of major psychiatric syndromes with a presumably strong biological basis.
- With the introduction of injectable intracavernosal preparations (e.g., alprostadil), and later of sildenafil and other phosphodiesterase inhibitors, most men with sexual dysfunction sought help from urologists and general practice physicians rather than psychiatrists.

Interestingly, the shift from treatment of "problems of living" and the lack of attention to them has led to perception of psychiatry as being less humanistic, or too medicalized (medicalization is preferred by some and detested by others in the field).

We feel that the recent heavy emphasis on biological aspects of management of various mental disorders, including sexual ones, constitutes a serious departure from the teaching and practice of clinical psychiatry in the past. Psychiatrists prided themselves on treating the "whole person," including all of the patient's ills and problems. Nowadays, psychiatrists treat mostly relatively narrow spectra of symptomatology. Issues such as a patient's sexuality or interpersonal relationship(s) are gradually disappearing from the repertoire of clinically oriented psychiatrists. We suspect that most young psychiatrists have not seen a couple for marital therapy or addressed their patients' sexual problems, other than those caused by medications. The teaching of human sexuality at medical schools is frequently limited and, at some schools, the subject is not even taught by psychiatrists. In our opinion, this is a sad state of affairs.

The shift to biology, the lack of training in psychological issues and in human sexuality, the lack of reimbursement for treatment of sexual dysfunction, and thus a lack of experience in the area of human sexuality may have led to another adverse consequence among psychiatrists: negative reactions when dealing with patients' sexuality. Because sexual disorders are not often seen in a general psychiatric practice nowadays, when they do present themselves they may evoke, in the psychiatrist who lacks clinical experience, intense reactions to the extremely intimate nature of the presented clinical material. Consequently, a psychiatrist may feel uneasy and view sexual matters as belonging to the patient's deeply personal realm and hesitate to inquire. Psychiatrists also may not know how to ask questions and may be concerned about showing their possible repugnance or excitement over the material being presented and inability to maintain neutrality. Managing one's countertransference in this situation may be difficult. Being aware of one's countertransferential feelings about patient's sexual problems, addressing them, and discussing them with colleagues or supervisors should become part of the comprehensive management of sexual dysfunction in clinical practice.

In spite of the shift from psychological to biological psychiatry and other mentioned issues, the recognition and treatment of sexual disorders remain important to a general psychiatric practice. Sexual problems have a high prevalence in the general population and a much higher prevalence in many psychiatric syndrome patient groups. Restoration of sexual function can improve the quality of life of many individuals with major psychiatric disorders, such as schizophrenia and bipolar disorder. Also, psychiatrists are becoming increasingly aware that many psychopharmacological agents cause sexual dysfunction and that this side effect may be an unspoken cause of treatment noncompliance.

A number of developments in the field of human sexuality are likely of interest to general psychiatrists. Knowledge is increasing concerning the prevalence of sexual dysfunction in major psychiatric syndromes, the psychopharmacological agents that are least likely to be associated with sexual side effects, and antidotes that are likely to reverse drug-induced sexual dysfunction. Other developments that should be of interest to general psychiatrists include psychopharmacological treatment of ejaculatory problems and optimization of treatment efficacy for erectile dysfunction by combining brief targeted psychological treatment with pharmacotherapy; the availability of the testosterone transdermal patch, which has been approved in the European Union, for the treatment of decreased libido in surgically postmenopausal women;

and investigations of a number of centrally active agents for the treatment of decreased libido in premenopausal women.

Also, a number of conceptual shifts have occurred within the field of human sexuality that may be of interest to the general psychiatrist. Conceptualization of the etiology of sexual disorders has been shifting in various ways: from an interpersonal to an individual model, and from a psychodynamic to a biological model. Many experts and therapists are questioning the relevance of the linear model of sexual response proposed by Masters and Johnson (1970) and Helen Kaplan (1974), and are advocating for the adoption of circular models of sexual responsiveness among women. In DSM-IV-TR (American Psychiatric Association 2000), a linear model of sexual response, in which desire precedes arousal and orgasm, has been adopted. Hypoactive sexual desire disorder is defined as an absence of desire for sexual activity and absence of sexual fantasies. Rosemary Basson (coauthor of Chapter 5, "Disorders of Sexual Desire and Subjective Arousal in Women," and Chapter 7, "Female Sexual Arousal Disorders," in this manual) and others have criticized this model, pointing out that many sexually functional women do not report sexual fantasies and may initially engage in sexual activity because of a desire for increased intimacy. Sexual arousal may precede sexual desire in such situations.

Cultural issues and factors in sexual dysfunction have been frequently mentioned in various textbooks and other publications. However, the research in this area has been scanty. We acknowledge that a culture and its values have a profound influence on its members' sexuality, and that the need for a clinician to be culturally competent is very important in the management of sexual dysfunction. Issues of culture and its impact on management of particular sexual dysfunctions may be discussed in individual chapters; however, very limited solid, clinically oriented data, beyond case reports and case studies, exist in this area. Nevertheless, although sexual dysfunctions are clearly present in all cultural, ethnic, and minority groups, the prevalence of sexual dysfunctions varies across cultures. Various cultures have different views and definitions of what is "normal" and what is deviant. Many cultures are predominantly male oriented and may ignore female sexuality. A male clinician with a male-oriented cultural background may find it extremely difficult to address the sexual problems of female patients. A culturally competent clinician should always consider the impact of culture when examining and treating patients from various cultures. Cultural stereotypes and biases should also be considered, explored, and addressed. Examples include views of human immunodeficiency virus (HIV) infection or homosexuality among some minorities. The clinician should not forget the impact of religion, religiosity, and spirituality on sexuality (e.g., that sex-negative cultures view sex as an act of procreation only and sex-positive cultures view sex also as a matter of pleasure and leisure). Treatment of sexual dysfunction in a couple in which partners are from different cultures may be especially difficult. Another important consideration is that psychological treatment modalities may be less acceptable or understandable for many members of non-Western cultures. We suggest that cultural issues need to be considered in evaluating and treating every patient with sexual dysfunction. Cultural formulation of cases of patients from different cultures may be particularly helpful.

Many psychiatrists in the area of human sexuality immediately recognize the relevance of the biopsychosocial model for the understanding and treatment of sexual dysfunction. This conceptual model allows the psychiatrist to incorporate biological and psychological interventions and to appreciate the importance of cultural factors in the expression of sexuality. This model has been a guiding principle for our manual and its chapters.

The goal of this edited text is to provide the general psychiatrist with a concise, clinically oriented guide to the management of sexual dysfunction. The reader may wonder why this clinical manual is organized as it is, why certain areas are covered and certain issues are not, and why we put together an international team of authors.

We conceptualize the text as being divided into three major parts. In Part I, "Assessment, Comorbidity, and Medication Effects," the first four chapters cover general areas relevant to the understanding of clinical aspects of human sexuality within the frame of psychiatry and to helping in integrating the rest of the volume into coherent clinical information useful for the management of sexual dysfunctions. In the first chapter the authors indicate that sexual dysfunctions are fairly common not only in the United States but around the globe. The second chapter presents the assessment of sexual function in clinical and research settings and should help the reader to understand the complexity of evaluating sexual functioning and all its facets. In the the following two chapters, the authors connect sexual disorders to the rest of clinical psychiatry and medicine; they discuss the complex comorbidity and coexistence of sexual dysfunction with various mental and physical illnesses, and the association of sexual dysfunction with numerous psychotropic and nonpsychotropic medications.

After the stage is set in Part I, the authors of the eight chapters of Part II, "Management of Sexual Disorders," review all major sexual dysfunctions. The chapter topics include management of female and male hyposexual disorders, female arousal disorder, male erectile disorder, female orgasmic disorders, delayed and premature ejaculation, dyspareunia, vaginismus, and paraphilias (which we consider to be dysfunction of "usual" human sexuality, as implied by the name *paraphilias*, which is derived from Greek and means "love beyond the usual"). To be relevant to the general psychiatrist, most chapters in this part are organized around diagnostic entities. We used DSM-IV-TR as a guide to determining the areas of sexual dysfunctions covered in this part. We believe that a clinically oriented management manual should be anchored in a meaningful nomenclature with which a clinically oriented psychiatrist is fairly familiar, and we hope that DSM-IV-TR is familiar if not to all then at least to many readers. The management of gender identity disorders is not included in this manual; we believe that the management of these disorders is beyond the scope of general psychiatric practice and should be referred to a specialist or a specialized institution. Thus, discussing anything beyond establishing the diagnosis of this disorder would be beyond the scope of this manual. Similarly, the fairly rare and easy-to-diagnose sexual aversion disorder is also not discussed in this manual; individuals with this disorder should be referred to a specialist for either individual therapy or sex therapy.

The final part of this manual, "Age-Related Sexual Issues," includes two chapters addressing management of sexual issues in children and adolescents and in elderly individuals. We believe that sexual issues in these two populations are very important, even for the clinician in general psychiatry practice. Many clinical psychiatrists are frequently faced with questions about what is and what is not "usual" or "normal" (whatever these words mean) in these areas and how to approach numerous issues regarding adolescent sexuality or sexuality in elderly patients. Both chapters are highly practical, clinically oriented, and pragmatic in their description of sexual problems in these populations.

We gathered a group of experts from various countries to address the topics covered in this manual. As we mentioned earlier, only a small number of psychiatrists in the United States devote their practice solely to the area of sexual dysfunction.

The field of human sexuality has undergone enormous development during the last several decades. Much of this development has unfortunately happened outside of psychiatry—in basic sciences, urology, obstetrics and gynecology, psychology, and other areas. Nevertheless, we believe that psychiatry is uniquely suited to be the central and unifying discipline in managing sexual dysfunctions. Psychiatrists, like all physicians, are trained in physiology, pharmacology, and other areas that are helpful in understanding the underpinnings of sexual functioning and its impairment. Psychiatrists are also trained in biological, psychological, and social aspects of mental disorders and dysfunctions, and therefore understand the biopsychosocial model that fits the area of sexual dysfunctions so well. They are also trained in various treatment modalities, both pharmacological and psychotherapeutic, used in the management of sexual dysfunctions. Last, but not least, they are trained to handle countertransference (transference), an issue of possible importance in the management of sexual dysfunction. Their education and training provide the best foundation for developing the most comprehensive management approach to sexual dysfunctions. Thus, we strongly believe that psychiatry should again bring the field of human sexuality within its purview. We hope that the *Clinical Manual of Sexual Disorders*, authored by specialists in the field of human sexuality and/or general psychiatry, will help the general psychiatrist in his or her management of sexual disorders.

References

American Psychiatric Association: Diagnostic and Statistical Manual of Mental Disorders, 4th Edition, Text Revision. Washington, DC, American Psychiatric Association, 2000

Freud S: Three essays on the theory of sexuality (1905), in Standard Edition of the Complete Psychological Works of Sigmund Freud, Vol 7. Translated and edited by Strachey J. London, Hogarth Press, 1953

Kaplan HS: The New Sex Therapy: Active Treatment of Sexual Dysfunctions. New York, Brunner/Mazel, 1974

Masters WH, Johnson V: Human Sexual Response. Boston, MA, Little, Brown, 1966

Masters WH, Johnson V: Human Sexual Inadequacy. Boston, MA, Little, Brown, 1970

PART I

Assessment, Comorbidity, and Medication Effects

Diagnosis, Epidemiology, and Course of Sexual Disorders

Rajeet Shrestha, M.D.

Robert Taylor Segraves, M.D., Ph.D.

In the last decade, research concerning the epidemiology of sexual problems has increased over the previous decades. Considerable evidence has shown that sexual disorders have a high prevalence in the general population and in certain psychiatric subpopulations. Research using varied methodology has been remarkably consistent in finding a high prevalence of sexual concerns in individuals in all countries studied. Studies have been less consistent, however, in identifying risk factors for sexual problems. The high prevalence of sexual concerns in the general population and in psychiatric patients indicates the importance of incorporating the identification and treatment of sexual concerns into psychiatric practices. Our purpose in this chapter is to briefly review the data concerning the prevalence of sexual difficulties in the general population, the correlates of these disorders, and major methodological issues that need to be considered when evaluating epidemiological data. Because this chapter is intended for the clinical psychiatrist, we focus on findings that may be of interest to a psychiatric practitioner.

Basic Methodological Issues

A basic knowledge of methodological issues is necessary for understanding the significance of the findings of various epidemiological studies. In epidemiological studies, a sample of a specified population is studied, and the data obtained from that sample are used to estimate population characteristics. Therefore, the sample selected for the study must indeed be representative of the population to which the results are generalized. For example, a study of the prevalence of sexual disorders in patients seen in a sample of psychiatric practices cannot be used to accurately estimate the prevalence of sexual disorders in the general population because sexual disorders may be more common in psychiatric populations than in the general population.

Probability sampling is employed to protect against bias in the process of sample selection and refers to the various methods of sample selection in which the probability of each element of the population being selected is known. However, no method of sampling the population is perfect. For example, in a large community-based study, some individuals may decide not to participate in the study. Selection bias might be introduced if the population refusing to respond is different in certain characteristics as a group from the population that responds to the study, in which case the respondent sample is nonrepresentative of the entire population. Increasing the sample size (or increasing the response rate) typically diminishes the selection bias.

Most epidemiological studies are cross-sectional—that is, the researchers attempt to study a cross-section of the population at a given time. Cross-sectional studies are employed more often than longitudinal studies (following a sample of the population over time) mainly because of time and cost considerations. Cross-sectional studies give information about the prevalence of a certain condition in the population (e.g., prevalence of erectile dysfunction) and the association between various factors of interest (e.g., the association between measures of depression and sexual complaints).

A prospective study is designed to examine the association of different factors over time. This approach would seem optimal for studying the association of age with the incidence of specific sexual disorders, but it has limitations. For example, if a study is conducted over 4 years, each year some individuals might decide to discontinue participation. Thus, bias may be introduced because the participating sample may differ in some significant way from the population of nonparticipants (and from the population the original sample was intended to represent).

Other important methodological issues include adequacy of the sample size, data collection method, quality of the data obtained, psychometric properties (reliability and validity) of the questionnaires employed, and response rate. Despite the great variation of research methodology across different studies of sexual dysfunctions, the major findings have been remarkably consistent across different cultures and time frames. Many seemingly inconsistent findings across different studies may actually be related to differences in ages sampled or in the way subjects were interviewed or the specific questions included. Another issue that is of particular relevance to studies of sexual disorders has been the epidemiological limitations of available nosological categories; this issue is discussed in the next section.

Definition and Classification

A major issue complicating the study of sexual dysfunctions is the absence of a set of commonly accepted operational definitions. According to DSM-IV-TR (American Psychiatric Association 2000), sexual dysfunction "is characterized by a disturbance in the processes that characterize the sexual response cycle or by pain associated with sexual intercourse" (p. 535). The diagnostic criteria consist of 1) persistent or recurrent symptoms in one of the four phases of the sexual response cycle (i.e., desire, excitement, orgasm, and resolution) that 2) cause "marked distress" and 3) are not better accounted for by another Axis I disorder or due exclusively to substance use or a general medical condition. DSM-IV-TR also provides for subtypes based on onset (lifelong vs. acquired), context (generalized vs. situational), and etiological factors (psychological vs. combined) associated with these symptoms. ICD-10 (World Health Organization 1992), states that sexual dysfunction "covers various ways in which an individual is unable to participate in a sexual relationship as he or she would wish" (p. 355). In contrast to DSM-IV-TR, ICD-10 does not mention distress in its definition of sexual dysfunctions.

DSM-IV-TR classifies sexual disorders based primarily on the first three phases of the sexual response cycle. Sexual disorders affecting the *desire phase* are hypoactive sexual desire disorder and sexual aversion disorder; those affecting the *excitement phase* are female sexual arousal disorder and male erectile disorder; and those involving the *orgasm phase* are female orgasmic disorder, male orgasmic disorder, and premature ejaculation. Dyspareunia and vaginismus are the sexual pain disorders. These primary sexual dysfunctions are diagnosed when they are significantly related etiologically to psychological factors. They are to be differentiated from substance-induced sexual dysfunction and sexual dysfunction due to a general medical condition, which are diagnosed when the symptoms are considered to be due exclusively to substance use or a general medical condition, respectively. Sexual dysfunctions that do not meet criteria for any of the above dysfunctions are categorized as sexual dysfunction not otherwise specified.

The definitions for sexual dysfunctions provided in DSM-IV-TR have been criticized by various investigators for a number of reasons. Because the diagnostic criteria do not specify frequency, severity, or duration required for diagnosis, distinguishing between minor sexual complaints and more serious dysfunctions is difficult. Sexual complaints are almost universal, often related to life stress or relationship issues; are usually transient; and typically remit without medical intervention. Sexual dysfunctions, on the other hand, tend to be more severe and persistent, and to require intervention. Graham and Bancroft (2007) argued eloquently for the need to differentiate minor sexual complaints from sexual dysfunctions. Some studies (Mercer et al. 2003) have found that most sexual complaints are of short duration (Segraves and Woodard 2006). Because DSM-IV-TR criteria for sexual dysfunctions do not specify the duration for which the symptoms need to be present to be diagnosed as a disorder, sexual complaints related to transient stress may be erroneously grouped together with disorders of longer duration.

Furthermore, DSM-IV-TR does not clarify what the words "persistent or recurrent" mean, thus leaving interpretation up to the individual clinician and thereby making the diagnostic process more arbitrary. For example, the DSM-IV-TR criteria for female orgasmic disorder include "persistent or recurrent delay in, or absence of, orgasm following a normal sexual excitement phase" (p. 549). If a woman enjoys sexual activity but reaches orgasm in only 30% of all sexual encounters, does she have the disorder? How long does this problem have to persist before it is diagnosed as a disorder or labeled as a case in an epidemiological study?

The diagnostic criteria for sexual dysfunctions in DSM-IV-TR have been criticized for being imprecise. This imprecision has important epidemiological implications. For example, the definition of premature ejaculation does not specify any time parameters and simply states that ejaculation must occur with minimal stimulation before the person wishes it. In one study, 13% of men diagnosed by expert clinicians as having premature ejaculation were found to have intravaginal ejaculatory latencies between 5 and 25 minutes in duration (Patrick et al. 2005). Clearly, the DSM-IV-TR criteria in practice are overinclusive when one realizes that multinational epidemiological studies have found that 97.5% of men in the general population have ejaculatory latencies of more than 1.5 minutes (Waldinger et al. 2005a, 2005b).

Similarly, the absence of specificity about severity or frequency in the criteria for sexual dysfunctions can give rise to misleading conclusions. Research by Laumann et al. (1994, 1999) has been quoted as finding that 43% of women in the United States have sexual dysfunction. In reality, this number included women with occasional, periodic, and frequent difficulties. If the estimate is limited to women with frequent complaints, the percentage of women having sexual dysfunction drops dramatically (Segraves and Woodard 2006). Other epidemiological studies have also found that the number of individuals complaining that sexual problems occur nearly all of the time was much lower than the number of individuals complaining of infrequent problems (Oberg et al. 2004). Investigators have also criticized the assumption of parallelism between male and female sexual disorders. Many of the suggested modifications will likely be incorporated in the upcoming DSM-V (Basson et al. 2000; Segraves et al. 2007).

Course

The discussion on the course of sexual dysfunctions is limited by lack of prospective studies. In general, situational disorders are more likely to be psychogenic in origin and are frequently episodic. These disorders may remit spontaneously under favorable circumstances. Generalized sexual disorders are more likely to be organic in etiology, and their course may be determined by the underlying pathological condition.

Mercer et al. (2003) showed that about 41% of women in their study reported lack of sexual interest lasting at least 1 month in the previous year, but only 10% of women had a persistent lack of sexual interest lasting at least 6 months in the previous year. Similar observations were made in the study for other sexual complaints of both men and women, which suggest that most sexual complaints may be of short duration. Similarly, other studies have found that most sexual problems are of short duration (Segraves and Woodard 2006).

Studies of Sexual Dysfunction in the General Population

The largest multinational, cross-sectional study of sexual behavior reported to date was the Global Study of Sexual Attitudes and Behavior (GSSAB) (Laumann et al. 2005; Nicolosi et al. 2004). This study involved 27,500 men and women ages 40–80 years in 29 countries; the individuals were grouped into seven clusters based on geographic region, cultural backgrounds, and data collection methods. A standard questionnaire was used, although sampling methods varied from country to country. The lack of a uniform sampling method across countries limits meaningful cross-cultural comparisons. Individuals were assessed for the presence of various sexual problems lasting at least 2 months within the previous 12 months. Severity was assessed by asking the respondents to stratify an affirmative response according to frequency of occurrence: *occasionally*, *sometimes*, or *frequently*. A number of variables that were likely to be associated with sexual problems were also studied. Those respondents who indicated having occasional sexual problems were not included in the analysis of prevalence rates or their association with various factors.

The worldwide prevalence of sexual dysfunctions occurring periodically or frequently has been estimated, from GSSAB data, at 38% for women and 29% for men. Women had a higher frequency of sexual problems than males in all seven clusters both individually and globally. Among women in the cluster containing North Americans, the prevalence of problems occurring at any frequency (and, in parentheses, the prevalence of problems occurring sometimes or frequently) were as follows: 32.9% (19.6%) for lack of sexual interest, 27.1% (18.7%) for lubrication difficulties, 25.2% (15.7%) for inability to reach orgasm, and 14.0% (8.1%) for pain during sex. Among the men in this cluster, the prevalence of problems occurring at any frequency (and, in parentheses, the prevalence of problems occurring sometimes or frequently) were as follows: 27.4% (15.7%) for early ejaculation, 20.6% (11.2%) for erectile difficulties, 17.6% (9.5%) for lack of sexual interest, and 14.5% (8.1%) for inability to reach orgasm at any frequency. A much lower percentage complained of frequent problems. For example, among men in this cluster, only 4.7% complained of frequent problems with early ejaculation, and those complaining of frequent problems with erectile difficulties, lack of sexual interest, and inability to reach orgasm were estimated at 4.5%, 2.7%, and 2.7%, respectively.

In most clusters, age was correlated with lubrication difficulties in women and with lack of interest, inability to reach orgasm, and erectile difficulties in men. Depression, financial problems, and relationship factors such as low expectations about the future of the relationship were also associated with different sexual problems for males and females. For the reader's convenience, GSSAB data concerning the prevalence of sexual problems in the Non-European West and in the United States are presented in Table 1–1. Findings of correlates of sexual problems from this study are summarized in Table 1–2.

Prevalence rates reported for North America in the GSSAB are similar overall to the results reported for other national population studies. The National Health and Social Life Survey (Laumann et al. 1994, 1999) contained data from a probability sample of the U.S. population ages 18–59 years. Again, lack of desire and difficulty achieving orgasm were the most common female complaints, and early climax, lack of interest, and erectile dysfunction were the most common male complaints. Problems with sexual desire and erection were related to age in males, whereas only problems with lubrication were related to age in women. A recent study of sexual function in men and women ages 57–85 years also found high prevalence of erectile dysfunction in men and problems with lubrication in women in this age group (Lindau et al. 2007).

Investigators in other countries have also found the prevalence of multiple sexual problems to increase with age in women (Hisasue et al. 2005; Safarinejad 2006). Decreased sexual desire with age in women has been reported in some but not all studies (Eplov et al. 2007). The prevalence of premature ejaculation has not been found to be age related.

Table 1–1.   Percentage of GSSAB study participants reporting that sexual problems occur sometimes or frequently

Sexual problem	Non-European West	United States
Males		
Early ejaculation	15.7	13
Erectile difficulties	11.2	10
Lack of sexual interest	9.5	6
Inability to reach orgasm	8.1	6
Females		
Lack of sexual interest	19.6	12
Lubrication difficulties	18.7	14
Inability to reach orgasm	15.7	12
Pain during sex	8.1	5

Note.   GSSAB = Global Study of Sexual Attitudes and Behavior.
Source.   Data from Laumann et al. 2005.

Longitudinal studies can be used to measure the differential effects of aging alone as opposed to specific age-related health events. The Melbourne Women's Midlife Health Project was a population-based longitudinal study of Australian women ages 45–55 years (Guthrie et al. 2004). Aging and relationship duration were both found to be associated with a decline in female sexual function. However, menopause itself was associated with an additional decrement in function, which appeared to be related to declining estradiol levels. The major factors influencing current sexual function were the prior level of sexual function and feelings toward the sexual partner (Dennerstein et al. 2005). Other studies have found that women with surgical menopause have even greater decrements in sexual function than women experiencing natural menopause (Dennerstein et al. 2006).

In general, health problems were found to be more highly correlated with male sexual problems than with female sexual concerns (Lewis et al. 2004). Longitudinal studies in males have shown clear associations between the development of erectile dysfunction and health and lifestyle factors such as obesity, lack of exercise, hyperlipidemia, and cigarette smoking (Rosen et al.

Table 1–2.   Correlates of sexual problems from GSSAB

	Men	Women
Increased age	Increased prevalence of erectile difficulties	Difficulty with lubrication
Depression	Erectile difficulties	Lack of sexual interest and lubrication difficulties
Interpersonal discord		Lack of sexual interest
Vascular diseases	Erectile difficulties	

Note.   GSSAB = Global Study of Sexual Attitudes and Behavior.
Source.   Data from Laumann et al. 2005.

2005). A number of other studies have also found positive correlations between the prevalence of erectile dysfunction and cigarette smoking (He et al. 2007), measures of depression (Low et al. 2006), medication usage, and markers of cardiovascular disease (Boyle 1999; Feldman et al. 1994). In the longitudinal Massachusetts Male Aging Study, scores indicating submissiveness on the Jackson Personality Research Form E predicted the later development of erectile dysfunction (Araujo et al. 2000).

The presence of female sexual distress has been correlated more often with measures of mental health and quality of relationships (Bancroft et al. 2003). Some evidence indicates that lifetime history of sexual abuse or assault may be related to an increased prevalence of sexual disorders in women (Fugl-Meyer and Fugl-Meyer 2006).

Psychopathology and Sexual Disorders

Sexual disorders frequently occur comorbidly with a number of psychiatric disorders. In a population study in Iceland, the lifetime prevalence of diagnosed sexual dysfunction was found to be 14.4%. Of those diagnosed as having a psychosexual disorder, 57% had a lifetime prevalence of another psychiatric disorder. The most common lifetime diagnosis was generalized anxiety disorder, but other disorders associated with sexual disorders included substance abuse and dependence, phobic disorders, dysthymia, and obsessive-compulsive disorder (Lindal and Stefansson 1993). Furthermore, a number of psychotropic medications are known to cause sexual side effects. Timely identification and management of coexisting or medication-induced sexual dysfunctions in psychiatric populations can have significant implications for quality of life and medication compliance issues. A brief review of sexual dysfunctions in psychiatric populations is offered here, and more detailed discussions follow in later chapters.

Depression has long been considered to be associated with impaired sexual function. Loss of libido is part of the constellation of symptoms characterizing depressive illness and may be one of the presenting symptoms. As mentioned in the preceding section, "Studies of Sexual Dysfunction in the General Population," epidemiological studies have found complaints of depression to be associated with loss of libido and erectile dysfunction. The Massachusetts Male Aging Study also showed that men with depressive symptoms were 1.82 times more likely to have erectile dysfunction than those without depressive symptoms (Araujo et al. 1998). A population-based study of depression in individuals ages 60 and older in Finland found that loss of libido was part of the depressive syndrome up to age 70 in females and in all ages in men (Kivela and Pahkala 1988).

Studies comparing patients diagnosed with depression and nondepressed control subjects have found that depression is associated with loss of libido. Casper et al. (1985) compared 132 patients hospitalized for depression with 80 patients without depression. An extensive battery of assessment instruments was utilized. Loss of libido was diagnosed in 72% of patients with unipolar depression and 77% of patients with bipolar disorder, but in only 5% of age- and sex-matched nondepressed control patients. Mathew and Weinman (1982) investigated the incidence of sexual dysfunction in 51 drug-free depressed outpatients and an age- and sex-matched control group. Feighner criteria for primary affective disorders (Feighner et al. 1972) were used to obtain a diagnostically homogeneous group. Loss of libido was noted in 31% of the depressed patients as opposed to 6% of the control group. Angst (1998), in a prospective cohort study, compared individuals ages 28–35 who scored high on questionnaire measures of depression versus those who had lower scores. Sexual problems were twice as common in patients diagnosed with depression than in those not depressed.

Kennedy et al. (1999) reported the results from a careful sexual interview of 134 patients with major depressive disorder not currently receiving antidepressant treatment. Although no control group was used for comparison, the findings are notable because 40% of patients reported no sexual activity in the preceding month and between 40% and 50% of patients reported decreased libido prior to starting treatment. Reynolds et al. (1988) compared the sexual function of men with depression, men with erectile dysfunction, and healthy control subjects and found that depressed men reported diminished thoughts about sex and decreased sexual activity. Another study found diminished nocturnal erections in men with depression (Thase et al. 1987).

Numerous clinicians, including Emil Kraepelin, Eugen Bleuler, and Wilhelm Mayer-Gross, have noted hypersexuality during manic episodes as well as decreased sexuality during depressive episodes. Studies have found increased libido, increased nudity, increased seductive behavior, increased frequency of sexual activity, unexplained promiscuity, and increased promiscuity during manic episodes (Goodwin and Jamison 1990). In addition, patients with bipolar disorder have been found to have more lifetime sexual partners than patients with unipolar depression (Spalt 1975). Many women report the increased sexual intensity experienced during hypomania to be an important and enjoyable change (Jamison et al. 1980).

A smaller number of studies have examined the frequency of sexual problems in patients with anxiety disorders, including posttraumatic stress disorder (PTSD), panic disorder, social phobia, and obsessive-compulsive disorder, and have produced evidence suggestive of a higher frequency of sexual problems in patients with these anxiety disorders. Kotler et al. (2000) found that patients with untreated PTSD had poorer sexual functioning than control subjects in the domains of desire, arousal, orgasm, activity, and satisfaction. Patients with PTSD who were also receiving selective serotonin reuptake inhibitors (SSRIs) had even greater impairment. Similar results were reported by Cosgrove et al. (2002); however, the fact that many of their subjects were being treated with SSRIs complicates the interpretation of their data.

A study of women with panic disorder or obsessive-compulsive disorder found a higher incidence of both hypoactive sexual desire disorder and sexual aversion disorder in these patients than in control subjects (Minnen and Kampman 2000). Another study found a high frequency of sexual aversion in both male and female patients with panic disorder (Figueira et al. 2001). Studies have not found a strong correlation between panic disorder and erectile dysfunction (Blumentals et al. 2004; Okulate et al. 2003). Aksaray et al.

(2001) found that sexual avoidance and anorgasmia were more common in women with obsessive-compulsive disorder than in women with generalized anxiety disorder. Fontenelle et al. (2007) found that patients with obsessive-compulsive disorder had less frequent effective erections and more difficulty achieving orgasms than did those with social phobia. Patients with social phobia have been found to have a high frequency of premature ejaculation (Figueira et al. 2001). Another study found a nonsignificant tendency for men with social phobia to have premature ejaculation as well as decreased frequency of orgasm. In general, patients of both sexes with social phobia tended to think about sex less often than did control subjects, and women with social phobia tended to have a decreased rate of sexual activity (Bodinger et al. 2002).

Although clinicians commonly observe sexual difficulties in patients with eating disorders, controlled studies relating to sexual problems in patients with eating disorders are limited. Available studies suggest the presence of a number of sexual difficulties in patients diagnosed with anorexia nervosa. In one study, women diagnosed with anorexia were more likely not to have had sexual intercourse, to have difficulties with orgasm, and to have low sexual desire compared with age- and education-matched controls (Raboch and Faltus 1991). Patients with anorexia have also been found to be less sexually active than patients with bulimia, and caloric intake and body mass index have been found to be related to sexual activity (Morgan et al. 1999; Wiederman et al. 1996).

A number of studies have found that patients diagnosed with schizophrenia have more sexual difficulties, including markedly decreased levels of sexual desire, less sexual satisfaction, and lower rates of orgasm, than psychiatrically healthy controls (Friedman and Harrison 1984; Kockott and Pfeiffer 1996; Lyketsos et al. 1983; Macdonald et al. 2003; Raboch 1984). Aizenberg et al. (1995) compared the sexual functions of three groups: patients with schizophrenia who were treated with antipsychotic medication, drug-free patients with schizophrenia, and a psychiatrically healthy control group. Sexual dysfunction was pervasive in both patient groups. An interesting finding in this study was that the patient group on antipsychotic medication had more desire for sexual activity than the drug-free patient group but at the cost of more difficulties with erection and ejaculation. Psychiatric conditions found to occur comorbidly with sexual disorders are summarized in Table 1–3.

Table 1–3.   Psychiatric comorbidity with sexual problems

Major depressive disorder

Social phobia

Obsessive-compulsive disorder

Generalized anxiety disorder

Posttraumatic stress disorder

Schizophrenia

Substance abuse and dependence

Bipolar disorder

Dysthymia

Eating disorders

Panic disorder

Although many clinicians suspect that a link exists between personality structure and sexual behavior, minimal systematic study has been done of this relationship. Some evidence of disturbed sexual function has been reported in patients diagnosed with borderline personality disorder. Patients with borderline personality disorder and a history of childhood sexual abuse appear to have a higher incidence of sexual difficulties (Zanarini et al 2003).

Conclusion

Sexual concerns are highly prevalent in all populations studied and tend to be more frequent in women than in men. Most sexual concerns appear to be of mild to moderate severity and of brief duration. The exact prevalence of sexual concerns that meet criteria for sexual disorders is unclear. Minimal epidemiological studies have been done of the prevalence of sexual disorders in psychiatric populations; however, the available evidence suggests that many psychiatric patient groups have an elevated prevalence of sexual disorders.

Key Points

- Sexual complaints are common in the general population.
- Females have more sexual complaints than do males.
- The most common female complaints include low sexual desire and difficulty achieving orgasm.
- The most common male complaints are premature ejaculation and erectile dysfunction.
- Female complaints of lack of lubrication and male complaints of erectile dysfunction increase with age.
- Exact estimates of the prevalence of sexual disorders in the general population are complicated by the lack of universally accepted operational definitions.
- A number of studies suggest that the incidence of sexual disorders is increased in many psychiatric subpopulations.
- An increased incidence of sexual dysfunction is reported in patients diagnosed with depression, generalized anxiety disorder, social phobia, obsessive-compulsive disorder, posttraumatic stress disorder, and schizophrenia.

References

Aizenberg D, Zemishlany Z, Dorfman-Etrog P, et al: Sexual dysfunction in male schizophrenic patients. J Clin Psychiatry 56:137–141, 1995

Aksaray G, Yelken B, Kaptanoglu C, et al: Sexuality in women with obsessive compulsive disorder. J Sex Marital Ther 27:273–277, 2001

American Psychiatric Association: Diagnostic and Statistical Manual of Mental Disorders, 4th Edition, Text Revision. Washington, DC, American Psychiatric Association, 2000

Angst J: Sexual problems in healthy and depressed persons. Int Clin Psychopharmacol 13 (suppl 6):S1–S4, 1998

Araujo AB, Durante R, Feldman HA, et al: The relationship between depressive symptoms and male erectile dysfunction: cross-sectional results from the Massachusetts Male Aging Study. Psychosom Med 60:458–465, 1998

Araujo AB, Johannes CB, Feldman HA, et al: Relation between psychosocial risk factors and incident erectile dysfunction: prospective results from the Massachusetts Male Aging Study. Am J Epidemiol 152:533–541, 2000

Bancroft J, Loftus J, Long JS: Distress about sex: a national survey of women in heterosexual relationships. Arch Sex Behav 32:193–208, 2003

Basson R, Berman J, Burnett A, et al: Report of the International Consensus Development Conference on Female Sexual Dysfunction: definition and classifications. J Urol 163:888–893, 2000

Blumentals WA, Gomez-Caminero A, Brown RR, et al: A case-control study of erectile dysfunction among men diagnosed with panic disorder. Int J Impot Res 16:299–302, 2004

Bodinger L, Hermesh H, Aizenberg D, et al: Sexual function and behavior in social phobia. J Clin Psychiatry 63:874–879, 2002

Boyle P: Epidemiology of erectile dysfunction, in Textbook of Erectile Dysfunction. Edited by Carson CC, Kirby RS, Goldstein I. Oxford, UK, Isis Medical Media, 1999, pp 15–24

Casper RC, Redmond DE Jr, Katz MM, et al: Somatic symptoms in primary affective disorder: presence and relationship to the classification of depression. Arch Gen Psychiatry 42:1098–1104, 1985

Cosgrove DJ, Gordon Z, Bernie JE, et al: Sexual dysfunction in combat veterans with post-traumatic stress disorder. Urology 60:881–884, 2002

Dennerstein L, Lehert P, Burger H: The relative effects of hormones and relationship factors on sexual function of women through the natural menopausal transition. Fertil Steril 84:174–180, 2005

Dennerstein L, Koochaki P, Barton I, et al: Hypoactive sexual desire disorder in menopausal women: a survey of Western European women. J Sex Med 3:212–222, 2006

Eplov L, Giraldi A, Davidsen M, et al: Sexual desire in a nationally representative Danish population. J Sex Med 4:47–56, 2007

Feighner JP, Robins E, Guze SB, et al: Diagnostic criteria for use in psychiatric research. Arch Gen Psychiatry 26:57–63, 1972

Feldman HA, Goldstein I, Hatzichristou DG, et al: Impotence and its medical and psychosocial correlates: results of the Massachusetts Male Aging Study. J Urol 151:54–61, 1994

Figueira I, Possidente E, Marques C, et al: Sexual dysfunction: a neglected complication of panic disorder and social phobia. Arch Sex Behav 30:369–377, 2001

Fontenelle LF, de Souza WF, de Menezes GB, et al: Sexual function and dysfunction in Brazilian patients with obsessive-compulsive disorder and social anxiety disorder. J Nerv Ment Dis 195:254–257, 2007

Friedman S, Harrison G: Sexual histories, attitudes, and behavior of schizophrenic and "normal" women. Arch Sex Behav 13:555–567, 1984

Fugl-Meyer A, Fugl-Meyer K: Prevalence data in Europe, in Women's Sexual Function and Dysfunction: Study, Diagnosis and Treatment. Edited by Goldstein I, Meston C, Davis S, et al. New York, Taylor & Francis, 2006, pp 34–41

Goodwin F, Jamison K: Manic-Depressive Illness. New York, Oxford University Press, 1990

Graham C, Bancroft J: Assessing the prevalence of female sexual dysfunction with surveys: what is feasible? in Women's Sexual Function and Dysfunction: Study, Diagnosis and Treatment. Edited by Goldstein I, Meston C, Davis S, et al. New York, Taylor & Francis, 2007, pp 520–562

Guthrie JR, Dennerstein L, Taffe JR, et al: The menopausal transition: a 9-year prospective population-based study. The Melbourne Women's Midlife Health Project. Climacteric 7:375–389, 2004

He J, Reynolds K, Chen J, et al: Cigarette smoking and erectile dysfunction among Chinese men without clinical vascular disease. Am J Epidemiol 166:803–809, 2007

Hisasue S, Kumamoto Y, Sato Y, et al: Prevalence of female sexual dysfunction symptoms and its relationship to quality of life: a Japanese female cohort study. Urology 65:143–148, 2005

Jamison KR, Gerner RH, Hammen C, et al: Clouds and silver linings: positive experiences associated with primary affective disorders. Am J Psychiatry 137:198–202, 1980

Kennedy SH, Dickens SE, Eisfeld BS, et al: Sexual dysfunction before antidepressant therapy in major depression. J Affect Disord 56:201–208, 1999

Kivela SL, Pahkala K: Clinician-rated symptoms and signs of depression in aged Finns. Int J Soc Psychiatry 34:274–284, 1988

Kockott G, Pfeiffer W: Sexual disorders in nonacute psychiatric outpatients. Compr Psychiatry 37:56–61, 1996

Kotler M, Cohen H, Aizenberg D, et al: Sexual dysfunction in male posttraumatic stress disorder patients. Psychother Psychosom 69:309–315, 2000

Laumann EO, Gagnon J, Michael RT, et al: The Social Organization of Sexuality: Sexual Practices in the United States. Chicago, IL, University of Chicago Press, 1994

Laumann EO, Paik A, Rosen RC: Sexual dysfunction in the United States: prevalence and predictors. JAMA 281:537–544, 1999

Laumann EO, Nicolosi A, Glasser DB, et al: Sexual problems among women and men aged 40–80 y: prevalence and correlates identified in the Global Study of Sexual Attitudes and Behaviors. Int J Impot Res 17:39–57, 2005

Lewis RW, Fugl-Meyer KS, Bosch R, et al: Epidemiology/risk factors of sexual dysfunction. J Sex Med 1:35–39, 2004

Lindal E, Stefansson JG: The lifetime prevalence of psychosexual dysfunction among 55- to 57-year-olds in Iceland. Soc Psychiatry Psychiatr Epidemiol 28:91–95, 1993

Lindau ST, Schumm LP, Laumann EO, et al: A study of sexuality and health among older adults in the United States. N Engl J Med 357:762–774, 2007

Low W, Khoo E, Tan H, et al: Depression, hormonal status and erectile dysfunction in the aging male: results from a community study in Malaysia. J Mens Health Gend 3:263–270, 2006

Lyketsos GC, Sakka P, Mailis A: The sexual adjustment of chronic schizophrenics: a preliminary study. Br J Psychiatry 143:376–382, 1983

Macdonald S, Halliday J, MacEwan T, et al: Nithsdale Schizophrenia Surveys 24: sexual dysfunction. Case-control study. Br J Psychiatry 182:50–56, 2003

Mathew RJ, Weinman ML: Sexual dysfunctions in depression. Arch Sex Behav 11:323–328, 1982

Mercer CH, Fenton KA, Johnson AM, et al: Sexual function problems and help seeking behavior in Britain: national probability sample survey. BMJ 327:426–427, 2003

Minnen A, Kampman M: The interaction between anxiety and sexual functioning: a controlled study of sexual functioning in women with anxiety disorders. Sexual and Relationship Therapy 15:47–57, 2000

Morgan JF, Lacey JH, Reid F: Anorexia nervosa: changes in sexuality during weight restoration. Psychosom Med 61:541–545, 1999

Nicolosi A, Laumann EO, Glasser DB, et al; Global Study of Sexual Attitudes and Behaviors Investigators' Group. Sexual behavior and sexual dysfunctions after age 40: the global study of sexual attitudes and behaviors. Urology 64: 991–997, 2004

Oberg K, Fugl-Meyer AR, Fugl-Meyer KS: On categorization and quantification of women's sexual dysfunctions: an epidemiological approach. Int J Impot Res 16:261–269, 2004

Okulate G, Olayinka O, Dogunro AS: Erectile dysfunction: prevalence and relationship to depression, alcohol abuse and panic disorder. Gen Hosp Psychiatry 25:209–213, 2003

Patrick DL, Althos SE, Pryor JL, et al: Premature ejaculation: an observational study of men and their partners. J Sex Med 2:358–367, 2005

Raboch J: The sexual development and life of female schizophrenic patients. Arch Sex Behav 13:341–349, 1984

Raboch J, Faltus F: Sexuality of women with anorexia nervosa. Acta Psychiatr Scand 84:9–11, 1991

Reynolds CF, Frank E, Thase ME, et al: Assessment of sexual function in depressed, impotent, and healthy men: factor analysis of a brief sexual function questionnaire for men. Psychiatry Res 24:231–250, 1988

Rosen RC, Wing R, Schneider S, et al: Epidemiology of erectile dysfunction: the role of medical comorbidities and lifestyle factors. Urol Clin North Am 32:403–417, 2005

Safarinejad MR: Female sexual dysfunction in a population-based study in Iran: prevalence and associated risk factors. Int J Impot Res 18:382–395, 2006

Segraves R, Woodard T: Female hypoactive sexual desire disorder: history and current status. J Sex Med 3:408–418, 2006

Segraves R, Balon R, Clayton A: Proposal for changes in diagnostic criteria for sexual dysfunctions. J Sex Med 4:567–580, 2007

Spalt L: Sexual behavior and affective disorders. Dis Nerv Syst 36:644–647, 1975

Thase ME, Reynolds CF, Jennings JR, et al: Do nocturnal penile tumescence recordings alter electroencephalographic sleep? Sleep 10:486–490, 1987

Waldinger MD, Quinn P, Dilleen M, et al: A multinational population survey of intravaginal ejaculation latency time. J Sex Med 2:492–497, 2005a

Waldinger MD, Zwinderman AH, Olivier B, et al: Proposal for a definition of lifelong premature ejaculation based on epidemiological stopwatch data. J Sex Med 2:498–507, 2005b

Wiederman MW, Pryor T, Morgan CD: The sexual experience of women diagnosed with anorexia nervosa or bulimia nervosa. Int J Eat Disord 19:109–118, 1996

World Health Organization: International Statistical Classification of Diseases and Related Health Problems, 10th Revision. Geneva, World Health Organization, 1992

Zanarini M, Parachini E, Frankenburg F, et al: Sexual relationship difficulties among borderline patients and Axis II comparison subjects. J Nerv Ment Dis 191:479–482, 2003

Recommended Readings

Kang J, Laumann E, Glasser D, et al: Worldwide prevalence and correlates, in Women's Sexual Function and Dysfunction: Study, Diagnosis and Treatment. Edited by Goldstein I, Meston C, Davis S, et al. New York, Taylor & Francis, 2006, pp 42–51

King M, Holt U, Nazareth Z: Women's view of their sexual difficulties: agreement and disagreement with clinical diagnosis. Arch Sex Behav 36:281–288, 2007

Nicolosi A, Buvat J, Glassr D, et al: Sexual behavior, sexual dysfunctions and related help seeking patterns in middle-aged and elderly Europeans: the global study of sexual attitudes and behaviors. World J Urol 24:423–428, 2006

Nicolosi A, Laumann E, Glaser D, et al: Sexual activity, sexual disorders and associated help-seeking behavior among mature adults in five Anglophone countries from the Global Survey of Sexual Attitudes and Behaviors (GSSAB). J Sex Marital Ther 32:331–342, 2006

2

Clinical Evaluation of Sexual Dysfunctions

Leonard R. Derogatis, Ph.D.

Richard Balon, M.D.

In the clinical context, an evaluation is typically an appraisal or assessment of an individual's health status, either generically or relative to some health domain or system. In the case of this text, the domain of interest is the individual's sexual functioning or sexual dysfunction. We define *evaluation* as a specified set of operations designed to examine and determine the state of an individual's health status, typically with the purpose(s) of defining a benchmark for status of functioning, conducting an assessment of morbidity (i.e., determining a diagnosis), or establishing a need for, or the optimal course of, a therapeutic intervention.

Evaluations of sexual dysfunction are of at least two different types: 1) those done for individual "clinical" purposes and 2) those done as part of a research protocol or trial. This distinction bears amplification because although there is definite overlap between the approaches to assessment employed in these two evaluative contexts, their perspectives, purposes, and goals are often quite dissimilar. Nevertheless, each type of evaluation can glean important information and ultimately benefit from the other.

The distinction between clinical and research evaluations of sexual dysfunction is also important because, traditionally, the techniques developed in a research modality are later transferred, often via a somewhat opaque translational process, into standard clinical practice. This being the case, we believe it is important to understand the nature and scope of the differences in the relative approaches to clinical evaluation in clinical versus research settings.

Clinical sexual evaluations focus on the nature and scope of an individual's sexual morbidity and are carried out within a broad overall health context. Patient medical, psychological, cultural, and/or relational complexities are factored into the assessment equation and resulting treatment recommendations. Therefore, clinical evaluations sometimes are of greater depth than research evaluations, although the sequential thorough follow-up evaluations built into typical research protocols are usually not part of the patient's routine clinical appraisal. The principal goal of most clinical evaluations is to determine the patient's sexual diagnosis and devise an optimal treatment regimen for his or her condition.

By contrast, the focus of research evaluations is typically on determining the presence or absence and the relative severity of a specified index condition in the patient. The condition and its treatment are typically the principal focus of the research program. Characteristically, a comprehensive baseline screening process rules out patients with comorbid conditions; prohibitive medications; laboratory values outside the normal range; medical histories positive for specific conditions (e.g., cancer, psychiatric disorders); and undesired physical, relational, or demographic status (e.g., body mass index>35, personal relationship impairment, age>70 years). Evaluations done as part of research protocols or trials are initiated at "baseline" and continued systematically throughout the course of the research study, although the baseline and final assessments are usually the most comprehensive. Evaluations for any treatment-emergent adverse events are added once treatment has been initiated. Research evaluations are typically bound by the context of the index condition and its treatment (i.e., they might focus on only one aspect of sexual functioning). Compared with a standard clinical sexual evaluation, the research sexual evaluation should be appreciated as having a relatively narrow focus and a highly defined sample of patients. However, the nature and sharp focus of the research evaluation may provide clinicians with guidance in their gathering of clinical information.

Although many of the same operations are involved in both research and clinical evaluations, the logistical and operational features of the assessments and their primary objectives are usually quite distinct. In research situations, the patient's diagnosis is usually specified a priori, as are the nature and dosage of any treatment being evaluated. Diagnosis is indicated by the protocol, with specific research or clinical criteria being provided, and the ultimate purpose of the evaluation is usually to help determine the efficacy and safety of a specified intervention in treating patients with the specific diagnosis in question. In clinical evaluations, examiners are usually working with patients de novo. Unless the individual is a patient in the clinician's practice, nothing is specified or known a priori except the patient's gender and presenting complaint. At the very least, in addition to a diagnostic interview (see Table 2–1 later in this chapter), a focused review of systems within the medical history and a comprehensive sexual history are necessary.

Regardless of whether an evaluation occurs within a clinical or research context, an examiner bases his or her conclusions on three fundamental sources of data: 1) clinical interview, including a review of systems; 2) psychometric assessment; and 3) physical examination, with or without laboratory assays and specialized tests. Most data in psychiatric evaluations derive from the first one or two sources, with occasional insights or clarification drawn from physical examinations and/or laboratory test results. In the sections that follow, we outline in some depth each of these evaluative resources and advance a paradigm for articulating the data developed from each source. Although some readers may be tempted to skip reading the research parts of this chapter, we encourage a careful reading of these parts to help sharpen clinical skills and possibly improve comprehension of scientific literature.

Clinical Interview

The clinical interview is the primary source of information about a patient's sexual functioning in clinical practice. This interview is extremely important in both clinical and research contexts; however, it is conducted somewhat differently in the two contexts.

Clinical Practice Interview

Patients seen in clinical practice may present with or without any previous screening information. When the patient is a regular patient of a health care provider, some critical information may be available either from previous examination(s) or from a wider data bank, such as electronic medical records and/or referral information (letter, notes). Also, some clinicians may routinely ask all patients (or certain types of patients) to complete standard questionnaires or self-rating scales (see "Psychometric Assessment" section later in this chapter) prior to the clinical interview. Clinicians may ask patients to complete these questionnaires or scales while in the waiting room or may mail these assessment instruments to patients to complete and return at their first appointment. The expectation is that these forms are reviewed with the patient during the clinical interview, either before the interview starts or preferably after the interview, during which time the information obtained during the interview and from the questionnaires or scales is compared and discussed. The clinician needs to realize that neither the clinical interview nor the psychometric evaluation can always be accepted at face value for various reasons (e.g., patient's hesitancy to talk about sexuality, Puritanism); therefore, comparing and discussing these two sources of information are likely to reveal the most useful set of information.

In clinical practice, the clinical evaluation never disqualifies the patient from participating in treatment, unless the evaluation leads to the discovery of a condition (e.g., acute hypertension, gynecological cancer) that takes precedence over the sexual problem and requires a more immediate intervention. Basically, the evaluation is designed to provide an ever-widening circle of accumulating evidence on health-related factors that, either together or independently, may represent feasible etiological factors regarding the patient's current condition.

Not all sexual problems meet the criteria for sexual *dysfunctions*; sometimes, patients experience sexual tribulations that do not qualify for formal diagnosis and are better characterized as sexual *difficulties*. For example, disagreements among partners concerning how often to have intercourse (given a reasonable normative range), or when during the day to have sex, or what positions or sexual activities to try, do not truly qualify as dysfunctions and are much more productively treated as difficulties. They reflect conflicting inclinations concerning sexual activities that are rooted not in pathophysiology or psychopathology but rather in differing personal preferences or behaviors. Invoking a medical model to try to address such issues has little value, because usually they can be resolved through negotiation between the partners involved. Occasionally, a clinician can communicate useful information or provide education in such instances, but the concept of *treatment* as such is not appropriate. The use of psychoeducation or counseling without a focus on treating dysfunction in cases like these is more appropriate.

An important consideration in working with patients is that etiological factors arising from numerous biological, psychological, interpersonal, and cultural origins can be operational in cases of sexual dysfunction. Furthermore, these factors do not necessarily operate independently or in a mutually exclusive manner. Rather, multiple factors usually contribute to any particular case of sexual dysfunction. A female sexual pain disorder with a basis in menopause-induced changes can give rise to a perception of "withholding" on the part of the male partner, which, if communicated, can induce anger and guilt in the female patient associated with the idea that she has failed to be "a good lover." Erectile dysfunction with origins in vascular endothelial lesions often presents with a secondary (ego-protective) manifestation of sexual disinterest, which can be interpreted by the female partner as evidence that the male has lost interest in her as a sexual partner. Arranged marriage may bring a host of culturally based sexual problems, as demonstrated in one of the cases later in this chapter. The point to be emphasized here is that even if the clinician can accurately identify a primary etiological agent in a particular case, it does not eliminate the possibility of corollary factors that need to be addressed.

In Figure 2–1, we have condensed the numerous potential sources that can have an etiological bearing on sexual functioning into three broad classes: biological, psychological, and interpersonal. In doing so, we are aware that influences from other spheres beyond these three can act causally relative to sexual dysfunction. However, we feel reasonably certain that the majority of causal agents are subsumed under these three broad categories and that more esoteric influences account for only a small proportion of the prevalence of sexual dysfunctions.

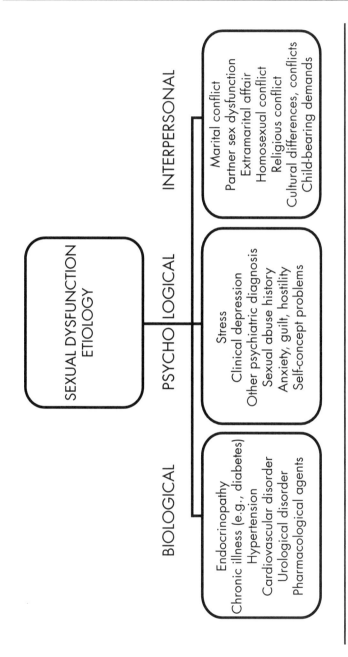

Figure 2–1.   Biological, psychological, and interpersonal factors that have etiological bearing on sexual dysfunction.

The first broad class of etiological causes outlined in Figure 2–1 is *biological.* An extremely large number of diseases, disorders, and biological derangements can act to impair sexual functioning. Causal agents include endocrinopathies, such as hyperprolactinemia and age-related hypogonadism; numerous chronic illnesses, such as diabetes and cardiovascular disorders; and medical conditions that directly affect the genital organs. In addition, a vast array of pharmacological agents, with selective serotonin reuptake inhibitors (SSRI) antidepressants and antihypertensives heading the list, possess the capacity to inhibit normal sexual functioning at every stage of the sexual response cycle. The potential magnitude of medication-induced dysfunction is underscored by the fact that the prevalence of sexual dysfunction associated with the SSRI antidepressants ranges from 35% to 65% (Clayton et al. 2002) (for further information, see Chapter 4, "Medications and Sexual Function and Dysfunction" in this manual). Whenever possible, the clinician needs to conduct a thorough physical examination and review of systems and take a careful history of medication use, paying particular attention to the temporal relationship between medication initiation and the onset of sexual symptoms. When present, biological etiologies tend to be primary in nature because they assault and undermine the fundamental biological matrix essential for the adequate performance of sexual behaviors. As we have emphasized, however, they are often not the sole etiological agent acting in any particular case.

The second main class of etiological precursors to sexual dysfunction is *psychological.* Stress (if it is of sufficient magnitude and duration), clinical depression, and other psychiatric disorders are all associated with precipitating sexual dysfunction. Of patients with clinical depression, 40%–50% have sexual dysfunction (Bonierbale et al. 2003). An individual does not have to be afflicted with a formal psychiatric disorder, however, for psychological factors to play a disruptive role in sexual function. Any strong negative affect state (e.g., anxiety, guilt, hostility) can be extremely disruptive to smooth, satisfying sexual function. Sex is most effortless when a person has a relaxed state of mind, whereas negative emotions distract the individual from integrating appropriate sexual cognitions and disrupt the smooth progression of sexual arousal from early, fleeting levels through high plateau and eventual orgasm. Often, such negative emotions are associated with chronic self-concept problems, in which the individual has heightened concern about some aspect of his or her physical or psychological person. Such conflicts can range widely, from concerns regarding physical adequacy and attractiveness (e.g., body image) to intrapsychic conflicts about fear of disease or pregnancy. The goal in the clinical interview is to ascertain that such conflicts exist, and treatment of such problems is often accomplished through referral to a specialist.

The final broad class of potential etiological agents in sexual dysfunction is termed *interpersonal* because they arise, for the most part, from conflicted interactions within the individual's interpersonal relationships. It goes without saying that such conflicts usually give rise to strong negative emotions. "Marital conflict" represents a more or less generic label for any of the hundreds, if not thousands, of controversies in which couples find themselves engaged from time to time. Usually, the sexual intimacy is disrupted not by the substantive aspect of the argument, but rather by the negative emotions that the partners harbor or direct at each other. At other times, the specific conflicted issue actually holds the disruptive potential. Conflicts revolving around extramarital liaisons or sexual disinterest arising from homosexual preferences are specific examples. In addition, child rearing may fall disproportionately to one or another parent, producing considerable dismay and resentment. Clinicians should also be sensitive to the possibility that a patient may not address a partner's sexual dysfunctions, often because of embarrassment or a misconstrued belief that the partner's dysfunction actually represents disinterest in the patient as a sexual partner.

Connected to both the psychological and interpersonal causes of sexual dysfunction are *cultural* factors. As Bullough (1976) pointed out, cultures can be sex positive (sex is viewed as life affirming and pleasurable) or sex negative (sex is considered an act of procreation only). Various cultures differ in their views of premarital sex (mostly forbidden, though frequently tolerated in men), masturbation (forbidden vs. tolerated or even encouraged), oral sex, or even some paraphilias (some cultures may tolerate some forms of zoophilia). Many cultures either ignore or view differently female sexuality and female participation in the sexual act (Bhugra and de Silva 2007). Thus, many members of these cultures may hesitate to bring their sexual partner for an evaluation of sexual problems.

The elements of a comprehensive clinical interview are summarized in Table 2–1.

Matrix for Interview With Focus on Sexual Dysfunction

The clinical interview with a focus on a possible sexual dysfunction can be conceptualized as a matrix of three sequential levels of questioning with the following goals:

> **Level 1:** Determine why the patient is seeing the clinician and what has prompted the visit or evaluation. Clarify whether the patient currently has or previously complained of sexual dysfunction. Partner questioning could be quite helpful at this level.

> **Level 2:** Determine the patient's sexual dysfunction(s) (e.g., hypoactive sexual desire disorder, erectile dysfunction). If the patient has more than one dysfunction, determine whether one can be identified as primary. Also, ascertain whether the dysfunction is transient, fluctuating, or permanent.

> **Level 3:** Seek information about the possible etiology of the patient's sexual dysfunction (e.g., marital discord, atherosclerosis, infection). Partner involvement could be also helpful at this level.

The clinician should also realize that a patient may present for an evaluation of problems or symptomatology seemingly unrelated to sexual issues, although issues related to sexual functioning may be underlying this symptomatology. Thorough questioning of sexual issues, as we emphasize frequently, should thus be part of any complete psychiatric evaluation.

Case Example 1

A 24-year-old woman is being evaluated for depression and anxiety. She reports that she has been stressed out about her husband because he "lost his business" and her parents "have always been really disapproving of him." She states that their marriage is good and that they "love each other very much." Later, when asked about her sexual functioning, she reveals that she has had sex with her husband only four or five times during the 6 months of their marriage. She admits that she has no desire to have sex, that she is not aroused during sex, and that she has never reached orgasm. She has never masturbated. Her husband was her first sexual partner. She has a complete aversion to any sexual activity and does not even like to have her breasts touched. She has been very distressed and depressed about the situation because she "loves her husband as a caring

Table 2–1.   Elements of a comprehensive clinical interview

1. Personal and general data	Age, marital status, having a sexual partner, being sexually active at present, sexual orientation, any recent change in sexual functioning
2. Reason for evaluation	Patient's vs. possible referral source's perception of reason for evaluation
3. Chief complaint in patient's own words	
4. Clarification/delineation of sexual dysfunction (see also section "Matrix for Interview With Focus on Sexual Dysfunction")	• Does patient have a sexual dysfunction or sexual difficulty? What dysfunction is it? • Do all parts of sexual cycle occur? What part of sexual cycle is afflicted (desire, arousal, libido, resolution)? • What are course, duration, and intensity/severity of the impairment? • Is existence of distress associated with the dysfunction? • What is frequency of the dysfunction (always, at times, influenced by stress)? • In which specific situations does the dysfunction occur (always, with regular partner only)? • Has sexual functioning changed over time? • Does patient masturbate? Does patient have any difficulties masturbating?
5. Sexual fantasies and dreams	• Does patient have sexual fantasies? If so, who is object of fantasies? • Does patient have sexual dreams or nightmares? If so, what is content and who is object? • Does patient have nocturnal ejaculations? • Does patient have recurrent dream themes? • Does patient have masturbation fantasies? • Does patient use books, magazines, or Internet for watching, masturbation, or stimulation?

Table 2–1. Elements of a comprehensive clinical interview *(continued)*

6. Interpersonal issues	• Is sex part of "love," romance, routine, or habit?
	• Who initiates sex? How is sex initiated?
	• What constitutes foreplay, and what is its quality and duration?
	• What are patient's and partner's preferences for type of sex (vaginal, oral, anal), position (missionary, on the top, etc.), techniques (manual stimulation, kissing of genitalia, mutual masturbation, etc.), and frequency, and what are the discrepancies between their preferences and expectations?
	• Is timing an issue (male coming too early or too late, orgasm at the same time)?
	• Is partner or couple involved in masochistic or sadistic practices?
	• What happens after sexual activity (spend any time together, demand for more sex from the partner, etc.)?
	• What is the relationship in general (marital discord, arguments, etc.)?
	• Does sex serve as any vehicle in interpersonal problems?
	• Does either partner avoid or feel aversion to sex?
	• Has patient had one (or repetitive) affairs outside of the relationship?
	• Does the dysfunction occur in that relationship? (If not, then it is not a true dysfunction, but an interpersonal problem.)
	• Does partner know of any affair and what is reaction to it?

Table 2–1. Elements of a comprehensive clinical interview (*continued*)

7. Developmental issues	• What was patient's age at first sexual experience?
	• What was type of first sexual experience (e.g., oral sex, mutual masturbation, vaginal sex, anal sex)?
	• Was the first experience voluntary or imposed (rape)?
	• What was patient's age at onset of menses or puberty, if known?
	• When and how was sexual knowledge acquired (parents, peers, school)?
	• Has patient had unusual sexual experiences?
	• What was the development of sexual orientation and identity?
8. Information about general mental and physical illness Include review of systems	Does patient have any of the following:
	• Presence of mental illness (depression, anxiety, psychosis)?
	• Presence of stress (problems with children, financial difficulties, job-related difficulties, family difficulties such as conflict with parents)?
	• Presence of physical illness (diabetes mellitus or other endocrine diseases; cardiovascular disease; sexually transmitted diseases such as genital herpes, gonorrhea, or HIV [also in partner?])?
	• Any pain during intercourse?
	• Is patient taking any medications (psychotropic medications, drugs for general medical conditions, over-the-counter preparations, medications for sexual difficulties previously prescribed) or herbal preparations?

Table 2–1. Elements of a comprehensive clinical interview *(continued)*

8. Information about general mental and physical illness *(continued)*	• Does patient abuse any substances (which substance, how much, how frequently, what impact on sexual functioning)?
	• Does patient use tobacco, alcohol, or caffeine?
	For males:
	• Does patient have morning erections?
	For females:
	• When was onset of menses? What is frequency?
	• Does patient have associated pain, cramping, or mood changes?
	• Is patient experiencing symptoms of menopause?
	For both:
	• What is method of contraception?
9. Cultural, moral, religious, and social values	• What is impact of patient's culture or ethnicity on sexuality?
	• What is impact of religious views (sex as a vehicle of procreation *vs.* sex as enjoyable activity with one's partner)?
	• What are religious attitudes toward contraception?
	• Do cultural and religious views influence patient's views of masturbation?
	• Do patient and partner differ in cultural, moral, religious, and social values?

Table 2–1.   Elements of a comprehensive clinical interview *(continued)*

10. Partner interview	• What are partner's views of relationship and of sexual dysfunction in question?
	• Do partner's views of sexuality and sexual functions differ from patient's views?
	• Does partner have difficulties (mental, physical, sexual) not revealed by patient (either due to lack of knowledge or out of respect/considerations of partner)?
	• Do partner and patient have cultural differences (e.g., arranged marriage)?
	• Do patient and partner accept each other's sexuality?

and loving husband." She further reveals that her lack of interest in sexual activity has become a source of tension in her relationship with her husband. Her sense of his disapproval of her as a wife and her fear of abandonment by him clearly are major precipitants of her anxiety and depressive symptoms.

This case demonstrates the importance of a thorough evaluation of all aspects of patient functioning because sexual functioning may be underlying other symptomatology.

Interviewing Tips

The interview should be semistructured yet tailored somewhat to the individual patient. The questions should be asked in a serious manner. The interviewer has to be comfortable about asking sex-related questions. The patient should be informed that some questions may not be completely comfortable and that if the patient feels uncomfortable, he or she should say so and refuse to answer (the interviewer may try to return to a topic later). The clinician should start with open-ended questioning and carefully listen to the patient's story and subsequently narrow the focus of questioning, following the cues. The questions need to be gradually more specific in all areas. General questions such as "How is your sex life?" are usually not very helpful. Questions should be specific to gender, sexual cycle (desire, arousal, orgasm, resolution), and dysfunction course. Examples of gender-specific questions include "Have you had any difficulties getting an erection during intercourse?" and "Are you lubricated enough during intercourse?" Questions related to sexual cycle include "Have you had problems reaching orgasm or ejaculating lately?" and "Has your sexual desire changed recently?" Examples of course-specific questions include "Does it take you too long to reach orgasm?" and "Do you or does your partner come too early?" Some examples of clinically oriented questions focused on sexual functioning are provided in Table 2–2.

Case Example 2

A 28-year-old physician who has been married for several months presents for an evaluation. He reports, "I have a problem with my sexual life. I have erectile dysfunction and may need Viagra." He further states, "We have not done anything sexually, really, yet. I come home from work, I am tired, I don't want to do anything. We try to have sex, nothing happens, so I just go to sleep." He claims that he gets an erection but that he cannot sustain a "good one" for

Table 2–2. Examples of clinically oriented questions about sexual functioning

General and introductory questions

1. I would like to ask you a few questions about your sex life now. I ask everybody about their sexual functioning during their initial evaluation, because I consider it to be a very important part of everybody's life.

2. Can you tell me whether you are satisfied with your sexual functioning? If not, why not?

3. How often do you have sex?

4. Is your partner satisfied with the frequency and quality of your sexual encounters?

5. Is your partner more or less inclined to have sex than you are? Is your partner more demanding about having sex? Is sex a source of any troubles in your relationship with your partner? If yes, why?

6. Who starts sex, you or your partner?

7. When did you start having sexual intercourse?

Questions about sexual desire/libido

1. Do you feel like having sex often?

2. Do you think about sex often?

3. Have there been any changes in your desire to have sex?

4. Do you feel that your partner has been more demanding of sex lately?

5. Are there any situations or things that increase your desire to have sex?

Questions about arousal/erection

For both genders:

1. Do you get easily aroused by your partner?

2. Do you get aroused by your partner even without any desire to have sex?

3. Have you observed any change in being aroused lately?

For women:

1. Do you get wet easily?

2. Have you had any problems with your lubrication lately?

3. Do you need more stimulation lately?

4. Do you think you are getting lubricated enough during intercourse?

Table 2–2. Examples of clinically oriented questions about sexual functioning *(continued)*

Questions about arousal/erection *(continued)*

For men:

1. Have you had any changes in getting hard or having an erection lately?

2. Are you getting hard enough during intercourse?

3. Are you having erections when you wake up?

4. Do you masturbate? If yes, are your erections easier or harder during masturbation than during intercourse?

Questions about orgasm

1. Do you have any difficulties reaching orgasm?

2. Do you reach orgasm at all?

3. Do you reach orgasm every time when having sex?

4. Do you need any additional stimulation to reach orgasm or to ejaculate?

5. Does it take you more time to come lately?

6. Do you have any pain during orgasm or ejaculation?

7. Does it take your partner too long to reach orgasm?

For women:

8. Does your partner reach orgasm too quickly?

Additional questions

1. Have you ever masturbated?

2. Do you masturbate now, in addition to having sex with your partner?

3. What (or whom) do you think about when masturbating?

4. Do you or your partner use any devices, such as a vibrator?

5. Do you have sex with anybody else? Do you find it more enjoyable than having sex with your partner?

6. Have you had sex with person(s) of the same sex? If yes, do you consider yourself heterosexual, bisexual, or homosexual? Does your partner know?

7. Have you ever been sexually abused?

a long enough time. He explains that he attempts to "enter" his wife but cannot, and then his erection slowly goes away. When asked whether his wife is relaxed and lubricated enough, he claims that she may not be lubricated and that she may have some pain, and may even be constricted. He claims that he wears condoms so he cannot feel whether she is lubricated. He states that "we almost did it once; I was in a little bit."

The patient has never been sexually active with anybody else; his wife is his first sexual partner. He states that he had spontaneous or manually evoked erections before marriage, but "not for a long time." He admits that he used to masturbate watching movies almost daily, and ejaculation occurred without any problems. He states that he becomes aroused by heterosexual scenes and denies any homosexual contacts or any fantasies. He still masturbates frequently.

His marriage was arranged, although he had known his wife for 18 months before marriage.

He denies depression, anxiety, suicidal or homicidal ideation, obsessions, or compulsions. He says that he is tired, he sleeps well, and his appetite is good. He works hard but does not feel unusually stressed at work. His wife only recently fully moved in; she spent some time with her family after their wedding.

The patient has never been seriously ill and has not had any surgeries. He does not take any medication. He denies use of drugs, alcohol, tobacco, or coffee.

Interview with wife (with patient in the room): Wife expressed unhappiness with their sexual life; she actually pressed the patient to get evaluated. She thinks that the husband does not pay enough attention to her needs. She claimed that during intimate moments, he sometimes gets up and goes to surf the Internet and comes back. "He watches TV while kissing me." She claimed that she has always been ready to have sex. She claimed to be lubricated, "but he does not know whether I am lubricated or not; he does not want to touch me there." She claimed that the reason they have had no vaginal intercourse is that "he does not want me to touch him and thus I cannot guide him to get inside," so he has been actually pressing his penis against her mons veneris or labia until the erection gets weaker. They have not tried oral sex or mutual masturbation.

This case demonstrates four important points regarding a clinical interview:

1. The importance of thorough, specific questioning and of following cues (e.g., to investigate why the patient was not able to maintain an erection)
2. The value of not assuming anything (e.g., that a physician who is also a patient knows what to do)

3. The importance of interviewing the partner (e.g., to gain more specific information about the patient's attitude toward his wife, her readiness, and her needs)

4. The significant role of cultural factors in sexual functioning (e.g., the fact that this marriage was arranged may have played some role in the couple's relationship and readiness to have sex)

Clinical Research Interview

In research trials, the so-called interview is almost always a series of interviews, usually done by different members of the research team to establish and verify each patient's status and qualification for the study being conducted. An initial screening interview, typically done by phone, frequently serves as a gross filter to establish certain patient characteristics (e.g., age, gender, education, marital status, length of relationship) and to confirm whether the patient does or does not meet study requisites (e.g., presence of inclusion criteria, absence of exclusionary characteristics). In subsequent in-person interviews, team members verify the data determined from the screening interview and establish certain patient physical parameters, such as height, weight, body mass index, blood pressure, medical history, drug history, and current health status. Usually, a sexual medicine expert then does a diagnostic interview to verify that the patient has the index condition and is free of any comorbid manifestations that might disqualify the patient from the study. Laboratory specimens are also collected at this time to be evaluated as further evidence of the patient's qualifications for entry into the study. Essentially, the research interview is conducted with the purpose of establishing that the patient indeed has the index condition of the study, meets all other study criteria, and is free of any medical, psychiatric, or sexual history or current condition that would prohibit him or her from study participation.

Psychometric Assessment

Psychometric assessment is an important source of potential information about a patient's sexual functioning. Psychometric assessment may take the form of self-report inventories, clinical rating scales, or structured interviews. Regardless of the particular measurement modality, all assessments are designed to enable the clinician to quantify the patient's report, usually across multiple domains or dimensions of sexual functioning (e.g., sexual desire, sexual arousal, orgasm), and some of these measures are used to generate an overall or aggregate sexual functioning score.

Because the tenets of psychological measurement are somewhat arcane and poorly understood, such measures are sometimes misconstrued as being "soft" or unscientific, a disapprobation that is clearly unwarranted in the case of *validated* psychological instruments. The design of such measures is as much governed by the laws of science as is the development of any form of physical measurement. The limitation of psychometrics has to do with its *precision*, not its science, primarily because psychometrics is predominantly used to quantify hypothetical constructs (e.g., sexual desire, depression, anxiety) instead of physical variables (e.g., weight, distance), using scales that are not as precise as those used with physical variables (Nunnally 1978). The validation of psychological measures is accomplished via a highly prescribed set of operations and stages. The validation process also tends to be programmatic in nature, constantly redefining and expanding, via evidence-based studies, the validation statement for each instrument (Derogatis and Laban 1998).

Most measures used to accomplish psychological assessment are self-report inventories, although structured interviews are sometimes employed. Self-report scales tend to be brief, inexpensive, and easy to use, and may be administered by nurses, technicians, or administrative personnel. Little or no specialized orientation or training is required to administer and process these measures, and many of them come with actuarial criteria to facilitate interpreting scores. In clinical research trials, self-report inventories are typically used as primary and secondary outcomes measures. In the context of clinical assessment, they are regularly used in primary care as screening devices for sexual dysfunction and in more specialized contexts as an additional mechanism to help understand the nature and magnitude of patients' sexual problems.

Specific Measures of Sexual Function

In this section and through the summary in Tables 2–3 and 2–4, we provide information on 11 contemporary instruments designed to assess and quantify the quality of an individual's sexual functioning. We have included the Female Sexual Distress Scale and its revision (FSDS/FSDS-R; Derogatis et al. 2002, 2008), which, although not strictly speaking a measure of sexual function or dysfunction, has become something of a standard in the field. The

FSDS/FSDS-R is a unidimensional measure of *sexually related personal distress* among women, the presence of which must be established before a diagnosis can be assigned using DSM-IV-TR (American Psychiatric Association 2000). All of the measures reviewed have been created relatively recently, with the majority having been developed and validated during the past decade. These instruments vary in terms of measurement modality, breadth of assessment, and gender relevance; however, all have accommodated themselves well against established psychometric criteria and have sound empirical evidence of reliability and validity. As explained later, none of these measures is a strictly diagnostic instrument of any particular sexual dysfunction. An important caveat is that none of these measures can replace the clinician's open, frank discussion of sexual issues with the patient.

The Arizona Sexual Experience Scale (ASEX) is a very brief, five-item self-report inventory that utilizes 6-point Likert scales for patients to record their sexual status. The scale was developed by McGahuey et al. (2000) to provide a mechanism for the rapid assessment of sexual functioning in patients being administered psychotropic drugs. The ASEX reflects sexual functioning in both men and women, and does so independently of sexual orientation and partner relationship. It measures sexual functioning in terms of five one-item domains: drive, arousal, penile erection/vaginal lubrication, ability to reach orgasm, and satisfaction from orgasm. ASEX domains were selected on the basis of those aspects of sexual functioning most affected by psychotropic drugs. The instrument has demonstrated good internal consistency and test-retest reliability, and it reflects the desirable characteristics of brevity and ease of administration.

The Changes in Sexual Functioning Questionnaire (CSFQ) is a 36-item structured interview designed with a focus on assessing sexual dysfunctions associated with psychiatric disorders and the pharmacological agents used to treat them (female version has 35 items, and male version has 36 items). The CSFQ comprises five dimensions: sexual desire–interest, sexual desire–frequency, sexual pleasure, sexual arousal, and orgasm. A total CSFQ score may also be derived. A self-report version of the instrument is also available. The instrument was initially standardized on a modest sample of medical students and psychiatric residents, and convergent validity was established with the domains of the Derogatis Interview for Sexual Functioning ($r=0.42$–0.76) (Clayton et al. 1997).

Table 2–3.   Descriptive properties of 11 contemporary measures of quality of sexual function

Inventory name	Modality/ gender	No. of items	Administration time (minutes)	Domains
Arizona Sexual Experience Scale (ASEX; McGahuey et al. 2000)	SR Male and female	5	<5	Drive, arousal, penile erection/vaginal lubrication, orgasm, satisfaction
Changes in Sexual Functioning Questionnaire (CSFQ; Clayton et al. 1997)	CI and SR Male and female	35 (F) 36 (M)[a]	<20	Desire–interest, desire–frequency, pleasure, arousal, orgasm, total score
Derogatis Interview for Sexual Functioning (DISF; Derogatis 1997)	CI and SR Male and female	25	12–15	Cognition/fantasy, arousal, behavior/ experience, orgasm, drive/ relationship, total score
Female Sexual Function Index (FSFI; Rosen et al. 2000)	SR Female only	19	15	Desire, arousal, lubrication, orgasm, satisfaction, pain
Index of Premature Ejaculation (IPE; Althof et al. 2006)	SR Male only	10	<10	Sexual satisfaction, control, distress
International Index of Erectile Function (IIEF; Rosen et al. 1997)	SR Male only	15	<15	Erectile function, orgasm, desire, intercourse satisfaction, overall satisfaction
Profile of Female Sexual Function (PFSF; Derogatis et al. 2004; McHorney et al. 2004)	SR Female only	37	<20	Desire, arousal, orgasm, pleasure, concerns, responsiveness, self-image

Table 2–3. Descriptive properties of 11 contemporary measures of quality of sexual function *(continued)*

Inventory name	Modality/ gender	No. of items	Administration time (minutes)	Domains
Sexual Function Questionnaire (SFQ; Quirk et al. 2002)	SR Female only	26	<15	Desire, arousal–sensation, arousal–lubrication, enjoyment, orgasm, dyspareunia, partner relationship, total
Sexual Interest and Desire Inventory (SIDI; Clayton et al. 2006)	CI Female only	13	<15	Overall total score
Short Personal Experiences Questionnaire (SPEQ; Dennerstein et al. 2001)	SR Female only	9	<5	Feelings for partner, sexual responsivity, sexual frequency, libido, distress/dyspareunia, partner problems
Female Sexual Distress Scale (FSDS; Derogatis et al. 2002) and revised version (FSDS-R; Derogatis et al. 2008)	SR Female only	12 (FSDS) 13 (FSDS-R)	<5	Unidimensional scale measuring sexually related personal distress; revised version has an additional desire item

Note.   See Table 2–4 for summary of psychometric properties of the measures described in this table. CI=clinical interview; SR=self-report.

[a]CSFQ has 35 items for females and 36 items for males.

Table 2–4. Psychometric properties of 11 contemporary measures of quality of sexual function

Inventory name	Reliability			Discriminative validity		Sensitivity/ specificity	Published norms?
	IC (α)	TRT (r)	IRR	Function/ dysfunction	Therapeutic change		
Arizona Sexual Experience Scale (ASEX)	0.91	0.80	—	Yes	Yes	0.82/0.90	No
Changes in Sexual Functioning Questionnaire (CSFQ)	0.64–0.80	0.66–0.86	—	Yes	Yes	—	Yes
Derogatis Interview for Sexual Functioning (DISF)	0.74–0.80	0.80–0.90	0.84–0.92	Yes	Yes	0.89/0.75	Yes
Female Sexual Function Index (FSFI)	0.82	0.79–0.86	—	Yes	Yes	—	Yes
Index of Premature Ejaculation (IPE)	0.74–0.91	0.70–0.90	—	Yes	Yes	—	No
International Index of Erectile Function (IIEF)	0.73–0.95	0.64–0.84	—	Yes	Yes	0.97/0.88	Yes

Table 2–4. Psychometric properties of 11 contemporary measures of quality of sexual function *(continued)*

| Inventory name | Reliability | | | Discriminative validity | | | Published norms? |
	IC (α)	TRT (r)	IRR	Function/ dysfunction	Therapeutic change	Sensitivity/ specificity	
Profile of Female Sexual Function (PFSF)	0.87–0.96	0.62–0.84	—	Yes	Yes	0.86/0.93	No
Sexual Function Questionnaire (SFQ)	0.79–0.91	0.42–0.78	—	Yes	Yes	—	Yes
Sexual Interest and Desire Inventory (SIDI)	0.90	—	—	Yes	Yes	—	No
Short Personal Experiences Questionnaire (SPEQ)	0.74–0.80	0.81–0.90	—	Yes	Yes	0.79/0.79	Yes
Female Sexual Distress Scale (FSDS) and revised version (FSDS-R)	0.93	0.87–0.93	—	Yes	Yes	0.93/0.93	Yes Cutoff score(s)

Note. See Table 2–3 for description of the measures summarized in this table. IC=internal consistency reliability; IRR=interrater reliability; TRT=test-retest reliability.

The Derogatis Interview for Sexual Functioning (DISF) is a coordinated set of brief, gender-specific instruments designed to provide an estimate of the quality of an individual's current sexual functioning (Derogatis 1997). The DISF includes a 25-item semistructured interview that represents quality of sexual functioning in a multidomain format and a matching self-report inventory (DISF-SR) designed to accomplish the same goal in a patient self-report mode. All instruments in the DISF series are designed to be interpreted at three distinct levels: discrete items, functional domains, and aggregate summary score. DISF items are arranged into five primary domains of sexual functioning: sexual cognition/fantasy, sexual arousal, sexual behavior/experience, orgasm, and sexual drive/relationship. In addition, an aggregate DISF total score is computed that summarizes quality of sexual functioning across the five primary DISF domains. The DISF interview and self-report together take approximately 12–15 minutes to administer, with the interview usually taking a few minutes longer than the self-report. The DISF is currently available in 12 foreign languages.

The Female Sexual Function Index (FSFI) is a 19-item self-report inventory designed to measure the quality of female sexual functioning. The FSFI represents sexual functioning on six primary dimensions of sexuality and has an aggregate total score. The FSFI was initially validated on a clinically diagnosed sample of women with female sexual arousal disorder. Subsequently, the validation statement was extended to include women with a primary clinical diagnosis of inhibited female orgasm disorder or hypoactive sexual desire disorder (HSDD) (Rosen et al. 2000).

The Index of Premature Ejaculation (IPE) is a 10-item self-report inventory that focuses on the subjective aspects of the premature ejaculation experience, serving as a complement to the elapsed time measures that form the basis of intravaginal ejaculatory latency time. As part of the psychometric analysis, the IPE was subjected to factor analysis, and three factors were identified: sexual satisfaction, control, and distress (Althof et al. 2006).

The International Index of Erectile Function (IIEF) is a 15-item self-report inventory developed by Rosen et al. (1997) with the principal purpose of making available a valid and reliable brief measure of erectile function and capacity. It has been frequently recommended as a primary endpoint in clinical trials of erectile dysfunction and has become a standard in that regard. The IIEF was developed in conjunction with the clinical trial program for sildenafil and has since served as a major endpoint in over 50 clinical trials (Rosen et al. 2002). At present, it has been linguistically validated in over 32 languages. The IIEF represents quality of male sexual function in terms of five domain scores: erectile function, orgasmic function, sexual desire, sexual satisfaction, and overall satisfaction. It does not possess a total score. More recently, a five-item brief form of the IIEF, termed the Sexual Health Inventory for Men, has been developed and validated (Rosen et al. 2002).

The Profile of Female Sexual Function (PFSF; Derogatis et al. 2004; McHorney et al. 2004) is a self-report inventory developed by Proctor & Gamble Pharmaceuticals to serve as a measure of major outcomes in their trials of a transdermal testosterone treatment system for women suffering from low sexual desire. Qualitative linguistic validation was conducted in women with HSDD and non-HSDD women in eight countries to ensure that items would have the same meaning across languages. The instrument consists of 37 items organized into seven domains (sexual desire, arousal, orgasm, sexual pleasure, sexual concerns, sexual responsiveness, and sexual self-image), which thoroughly describe female sexual function in menopausal women with HSDD. The PFSF was designed specifically for measurement of sexual desire in women with low libido. A brief form of the PFSF has also recently been developed (Rust et al. 2007).

The Sexual Function Questionnaire (SFQ) is a self-report inventory designed as an outcome measure of female sexual function (Quirk et al. 2002). It comprises 26 items reflecting all aspects of the sexual response cycle—desire, arousal, and orgasm—as well as dyspareunia. Factor analysis yielded seven domains of female sexual function: desire, physical arousal–sensation, physical arousal–lubrication, enjoyment, orgasm, dyspareunia, and partner relationship.

The Sexual Interest and Desire Inventory (SIDI; Sills et al. 2005; see also Clayton et al. 2006) is a brief, 13-item clinician-administered rating scale focused on measuring severity and change in response to treatment of HSDD in premenopausal women. The SIDI boasts a unique measurement format in that items address both intensity and frequency of sexual events in a matrix arrangement. An overall total score is provided.

The Short Personal Experiences Questionnaire (SPEQ) is a questionnaire developed by Dennerstein et al. (2001) with a specific focus on assessing the sexual functioning of middle-aged and older females. The optimization analysis finalized the number of items in the SPEQ to eight. Subsequently, an additional item on orgasm was added, bringing the total number of SPEQ items to nine.

The Female Sexual Distress Scale is a 12-item self-report inventory that was developed to quantify and measure the construct of sexually related personal distress (Derogatis et al. 2002). The presence of manifest distress in presenting patients has been a required criterion for a diagnosis of female sexual distress in the DSM-IV system; however, no operational mechanism for quantifying distress had been previously described. Additionally, in the U.S. Food and Drug Administration's most recent guidance on clinical drug trials in female sexual distress (U.S. Food and Drug Administration, Center for Drug Evaluation and Research 2001), the agency has required documentation of manifest personal distress for patient inclusion in clinical treatment trials.

Recently, a revised 13-item version of the instrument, the FSDS-R, has been developed and validated with a focus on greater sensitivity in women with HSDD (Derogatis et al. 2008). This psychometrically sound instrument is brief (taking less than 5 minutes to administer) and very easy to use. The FSDS-R has been shown to have excellent ability to discriminate between patients with and without female sexual distress and to be sensitive to therapeutically induced change.

Psychometric Assessment and Diagnosis

A word of caution should be introduced at this point regarding psychometric instruments: although diagnostic-like domain labels and dimension names may suggest that diagnosis can be accomplished via these brief scales, this is not the case. Psychometric assessment of the kind described here is designed to provide a quantitative snapshot of the individual's quality of sexual functioning. In most instances, it will enable the professional to appreciate an outline of the person's sexual function profile and/or suggest whether or not the individual manifests sexual symptoms consistent with a diagnosable condition. In research assessments, psychometric assessment represents a quantification along a dimension of functioning that, although it is clearly related to diagnosis, is not synonymous with it. Formal diagnosis of sexual dysfunction requires, in addition to a presenting complaint, both historical and contemporary perspectives on such important factors as medical history, drug history, psychological and affective status, quality of relationship(s), and psychiatric history. These comprehensive data cannot be ascertained via brief inventories, but must be determined through comprehensive clinical interview.

Nonetheless, psychometric assessment is essential to clinical trials outcomes research, and it can also be very useful to the busy clinician attempting to identify sexual dysfunction in his or her practice. In this review, we have tried to provide a sampling of the psychometric instruments currently available to measure and quantify the status of an individual's sexual functioning. Psychometrics has progressed dramatically in sexual medicine during the past decade, and a great deal of new development has taken place. Psychometric evaluation represents a potentially useful source of information about an individual's sexual functioning, particularly in light of the small expense and brief effort required to conduct the assessment.

Physical Examination, Laboratory Tests, and Other Specialized Tests

Physical Examination

A general physical examination, in addition to a good review of systems, can provide information about either general physical illness (cardiovascular, endocrinological, neurological) or some specific genital issues, such as genital anomalies (e.g., cryptorchidism, hypospadias, phimosis, underdeveloped genitalia, varicocele) or infections (urethritis, prostatitis, epididymitis, orchitis). Pelvic examination may be indicated in some sexual dysfunctions. Physical evaluation of genitalia and/or pelvic examination should be performed by a specialist (e.g., gynecologist).

Laboratory Tests

Although laboratory assays are occasionally definitive in determining the etiological picture (e.g., hyperprolactinemia associated with a pituitary adenoma), for the most part they indicate whether biological factors contribute to the diagnostic equation. The critical question about whether to perform laboratory assays often comes down to cost/benefit in the broadest sense of that concept: What is the incremental value of adding a particular test to the laboratory request, and what is the probability that the test will identify a significant causal agent? This increment must be weighed against the cost in time and energy required to obtain and interpret the test result, as well as the dollar cost associated with the assay.

Often, clinicians are discouraged from ordering any but the most basic laboratory tests because published data based on the general population show that the probability of a positive result is relatively small for any particular test. However, by virtue of their presenting complaint, patients with sexual dysfunction no longer represent the general population and instead are members of a specific subset of individuals in whom the probability (i.e., the base rate) of a sexually related biological dysregulation is much higher. This probability is particularly increased if the individual under evaluation is age 50 years or older.

One can find almost as many different lists of recommended laboratory tests as there are experts. Some of this variation is a result of the recommending expert's particular specialty and the nature of the patients seen in his or her practice. Also, the patient's gender obviously plays a role in the specific labs requested, as does the patient's presenting complaint, its duration (lifelong vs. acquired), and its specificity (situational vs. generalized). In some cases, little can be gained from laboratory assays, such as when a woman experiences low sexual desire with her husband but has no problems with her lover. Such manifestly interpersonal etiologies tend to be rare, however, and often difficult to ascertain. Nonetheless, the clinician needs to make an effort to probe all such areas. Selection of laboratory tests should always be guided by clinical context. For instance, a test for testosterone level would be indicated in a middle-aged male who suddenly lost sexual desire and in whom hypogonadism is suspected, or a test for thyroid-stimulating hormone level would be indicated in a middle-aged female who gradually developed lack of sexual desire, has a low energy level, and is gaining weight, though she takes no medications.

Table 2–5 includes a relatively generic inventory of laboratory assays that can be used in both male and female patients to determine if any "first-line" (relative to sexual functioning) biological functions appear abnormal. We have divided tests into "recommended" and "optional," based on what we personally do. Many more assays could be added, a few could be subtracted, and others could be shifted from one list to the other. Usually, laboratory tests do not provide a definitive etiology for a disorder; they more often provide a signal of where to look further.

Table 2–5.   Recommended laboratory assays useful in the diagnosis of sexual dysfunctions

Recommended diagnostic assays	Optional diagnostic assays
Plasma estradiol	Lipid profile
Total testosterone	Dehydroepiandrosterone
Free testosterone	Fasting glucose
Sex hormone–binding globulin	Glycosylated hemoglobin A_{1C}
Thyroid-stimulating hormone	Thyroid panel
Prolactin	Luteinizing hormone and follicle-stimulating hormone
	Complete blood count

Specialized Tests

A number of specialized tests or assessment methods are available; these are usually ordered by specialists. These tests include, for instance, Doppler sonography, phaloarteriography, dynamic cavernosometry, phalloplethysmography, various evaluations of nocturnal penile tumescence (e.g., Rigi-Scan), and other methods used to evaluate the vascular component of erectile dysfunction. Other examples include a host of assessment methods used in the evaluation of some paraphilic behaviors (e.g., penile plethysmography during projection of various images or during special audiotapes, Viewing Time; see Chapter 12, "Paraphilic Disorders").

Assimilation and Integration of Data

The clinical evaluation process essentially represents an iterative progression with ever-increasing quantities of data concerning the patient's presenting complaint; sexual, medical, and interpersonal histories; and assessment results. The clinician's principal task is to assimilate these data and integrate the multiple elements into a cohesive assessment and explanation of the patient's sexual dysfunction and its probable cause(s). Clinicians need to keep in mind a number of important issues during this process.

First, the evaluation should be perceived by the clinician, and explained to the patient, as being a programmatic endeavor; it is not a one-shot, all-or-none process, but rather a complementary series of assessments that will, it is hoped, result in a comprehensive understanding of the patient's problem and an optimal approach to treatment. This being the case, whenever possible, the patient's partner should be involved in the evaluation so that he or she can provide verification and corroboration of the facts of the case and, at the time of treatment recommendations or referral, help confirm the rationale for the clinician's recommendations.

Second, in the current era of patient-based medicine, the clinician should perceive and treat the patient (and the patient's partner whenever possible) as important decision makers in the evaluation and treatment process. The clinician should be careful not to assume an authoritarian posture, but rather take on the role of an expert guide by informing, educating, and sharing knowledge and experience with the patient, and ultimately conveying details concerning recommendations about the case (e.g., the reasons for referral to a specialist or for initiating a particular treatment regimen). Because education represents a critical aspect of the evaluation process, the clinician should discuss with the patient the data from the various clinical assessments and the processes whereby these data affect the clinician's decision-making process and recommendations regarding the case.

Data from the clinical interview, any psychometric assessments, and the physical examination or laboratory assays should be shared with the patient in an effort to help him or her understand the basis for the clinician's conclusions. These data and their assimilation by the clinician will form the platform for the clinician's treatment recommendations. Because the patient should be an active participant in decisions to accept or reject specific treatment recommendations, the patient needs to understand the nature of the data used by the clinician in decision making and be "on board" with recommendations being made.

In many cases, the patient's primary care provider can initiate and maintain effective treatment for the patient's sexual dysfunction, but this is not always possible. Referrals may be necessary for patients with underlying cardiovascular or endocrinological conditions, male or female disorders requiring surgery for optimal resolution, and psychiatric or interpersonal conflicts that demand specialized treatment knowledge. If a patient is referred to a specialist, the primary care provider needs to maintain communication with both the patient and the specialist about how treatment has progressed.

Optimal treatment is the ultimate goal of the clinical evaluation process, whether it is delivered by the primary care clinician or a specialized health care provider. The more relevant the information is that can be brought to bear in the evaluation process, the greater the likelihood that the most appropriate treatment and problem resolution will be achieved.

Key Points

- Comprehensive evaluation of the patient's sexuality and sexual dysfunction provides a benchmark for diagnosis and treatment.

- Clinical and research evaluations may differ in context, goals, perspective, purpose, and structure. These evaluations may overlap and also may serve as a source of information for each other.

- The clinical interview is the cornerstone of a thorough evaluation of sexual dysfunction.

- A comprehensive clinical interview should include elements focused on the specifics of the dysfunction, as well as information about developmental, interpersonal, mental, and physical health; medications; and value system issues, including cultural and religious ones.

- Interviewing the partner is usually very useful and, in fact, could be invaluable.

- The interviewer should create a comfortable atmosphere. Both the interviewer and the interviewee should be comfortable with the discussion of sexual issues.

- Comprehensive evaluation of sexual dysfunction frequently includes psychometric assessment, physical examination, and laboratory testing, in addition to a comprehensive clinical interview.

- Psychometric instruments administered prior to the clinical interview may provide valuable and clinically useful information.

- Findings from the interview, psychometric assessment, physical examination, and laboratory and other tests should be properly integrated. The integrated findings should serve as a basis for diagnosis and treatment planning.

- The clinician should share integrated findings and his or her conclusions with the patient in an open, understandable, courteous, and comfortable manner.

References

Althof S, Rosen R, Symonds T, et al: Development and validation of a new questionnaire to assess sexual satisfaction, control and distress associated with premature ejaculation. J Sex Med 3:465–475, 2006

American Psychiatric Association: Diagnostic and Statistical Manual of Mental Disorders, 4th Edition, Text Revision. Washington, DC, American Psychiatric Association, 2000

Bhugra D, de Silva P: Management of sexual dysfunction across cultures, in Textbook of Cultural Psychiatry. Edited by Bhugra D, Bhui K. New York, Cambridge University Press, 2007, pp 484–502

Bonierbale M, Lancon C, Tignol J: The ELIXIR study: evaluation of sexual dysfunction in 4557 depressed patients in France. Curr Med Res Opin 19:114–124, 2003

Bullough V: Sexual Variance in Society and History. Chicago, IL, University of Chicago Press, 1976. Cited by: Bhugra D, de Silva P: Sexual dysfunction across cultures, in Textbook of Cultural Psychiatry. Edited by Bhugra D, Bhui K. New York, Cambridge University Press, 2007, pp 364–378

Clayton AH, McGarvey EL, Clavet GJ, et al: Comparison of sexual functioning in clinical and nonclinical populations using the Changes in Sexual Functioning Questionnaire (CSFQ). Psychopharmacol Bull 33:747–753, 1997

Clayton A, Pradko JF, Croft HA, et al: Prevalence of sexual dysfunction among newer antidepressants. J Clin Psychiatry 63:357–366, 2002

Clayton AH, Segraves RT, Leiblum S, et al: Reliability and validity of the Sexual Interest and Desire Inventory—Female (SIDI-F), a scale designed to measure severity of female hypoactive sexual desire disorder. J Sex Marital Ther 32:115–135, 2006

Dennerstein L, Lehert P, Dudley E: Short scale to measure female sexuality: adapted from McCoy Female Sexuality Questionnaire. J Sex Marital Ther 27:339–351, 2001

Derogatis LR: The Derogatis Interview for Sexual Functioning (DISF/DISF-SR): an introductory report. J Sex Marital Ther 23:291–304, 1997

Derogatis LR, Laban MP: Psychological assessment measures of human sexual functioning in clinical trials. Int J Impot Res 10 (suppl 2):513–520, 1998

Derogatis LR, Rosen RC, Leiblum S, et al: The Female Sexual Distress Scale (FSDS): initial validation of a standardized scale for the assessment of sexually related personal distress in women. J Sex Marital Ther 28:317–330, 2002

Derogatis LR, Rust J, Golombok S, et al: Validation of the Profile of Female Sexual Function (PFSF) in surgically and naturally menopausal women. J Sex Marital Ther 30:25–36, 2004

Derogatis LR, Clayton A, Lewis-D'Agostino D, et al: Validation of the Female Sexual Distress Scale—Revised (FSDS-R) for assessing distress in women with hypoactive sexual desire disorder. J Sex Med 5:357–364, 2008

McGahuey CA, Gelenberg AJ, Laukes CA, et al: The Arizona Sexual Experience Scale (ASEX): reliability and validity. J Sex Marital Ther 26:25–40, 2000

McHorney CA, Rust J, Golombok S, et al: Profile of Female Sexual Function: a patient-based, international, psychometric instrument for the assessment of hypoactive sexual desire in oophorectomized women. Menopause 11:474–483, 2004

Nunnally JC: Psychometric Theory. New York, McGraw-Hill, 1978

Quirk FH, Heiman J, Rosen RC, et al: Development of a sexual function questionnaire for clinical trials of female sexual function. J Womens Health Gend Based Med 11:277–285, 2002

Rosen RC, Riley A, Wagner G, et al: The International Index of Erectile Function (IIEF): a multidimensional scale for assessment of sexual dysfunction. Urology 49:822–830, 1997

Rosen R, Brown C, Heiman J, et al: The Female Sexual Function Index (FSFI): a multidimensional self-report instrument for the assessment of female sexual function. J Sex Marital Ther 26:191–208, 2000

Rosen RC, Cappelleri JC, Gendrano N 3rd: The International Index of Erectile Function (IIEF): a state-of-the-science review. Int J Impot Res 14:226–244, 2002

Rust J, Derogatis LR, Rodenberg C, et al: Development and validation of a new screening tool for hypoactive sexual desire disorder: The Brief Profile of Female Sexual Function (B-PFSF). Gynecol Endocrinol 23:638–644, 2007

Sills T, Wunderlich G, Ryke R, et al: The Sexual Interest and Desire Inventory—Female (SIDI-F): item response analysis of data from women diagnosed with hypoactive sexual desire disorder. J Sex Med 2:801–818, 2005

U.S. Food and Drug Administration, Center for Drug Evaluation and Research: Guidance for industry: female sexual dysfunction: clinical development of drug products for treatment. March 8, 2001. Available at: http://www.fda.gov/cder/guidance/3312dft.htm. Accessed February 4, 2009.

3

Sexual Disorders With Comorbid Psychiatric or Physical Illness

Ronald Stevenson, M.D., FRCPC

Stacy Elliott, M.D.

Human sexuality is an excellent example of the fundamental, inescapable link between psyche and soma, reflecting the balance between wellness and illness, function and dysfunction, thought and behavior, isolation and relationship, self-worth and self-denigration, despair and joy. The sexuality of patients inevitably permeates nearly every kind of psychiatric practice in some way, either as cause or consequence of distress.

We gratefully acknowledge the sustaining influence of our clinical mentors, George Szasz, M.D., and William Maurice, M.D., and express thanks to our primary teachers—our patients.

A clinician can feel challenged, even intimidated, when confronted with a complicated patient whose sexual disorder reflects a combination of cognitive, behavioral, emotional, interpersonal, and physical etiologies. In this chapter, we outline a framework and a model to help psychiatrists, with appropriate medical consultations as necessary, provide effective interventions for such patients.

Relevance of Comorbid Sexual Disorders in Psychiatry

Inevitably, psychiatrists deal with patients who have other health problems. Indeed, chronic illness is associated with a 41% increase in recent psychiatric disorders (Blazer 2003). Similarly, sexual dysfunctions are highly comorbid with many illnesses and traumas, with the prevalence reaching 93% in some surveys of family practice patients (Aschka et al. 2001). A sexual disorder may be either a symptom or a cause of other treatable illnesses, such as anxiety, depression, pain, urinary tract infection, fatigue, infertility, and so on. Erectile dysfunction can be the harbinger of small blood vessel problems associated with serious cardiovascular disease, hypertension, and diabetes (Shabsigh et al. 2008). In particular, a mutually reinforcing comorbidity exists between erectile dysfunction, cardiovascular disease, and depression, and a problem in any one of these areas should prompt evaluation of the others (Goldstein 2000). Sexual problems can complicate recovery from illness. Conversely, some men with depression and erectile dysfunction experience resolution of mood symptoms when their sexual dysfunction is successfully treated (Seidman et al. 2001). Similarly, attention to sexual issues helps speed recovery in cardiac rehabilitation programs because it has beneficial effects on mood and relationships and because it promotes compliance with treatment (Muller 1999). As one final example of the ubiquity and relevance of sexual dysfunctions, sexual side effects are often the cause of medication noncompliance (Thomas 2003), perhaps most notably in psychiatry.

Role of the Psychiatrist

Nearly all sexual problems ultimately involve complex interactions of biological and psychological factors. Physical illness affects one's thoughts, feelings, and behaviors, just as emotional or other psychiatric illness manifests with somatic symptoms. Accordingly, perhaps more than any other medical discipline, psychiatry, by virtue of its roots in both biology and psychology, seems quintessentially well suited to the study and treatment of sexual disorders. Furthermore, most psychiatrists are able to devote the necessary time over a series of visits to talk with patients about personal and sensitive issues in an unhurried, respectful, objective, empathic, and compassionate manner—exactly the professional skill set needed to manage many sexual problems.

Nevertheless, more than three decades after Helen Singer Kaplan (1974) first emphasized mind-body links in her seminal text on sexual disorders, the biological aspects of clinical sexuality have been largely usurped by urology and gynecology, the psychological and relational aspects are often relinquished to nonphysician therapists and counselors, and the majority of psychiatrists seem unaware of their sensible role as key diagnostic, management, and research thought leaders in this profoundly important biopsychosocial area of clinical service. Indeed, if meaningful training in sexual medicine is offered at all in psychiatry residency programs, it is usually only as an elective experience.

The impact of sexual problems varies from personal embarrassment, unhappiness, and frustration, to a more pervasive loss of self-esteem and function. Relationships with the partner and with other family members can suffer, and some patients avoid friends or social opportunities. Distress and preoccupation can impair performance in educational or occupational settings. Given this potential cascade of individual and interpersonal damage, intermixed with the biopsychosocial causation, the psychiatrist is the ideal professional to discuss sexual issues in the context of a patient's overall emotional and physical health, concurrent medications, recreational drug use, general life circumstances, and sexual behaviors. Sexuality is not a lifestyle issue; it is a quality-of-life issue. The psychiatrist's goal is to maintain, restore, or improve a patient's quality of life, and sexual function should be a routine part of that clinical service mandate.

Specific Areas of Comorbidity: Extent of the Problem

Given the ubiquitous nature of sexuality, we can provide only a few brief examples of the types of conditions in which sexual problems overlap with medical and psychiatric illness.

Anxiety

Patients with anxiety (including phobic and obsessional) syndromes may experience heightened sexual performance fears or vulnerabilities to distraction, which may result in problems with interest, arousal, or orgasm. Figueira et al. (2001) found premature ejaculation in 47% of men with social phobia, as well as very high sexual aversion rates in patients with panic disorder (35.7% of men; 50% of women). Anxiety can lead to sexual avoidance even when libido is relatively intact. Conversely, anxiety, obsessionality, or insecurity can be reflected in sexual acting-out or compulsive sexual behaviors (Bancroft and Vukadinovic 2004).

Bipolar Affective Disorder

Sexual activity may escalate during hypomanic relapses. Impulsive sexual behavior can contravene a patient's personal, cultural, or religious beliefs, later causing distress to the patient and significant others as they reflect on the impact of any sexual indiscretions or deal with the consequences of sexually transmitted infections (Raja and Azzoni 2003).

Cancer

In both men and women with cancer, sexuality can be adversely affected by depression, anxiety, relationship stress, and loss of independence and work identity. The location of the tumor or metastases, as well as the intensity, duration, and form of treatment (surgery, radiation, chemotherapy), can have varying and profound effects on sexuality due to fatigue, pain, nausea, the effects of chemotherapy or radiation, and so forth. Sexual consequences are not limited to the active treatment phase; survivors may have long-term sexual problems, including decreased libido, dyspareunia, erectile dysfunction, and body image changes, sometimes leading to generalized sexual dysfunction. Women whose cancer treatments lead to ovarian failure have decreased levels of estrogen and testosterone, resulting in vaginal atrophy, decreased vaginal lubrication, and loss of libido. Hormonal replacement may not always be possible due to the type of malignancy (e.g., women with estrogen-sensitive breast cancer). Surgery or radiation to the female genitalia or bladder can lead to vaginal shortening, stenosis, or dryness, making sexual intercourse painful or even impossible (McKee and Schover 2001). Fertility also can be affected by hormonal changes or by direct toxicity of chemotherapy or radiation to the gonads.

Approximately 70% of men who undergo treatment for prostate cancer report impaired sexual function. Radical prostatectomy can damage one or both of the two neurovascular bundles critical for erection, although nerve sparing at the time of surgery, normal tumescence premorbidly, and younger age are all predictors of good postoperative erectile function (Smith and Christmas 1999). Although no ejaculatory fluid remains after removal of the prostate and seminal vesicles, male orgasm still occurs but may be altered, unchanged, or painful (Elliott 2002). Chemical or surgical castration results in loss of sexual desire, erectile dysfunction, and difficulty reaching orgasm; treatment with estrogens results in gynecomastia and other features of feminization (Kumar et al. 2005).

Other prostate diseases, such as benign prostatic hypertrophy causing lower urinary tract symptoms, are common in middle-aged and elderly men and contribute to a slightly higher prevalence of sexual dysfunction (Morant et al. 2009).

Cardiovascular Disease

Patients with major psychiatric illness (e.g., schizophrenia, bipolar disorder, major depression) are at higher risk for developing cardiovascular disease (Fleischhacker et al. 2008). Following a heart attack, 75% of patients either decrease or stop sexual activity, and 80% of patients with congestive heart failure report either marked problems with or an inability to engage in sexual activity (Taylor 1999). Men with chronic coronary artery disease experience some degree of erectile dysfunction, which is not surprising given that atherosclerosis affects the blood supply to the genitals as well as the heart. Cardiac medications may also contribute to sexual problems.

The reasons that patients and partners give for the decline in intimacy are more complicated than mere loss of interest or an inability to respond, instead often reflecting the multiple preoccupations and stresses of a chronic disease, as well as unwarranted fears of experiencing a heart attack during sex. In fact, sexual activity requires a fairly low energy output—about the same as climbing two flights of stairs or walking a mile in 20 minutes, and less than 0.2% of patients suffer a fatal heart attack during sexual activity (Parzeller et al.

2001). Accordingly, the vast majority of heart patients can be encouraged to engage in noncoital, non-goal-oriented caressing and pleasuring from the earliest rehabilitation stages and are safe to return to full sexual activity with intercourse when they are comfortable with the stair climbing test. For the seriously compromised cardiac patient, sexual activities should be deferred until proper risk stratification and resolution of any unstable cardiac condition (Jackson et al. 2006). In patients with cardiovascular disease and erectile dysfunction, treatment with a phosphodiesterase type 5 (PDE5) inhibitor might be an excellent option, although concurrent use of nitroglycerin for angina is contraindicated. Again, to forestall such drug combinations, psychiatrists need to be able to address sexual topics with patients.

Depression

Although antidepressants can cause sexual dysfunctions (see Chapter 4, "Medications and Sexual Function and Dysfunction"), sexual disinterest or arousal problems also arise in untreated depression in 50% of women and 40% of men (Kennedy et al. 1999). The incidence of erectile dysfunction may approach 100% in older men with more severe degrees of depression (Feldman et al. 1994). Yet, despite the presence of disinterest, sexual anhedonia, or other sexual dysfunction, actual sexual behavior may not decrease. Depressed women may remain sexually active at a frequency that is unrelated to their own loss of interest, instead matching the level of the partner's libido or the couple's established pattern of sexual interaction (Cyranowski et al. 2004). Accordingly, merely asking if a depressed patient is sexually active can miss the presence of a significant sexual dysfunction.

Diabetes

Diabetic patients with depression have a higher rate of diabetic complications, including sexual dysfunction (de Groot et al. 2001). In males with diabetes, the prevalence of erectile dysfunction (20%–85%) is three to five times higher than in the general population; this risk increases with age and is most strongly correlated with autonomic neuropathy, vascular disease, and poor glycemic control (Romeo et al. 2000). Less frequently, retrograde ejaculation occurs. Conflicting reports have been published on the sexual function of women with diabetes, but decreased lubrication is perhaps the most frequent complaint. Sexual dissatisfaction is also correlated with relationship and self-esteem problems, and is further complicated by reactions to catastrophic effects of diabetes, such as limb amputation (Tilton 1997).

Multiple Sclerosis

Demyelinating diseases of the central nervous system can affect cognitive, motor, and sensory function, depending on the area of brain or spinal cord involved. Furthermore, spasticity, fatigue, and muscle weakness can affect the ability to engage in certain sexual acts, including intercourse. DasGupta and Fowler (2003) estimated that more than 70% of men and women with multiple sclerosis experience some form of sexual dysfunction during their disease. Because multiple sclerosis is a neurologically disruptive disease, it is usually associated with diminution or loss of libido, arousal, and orgasmic capacity, all of which are compounded if the patient also has depression. Less commonly, some patients experience increased libido, possibly associated with mood elevations, even engaging in uncharacteristic sexual indiscretions that can be associated with significant stress, anxiety, or shame.

Parkinson's Disease

Parkinson's disease is associated with sexual dysfunction in both sexes, and sexual dysfunction can be one of the most demoralizing and disabling features of the disease. At least 75% of women with Parkinson's disease report difficulties with arousal and orgasm and 50% experience low sexual desire. About 70% of men with Parkinson's disease experience erectile difficulties. In addition, 40% have premature ejaculation and 40% have delayed orgasm (Bronner et al. 2004).

Personality Disorders

Patients with major personality disturbances can experience varying kinds of sexual difficulties, ranging from promiscuity to avoidance. In patients with borderline personality disorder, Zanarini et al. (2003) found 65% of women and 43% of men avoided sexual intimacy due to fears of becoming symptomatic as a result of relationship volatility, indicating that this could be an important area for therapeutic exploration and treatment.

Psychotic Disorders

In patients with schizophrenia or schizoaffective disorder, sexual function is usually impaired. Teusch et al. (1995) found that patients with schizophrenia had significantly more dysfunctions of interest, arousal, performance, and orgasm than did control subjects. Furthermore, their sexual satisfaction was lower. Antipsychotic medications compound these problems because of their significant sexual side effects.

Renal Disease

A significant decline in physical function occurs with chronic renal disease and is associated with depression in at least 25% of patients (Son et al. 2009). Hormonal alterations can affect sexual function in both genders, as well as semen quality in men. Subtle disturbances in the hypothalamic-pituitary-gonadal axis and impaired gonadal function are most notable in males, whereas central disturbances are more prominent in women (Leavy and Weitzel 2002). Hyperprolactinemia in both men and women results in decreased libido, decreased sexual intercourse rates, orgasmic difficulties, and abbreviated longevity of sexual life (Weizman et al. 1983). Anemia, fatigue, and medication side effects also impair sexual interest and function. Sexual function may or may not improve following transplantation (Chen et al. 2003; Tsujimura et al. 2002). Peritoneal dialysis may be associated with fewer sexual problems than hemodialysis (Kettas et al. 2008).

Spinal Cord Injury

Spinal cord injury can be associated with some degree of depression in 15%–20% of patients, regardless of gender or the characteristics of the injury (Kalpakjian and Albright 2006). However, with respect to sexual function, the level and completeness of the spinal cord lesion are critical in predicting the remaining potential. Mentally induced ("psychogenic") erections and vaginal lubrication are lost if the injury is complete and above the 10th thoracic neurological level (T10), whereas genital touch–induced "reflexogenic" arousal potential is lost if the sacral cord is damaged (Elliott 2003). Although women's fertility is unaffected by spinal cord injury, men experience changes to erection and ejaculation, and their semen quality is poor (Elliott 2003). However, approximately 45% of men and 50% of women report orgasmic ability after spinal cord injury, regardless of the level or nature of the injury (Elliott 2009).

Sexual activity is not without risk for persons with spinal cord injury. Autonomic dysreflexia, a potentially life-threatening condition of acute hypertension from unopposed sympathetically mediated influences, can be triggered by sexual activity—especially ejaculation—in persons with spinal cord injury above the T6 neurological level, and must be prevented or managed in private sexual or clinical sperm-retrieval situations (Ekland et al. 2008).

Substance Abuse

In women, sexual response tends to be impaired by use of alcohol, especially by chronic use. Blume (1998) found that alcohol interfered with women's sex hormones and was associated with irregular menstruation, infertility, early menopause, lack of sexual interest, and painful intercourse. O'Farrell et al. (1997) found that alcoholic men had problems with erectile dysfunction, delayed ejaculation, and less frequent intercourse as they aged. Evidence indicates that erectile dysfunction secondary to the polyneuropathy from thiamine deficiency resolves with vitamin B_1 treatment (Tjandra and Janknegt 1997). However, alcohol-related sexual problems may be less solvable because of adverse effects on the liver and the gonads (Gumus et al. 1998).

Use of street drugs can cause impulsivity or heightened libido, resulting in a greater number of sexual partners and a concomitant increase in the risk of acquiring a sexually transmitted disease (Colfax et al. 2005). Subjective reports vary concerning sexual function effects. Many men using stimulants such as amphetamines report increased sexual excitement, intensified orgasm, and longer duration of intercourse when using the drug. However, female polysubstance abusers report that crack cocaine inhibits their sexual performance and desire (El-Bassel et al. 2003). The majority of heroin addicts, as well as men treated with opioids for chronic pain, experience hypogonadism and erectile dysfunction or diminished libido (Daniell 2002). The literature does not yet support definitive conclusions about sexual dysfunctions in methadone users, but buprenorphine treatment of opioid addiction may be an option associated with fewer sexual problems (Hallinan et al. 2008). Finally, up to 71% of drug abusers noted that their decision to start taking drugs was an attempt to self-medicate a sexual difficulty or trauma (La Pera et al. 2008).

Traumatic Brain Injury

Traumatic brain injury commonly leads to fatigue, as well as disturbed sleep, depression, and pain (Bushnik et al. 2008). With respect to sexual function, in contrast to uninjured control subjects, persons with traumatic brain injury report lower energy and interest in initiating sexual activity (whether due to low testosterone or, perhaps, low motivation), difficulties with arousal (erection or lubrication), and difficulties reaching orgasm (Hibbard et al. 2000). Women may have difficulties with vaginal dryness, causing pain during sexual activity. Both genders report physical difficulties with body position, movement, and sensation, as well as body image changes that influence feelings of attractiveness and comfort.

Evaluation of Sexual Problems in Chronic Illness

As outlined in Table 3–1, the approach to evaluation is organized within three categories: 1) general mechanisms through which illness impairs sexual function, 2) a framework for outlining the assessment areas deserving attention, and 3) key principles informing both the evaluation and the treatment goals when sexual rehabilitation is being considered.

General Etiological Mechanisms

Illness or treatments contribute to sexual problems in any of four ways (Stevenson and Elliott 2007):

1. *Direct* effects of vascular, neurological (including pain), hormonal, anatomical, or other damage to an area functionally connected to sexual response
2. *Indirect* effects of a medical or psychiatric condition, such as changes to perception or judgment, mood or behavioral volatility, sensory or motor alterations, bladder and bowel incontinence, spasticity, tremor, fatigue, anxiety, depression, chronic pain, and so on
3. *Iatrogenic* effects of treatment (e.g., radiation, surgery, medication)
4. *Contextual* effects (i.e., due to biopsychosocial complexity and situational components)

Table 3–1.   Evaluation of sexual problems in patients with chronic illness

General etiological mechanisms

Direct

Indirect

Iatrogenic

Contextual

Sexual framework for assessment

Sexual interest changes

Sexual response changes

Factors related to the condition

Sensation

Pain

Movement and motor function

Hygiene and continence

Changes to body image

Fertility and parenting concerns

Relationship issues

General psychological effects

Principles of sexual rehabilitation

Maximize remaining capacity

Adapt to residual limitations

Persist with openness and optimism

Case Example 1

A 39-year-old married woman with two preteen children was diagnosed with progressive multiple sclerosis 5 years ago. A former teacher, she has been receiving disability benefits for 3 years and has recently begun using a wheelchair. She has three sexual concerns: disinterest, arousal disorder, and anorgasmia. The etiology of these problems could stem from 1) *direct* neurological changes in her brain or pelvis (altered neural signals; poor genital sensation), 2) *indirect* influences of multiple sclerosis (adductor spasm, making intercourse difficult; problems with positioning and weakness; concerns about incontinence with sexual activity; fatigue), 3) effects of multiple sclerosis *treatments* (use of antispasmodics and antidepressants), and 4) a broad range of *contextual* factors. Despite afternoon naps, she is exhausted by the end of the day from trying to maintain roles as mother and homemaker, and feeling inadequate at both. She is worried about the loss of her contribution to the family income and is frustrated by her restricted physical independence and unaccustomed social inaccessibility. Her sexual self-image has diminished, and she is feeling more depressed. Her reduced genital sensation makes it harder for her to reach orgasm, but she hesitates to ask her husband to spend more time caressing her, especially as she feels less able to please him sexually.

Each of these areas has a sexual consequence that needs individualized attention. The primary therapeutic goals may be to help her to minimize her fatigue (e.g., get a housecleaner; have someone else pick up the kids from school) so she can focus her energy on the loving relationships with her children and husband. Stress reduction through massage or meditation may also help. Time spent alone, perhaps in a warm bath, to reexplore her body could help her to discover potential new areas of eroticism or to use mindfulness and fantasy to amplify sensations from familiar areas. Use of a vibrator may also be helpful. Planning sexual times, rather than depending on spontaneity, will help ensure optimal energy levels.

Sexual Assessment Framework

As described in the following sections, the clinician can evaluate a variety of potential etiological elements using a patient-centered sexual assessment framework (Szasz 1992; see also Elliott, in press).

Sexual Interest

The clinician should determine whether the patient's current libido is higher or lower than premorbid libido. Does the patient have reversible etiologies (e.g., medication side effects, hormone imbalance, depression, mania, anxiety)? Are the emotional, relationship, and physical outcomes of sexual activity positive or negative? Some factors are amenable to individual or couples psychotherapy, and others to medical therapies (e.g., relief of pain, muscle strengthening, hormone replacement, pharmacotherapy for psychiatric symptoms).

Sexual Response

The clinician should elicit a description of the couple's approach to a typical sexual encounter. Are there manifestations of arousal (erection; vaginal lubrication and accommodation; awareness of neuromuscular tension in the pelvis; feelings of emotional excitement)? Does any activity reliably lead to orgasm, and are there noncoital options for achieving orgasm (with partner or alone)? Has either partner experienced changes in orgasmic capacity or intensity (e.g., suggesting either an emotionally based anhedonia or a problem of low testosterone)?

Factors Associated With the Condition

The clinician should ask about the patient's overall medical status and sense of wellness. Medications or other treatments can directly affect sexual function. The symptoms of the patient's condition (e.g., feeling unwell, nausea, fatigue, depression, excessive nighttime sweating, halitosis) can indirectly impair sexual response and the willingness to be sexual. Sexual self-image (and attractiveness) can be affected by the ability to independently manage oral, genital, or menstrual hygiene. Comorbid conditions can exacerbate any sexual problem. For example, a man with diabetes may already have several contributors to his erection difficulties (vasculopathy, neuropathy, endothelial dysfunction), but if he then has a radical prostatectomy for prostate cancer, his sexual functioning is further disadvantaged due to direct nerve damage. Feelings of loss, fears for the future, and other psychological reactions can then overwhelm the remaining potential.

Sensory Alterations

Injuries to brain areas associated with memory or fantasy, with visual sexual stimulation, or with perception of arousal and orgasm can have profound effects on sexual function, as can damage to the spinal cord and peripheral nerves that provide sensory information from genitalia and other erogenous areas. Postsurgically, genital sensory potential may continue to improve with nerve regeneration. Appreciation of sexual touch is affected by any loss of sensation in the genital area (e.g., due to multiple sclerosis or surgery) or other erogenous areas (e.g., loss of breast sensitivity after mastectomy). For patients with permanent neurological changes, positive sexual adaptation can still occur by learning to recruit new erogenous zones.

Pain

Unpleasant hypersensitivity can occur as a result of neurological changes, scarring, medication, or effects of chemotherapy, or can occur secondary to neuropathic pain. The patient may have genital discomfort (i.e., with touch or intercourse, or with ejaculation) or more generalized symptoms (e.g., from arthritis, fibromyalgia, or cancer). Sexual problems are twice as common in chronic pain patients than in the general population, and chronic pain can result in depression, weight loss or gain, physical deconditioning, and loss of self-image, resulting in decreased mental, physical, and sexual functioning (Ambler et al. 2001). Not only can pain be a serious sexual deterrent for a patient, but his or her partner may also be inhibited by the concern that sexual activity could aggravate the pain. Also, hypervigilance (by either partner) for possible cardiac pain (or symptoms or sensations that remind them of a cardiac event) can become a preoccupation that blocks sexual excitement.

Movement and Motor Function

The clinician should assess the patient's ability to undress independently, to get into bed, to reposition oneself or one's partner, and to caress and hold a partner. Spasm, tremor, and other motor problems limit the options for sexual activity. Application of birth control may be problematic. For men, the use of erection enhancement methods that require good visual acuity or hand function may require the assistance of a willing partner. Motor loss and dependency on wheelchairs or caretakers can also limit access to certain social venues and opportunities.

Continence and Related Hygiene

Bladder and bowel issues associated with aging, disability, or medication can influence a patient's willingness to be social or to leave the security and privacy of home; even the ability or wish to be sexual with a familiar partner can be affected. Potential odors or incontinence, a visible external collection apparatus, the duration of time needed for presexual hygiene or catheterization, and/or the need for assistance (e.g., a nurse or aide) can impede spontaneity, social comfort, and the opportunities for sexual expression.

Changes to Body Image

Illness or trauma can accelerate normal age-related changes in tissue elasticity, blood vessel capacity, nerve response, and genital function, especially vaginal lubrication and erectile capacities, with consequent effects on self-esteem and body image. The onset of depression in elderly individuals can blunt almost all aspects of sexual functioning. With surgery, scarring, or limb amputation, notwithstanding possible preservation of genital function, the effects on self-esteem can be significant, and depression may persist for years (Rybarczyk et al. 1995). A preoccupation with hiding body parts, deformities, or rehabilitative devices, or having reduced strength or balance, will affect physical comfort and positioning options for sex.

Fertility and Parenting Concerns

Apart from sexual functioning problems that interfere with the ability to have intercourse (e.g., vaginismus, erection or ejaculation problems), infertility may be associated with hormonal abnormalities due to the condition (e.g., head injury) or treatment (e.g., chemotherapy or radiation) or to the use of medications affecting the viability of oocytes or spermatozoa. Many medical fertility problems can be overcome with newer technology (e.g., in vitro fertilization, intracytoplasmic sperm injection, sperm banking, oocyte donation). More abstract issues of parenting capacity may also need to be addressed, such as in disorders that affect executive skills (planning, attention, judgment), as well as practical matters related to mobility, accessibility, and energy. Some couples may want information and guidance concerning the degree of inheritability of psychiatric or physical illnesses, so as to better inform their decisions about conception.

The clinician also should assess the safety of, and the patient's ability to utilize, certain birth control methods (e.g., a woman with mood or psychotic disorders may have motivational or attentional issues that interfere with consistent use of oral contraceptives; an individual with a hand function disability may be unable to place a barrier method of contraception; a person with immobility might be at higher risk for blood clots with hormonal birth control).

Relationship Issues

Being the partner to someone with a chronic mental disorder can be fatiguing, frustrating, and/or alienating. Being the caretaker as well as the partner for someone with a chronic medical condition or disability presents additional challenges. Both persons may find it awkward and anxiety provoking to be sexual in the broader context of attending to basic body functions or physical needs. For single people, accessing social and sexual opportunities may be problematic, particularly if the medical condition is visible (e.g., motor impairments, wheelchair dependence, disfigurement). However, hidden disability (e.g., brain injury, depression, anxiety disorders) can be just as devastating to one's sense of social and sexual confidence.

General Psychological Effects

Chronic illness may require physical, emotional, interpersonal, and economic adjustments. If sexuality had previously been a significant aspect of a person's self-esteem or self-image, the disruption occurring from illness can be profound. The pace of deterioration can be important because readiness to address the issue has to be balanced with other life priorities, such as recovery or financial losses. Unrealistic goals about future function can lead to despair when the true degree of impairment is acknowledged (Turvey and Klein 2008). The individual has to achieve a level of self-acceptance and confidence, or a state of "readiness," to reenter the sexual arena with a current partner or to consider meeting new partners, to explore the limitations and potentials of a changed body, or to contemplate the use of sexual aids.

Anxiety often results in diminished interest, arousal, and orgasmic capacity, but can also lead to heightened arousal (despite frustration from the sexual problem). The couple may experience a reversal of traditional masculine and feminine roles or a loss of economic security. Other important variables include privacy (e.g., from other persons in the house); the availability and loyalty of extended family, friends, and other supports; and the level of independence in daily living. Unanticipated changes in life goals may lead to feelings of partner incompatibility. With terminal or life-threatening illness (or associated treatments), some persons focus on survival, losing interest in sex, whereas others embrace sexuality as a positive, life-affirming issue, limited only by partner availability and support.

Principles of Sexual Rehabilitation

Treatment of medically related sexual disorders is most successful when three principles are followed (Elliott 2003):

- *Maximize* the remaining physiological capacities of the total body; similarly, maximize stability of mood, thought, and behavior.
- *Adapt* to residual limitations by utilizing specialized therapies (e.g., positioning options or specialized support cushioning, vibrators, erection enhancement medications or devices). Adaptation to psychiatric illness will depend on the patient's own resilience, as well as the nature, extent, and reliability of external supports, including that from partners.
- *Persist* in rehabilitation efforts with an exploratory, optimistic outlook. Sexuality has the potential for improvements even after the physical body has reached its maximum recovery.

A Sexual Response Model for Evaluating and Treating Sexual Disorders

Sexual response has long been conceptualized as a feedback loop or circuit that relies on the mind-body connection (Whalen and Roth 1987). Cognitions and emotions create physical reactions that depend on anatomical and neurophysiological integrity. In turn, the body's sensations and responses induce thoughts and feelings that prompt release of neurochemicals that either facilitate or inhibit both mental and physical arousal. Patients can learn to focus on positive, intimacy-enhancing, pleasurable interactions and capacities, or they can ruminate on disappointing, embarrassing, deficit-oriented experiences that limit enjoyment, exacerbate dysfunction, and foster avoidance of intimacy.

A diagram that illustrates these issues can clarify the targets and potentials for effective intervention. Patients and/or couples can then feel less stigmatized, better informed, and more engaged in a therapy that has been personalized for their situation. Our approach is to explain a patient's sexual dysfunction within the biopsychosocial context of their illness and life experience by using a model with five interacting levels: signal, evaluation, response, feedback, and outcome (see Figure 3–1). The details of the first four levels, as described below, including their impact on sexual interest, are presented in Figure 3–2.

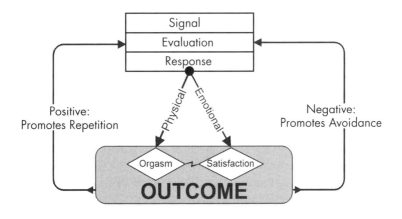

Figure 3–1.   Sexual response: levels of potential intervention.
Source.   Adapted from Stevenson and Elliott 2007.

Signal

The capacity to register a signal as sexual depends on biological factors (e.g., testosterone, sensory pathways) and psychological receptivity (e.g., attention/sedation, comfort/pain). If the signal is missing, inadequate, or unacceptable, or if reception is dulled or disabled, then the lack of any sexual response is predictable and explicable.

> *Examples:* A man with depression no longer notices his partner's invitations to be sexual. A woman with multiple sclerosis has diminished genital sensation and no longer finds clitoral stimulation to be exciting. A woman agrees to explore mild bondage but finds it disquietingly submissive and nonerotic.

Disinhibited patients may experience hyperreceptivity to previously neutral stimuli. In general, if a signal is present, recognized, and acceptable to the person, it prompts a rapid, but often complex, evaluation.

Evaluation

Sexual response is normally under steady-state inhibition mediated by the brainstem. In a theoretical sense, a complicated, often subliminal, assessment

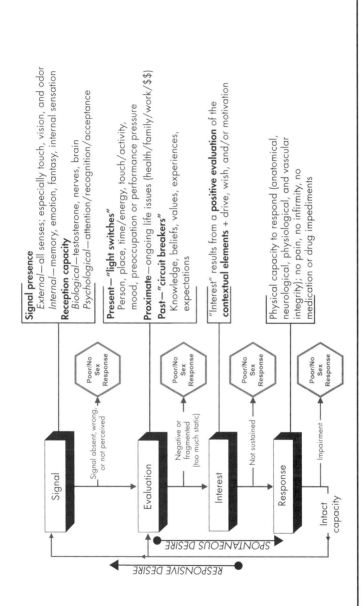

Figure 3–2. A biopsychosocial sexual response model.
Source. Adapted from Stevenson and Elliott 2007.

of immediate, current, and past issues determines whether that inhibition is removed.

Example: A shy young man, ridiculed by a former partner for ejaculating too quickly, has developed performance anxiety and erectile dysfunction; the anticipation of further failure (negative evaluation) maintains the brainstem inhibition, which impedes genital response, thereby perpetuating the erectile dysfunction. Anxiety and preoccupation would also likely interfere with perception of sensations that could improve his control over the timing of his orgasm, thereby exacerbating the rapid ejaculation.

In explaining the role of *present* issues (i.e., those of immediate concern) to patients, we use the analogy of a personalized bank of labeled light switches, operating during every moment of a sexual experience to turn sexual response "on" or "off" (Figure 3–1). Patients easily identify with the wish to 1) be with a partner whom they find attractive, who is attracted to them, and who provides feelings of sexual safety and security; 2) be in a setting that is comfortable and erotic; 3) be intimate when there are no other obligations and when pain, fatigue, or medication side effects are minimized; 4) experience a certain variety, site, intensity, rhythm, and pressure of touch or activity; 5) be in a happy, enthusiastic, and receptive mood (rather than angry, sad, or anxious mood); and 6) be free from preoccupations or distractions, especially about sex itself (performance anxiety). If too many light switches are "off" (i.e., if too much "electrical interference" or "static" is in the system), a sexual response does not happen.

Examples: Months after a bilateral mastectomy, a woman is distracted both by the loss of an important erogenous area and by concerns that her partner might find her scars unattractive. A man with a colostomy feels self-conscious about his abdominal appliance. A woman with multiple sclerosis is preoccupied with possible incontinence. A woman with arthritis experiences discomfort with sexual positions that had always been enjoyable, and now feels awkward and unfocused as she explores new options.

Communication between partners about these issues is critical. Through respectful discussion about effective signals and light switches, partners can avoid many misunderstandings.

Along with the potential immediate distractions are the *proximate* or adjacent ongoing life issues (health, finances, family, work, etc.) that may be more subtle but are still intrusive.

Past issues are likened to circuit breakers because each one potentially affects many light switches. As for the light switches, labels for the circuit breakers can be helpful: 1) knowledge about sex (often inaccurate or mistaken); 2) personal beliefs and values—all the "should do's" about appropriate sexual behavior from family, culture, religion, or the media; 3) past sexual experiences (good, bad, abusive); and 4) attitudes and expectations about sex and about relationships.

Examples: A man is discomfited by a sexually assertive female partner. A woman whose husband was disabled becomes resentful and sexually disinterested when she is forced to assume the unexpected role of caregiver and primary breadwinner.

An adult survivor of childhood sexual abuse, now in an otherwise loving relationship, finds that unpleasant and intrusive images of that distant trauma completely turn him off when his partner wants to give him oral sex.

Light switches and circuit breakers work independently, with no predictable interaction between them. If all the light switches are on in the moment of a sexual experience, a patient might be able to disregard a difficult history and still function well sexually. Alternatively, despite the lights being on in the moment, background factors can still intrude, inhibiting sexual response. It does not matter if the light switches or background issues are mundane or intricate—the amount and effect of the static depends on the individual—but for that person, in that context, the effect is predictable and comprehensible, a perspective that often helps engage the patient in recovery.

When evaluation is positive, conscious awareness of sexual interest begins, including one or more of three elements (Levine 1987): *drive*—the testosterone-dependent urge colloquially referred to as being horny; *wish*—for closeness, affection, or sensual touch; and *motivation*—a deliberate choice to be sexual (e.g., a sense of commitment, obligation, or routine; a wish to assist a partner with his or her sexual needs; nonsexual reasons). As interest evolves from a positive evaluation, so too does the body's sexual response.

Response

Removal of the brainstem inhibition allows stimulation of the lower spinal reflex centers, which triggers a cascade of responses: smooth muscles relax, vessels dilate, tissues engorge, and sensations intensify. As noted earlier, illness or treatments (e.g., changes to anatomy, nerves, blood supply, and hormones; immobility; peripheral effects of sedation, pain, or fatigue) can directly and indirectly compromise the body's capacity to respond. Patients are advised that, given their specific medical-psychiatric context, the lack of response is not unexpected. Therapeutic efforts can then target the various specific impediments to sexual function.

Examples: Employing a vibrator to compensate for diminished sensation from diabetic neuropathy; exploring other body areas for possible recruitment as erogenous zones following mastectomy; timing medication to optimize analgesic effect; treating medication-induced erectile dysfunction with a PDE5 inhibitor.

Feedback Loop

The mind continually assesses whether the sexual response is satisfactory and desirable, or incomplete, uncomfortable, disappointing, embarrassing, and so on. That critical secondary evaluation then maintains or inhibits the reflex somatic responses, thus completing a continuous feedback loop operating throughout a sexual experience. Younger, healthier persons may have greater resilience to ignore any static in the system. Age, physical or psychiatric illness, and pain or disability can affect all levels of the loop. Sexual self-confidence and identity (body image, self-esteem) can be especially vulnerable to chronic illness and/or treatment. An accepting partner can help reinforce the positive feedback elements for those whose capacities are altered.

Because urges for sex often decrease when health issues intrude, patients can be encouraged to rely less on *spontaneous desire* ("horny" feelings) and more on *responsive desire* (allowing sexual interest to kindle as a *consequence* of pleasant touching rather than as a *prerequisite* to it). Patients can be relieved and reassured to hear that such responsive desire, with or without spontaneous sexual urges, is common and, in a sense, quite "normal" (Basson 2001). Similarly, the motivation to be sexual might be related to a wish for closeness or connection, relaxation, tending to a partner's needs, or planned attempts at conception, rather than spontaneous erotic urges. Sexual activity might even be initiated for nonsexual reasons, such as material gain or other motives. Regardless of the incentive, being open to the possibility of responsive arousal can have pleasantly surprising results.

Case Example 2

A man with kidney failure was receiving dialysis three times per week in a hospital. The treatments gave him some relief from the symptoms of uremia and anemia, but he still had sleep apnea, hypertension, and erectile dysfunction, all of which made him fatigued and depressed. With his wife's assistance, he changed to home dialysis, but the bedroom then became his treatment center rather than the place in which he felt sexual. Dialysis was time-consuming, leaving him with little energy or motivation for his formerly active social life, further upsetting him and his partner. A PDE5 inhibitor had previously been effective for his erectile dysfunction but no longer seemed to work. His mood dropped even further, as did his sexual drive.

While on the transplant waitlist, he was referred to a psychiatrist, to whom he acknowledged the stress of the illness but identified the sexual problem as a priority. Laboratory tests indicated anemia and hypotestosteronemia, both potential major contributors to the sexual problem. Testosterone replacement improved his serum levels and increased his hematocrit, resulting in better energy, outlook, and mood, as well as restoring the efficacy of the PDE5 inhibitor. He removed his dialysis paraphernalia from the bedroom, and his wife's previous role in helping with her husband's basic needs was assumed by a home care nurse. The couple planned sex for times of maximum energy and convenience, and as they began having fun with creative non-goal-oriented sensuality experiences, both found themselves responding with more erotic excitement, as well as simply feeling close again as a couple.

Outcome

To emphasize their parallel but distinct qualities, we depict orgasm and satisfaction in a separate diagram (Figure 3–2) as the *physical* and *emotional* outcomes, respectively, of a sexual experience. Although the objective is often to achieve both, either can occur alone; that is, an orgasm may occur even though the experience does not generate a feeling of intimacy or satisfaction, or a sexual encounter can be intimate and emotionally satisfying without involving orgasm.

Case Example 3

A 40-year-old man with severe, treatment-resistant depression was taking a combination of medications, including antipsychotics and a selective serotonin reuptake inhibitor antidepressant. He believed the latter was the cause of his erectile dysfunction, so he periodically stopped the medication, unbeknownst to his wife, to function better sexually. He was very persistent in his overtures, despite her frequent refusals of his sexual advances. His wife also struggled with depression, in large part a reaction to the overwhelming stress of her husband's illness and its effect on their economic stability, on their relationship with their children, and on their marriage. Her own interest in sex had been virtually nonexistent for several years. However, notwithstanding her rejection of her husband's insistent advances, it was she who initiated the actual encounters when the couple did engage in sex, up to twice weekly. When this situation was clarified, the husband disclosed that his own interest was, in fact, quite low, but he was struggling to recapture the feelings of health and happiness that he recalled were once associated with being sexual; in effect, he was striving for normalcy by engaging in a so-called normal behavior. His wife revealed that her twice-weekly sexual invitations were not indicative of desire, but rather were a means to forestall the volatile mood swings that she observed in him when his advances were postponed too long. As the couple saw this dynamic exposed in the sexual response model, they quickly recognized that the route back to genuine intimacy, however challenging it still might be, would be through non-goal-oriented, noncoital pleasuring experiences that could rekindle some of their forgotten trust and joy.

Treatment

Clinical Utility of the Sexual Response Model

The sexual response model identifies five targets for assessment and possible intervention: 1) signal presence and reception capacity, 2) evaluation, 3) response capacity, 4) feedback enhancement, and 5) outcome. Depending on the predominance of biological or psychological factors, the patient and clinician can focus on one or more of these areas with various combinations of treatment, whether supportive counseling, cognitive-behavioral or insight-oriented psychotherapy (including "mindfulness" training), medication, sexual aids, surgery, and so forth. For patients with a sexual dysfunction due predominantly to biological or physical factors, the clinician can emphasize and legitimize the importance of contextual and emotional elements. This focus can be critical in maximizing recovery because application of some treatments, such as medications or sexual aids ("toys"), may be either used incorrectly or abandoned unless the contextual elements are addressed. For patients with more psychologically based dysfunctions, use of the model helps remove the stigma that the problem is "all in their head" by giving equal importance to the mind and the body. The use of the model contributes to a more comprehensive, humanistic assessment and diagnosis, engaging the patient in understanding the complexities of his or her sexual response, as well as the targets and the possibilities for improvement, hopefully leading to more enduring therapeutic success. Throughout, we emphasize three critical themes: *empowerment* (what happens to one's body should be solely at his or her invitation or request), *communication* (of one's needs to his or her partner), and *responsibility* (for exploring how to maximize one's own sexual response).

For psychiatrists, the time required to describe, or simply sketch out, a model like this will vary both with the patient's level of sophistication and comprehension and with the clinician's confidence and familiarity with the model. In general, 10–20 minutes is sufficient to present the diagram in varying degrees of detail and to solicit the patient's understanding and insights. In our experience, the vast majority of patients and couples find that the model reflects and explains their sexual problems in specific and useful ways. A separate appointment or series of visits can be arranged to discuss the implications and treatment options.

With a full sexual functioning and development history in hand (see Chapter 2, "Clinical Evaluation of Sexual Dysfunctions"), the clinician can integrate the sexual framework and rehabilitation principles described earlier in this chapter with this kind of sexual response model to provide enough information to dictate precise targets for therapeutic effort (or further investigation), emphasizing the patient's or couple's specific strengths or challenges, including medical, psychiatric, and relationship health, as well as other individual contextual issues that facilitate or inhibit arousal for the individual or partners.

Case Example 4

When he was 71 years old, Eric's wife died after a prolonged illness. The couple had been affectionate but not sexual during the later years, and Eric had masturbated only occasionally, setting aside his own sexual needs and devoting his time and attentions to his wife's care and comfort until her death. Two years later, though still missing her a great deal, he gradually became more active in community activities. His new friendships included 69-year-old Dolores. Eric felt confused at not sharing her evident interest in romance. He wondered if his sexually active years were behind him. Perfunctory experimentation with masturbation resulted in erectile failure, and his sexual drive and overall energy were low.

Eric saw his doctor about the erectile dysfunction and confirmed that, despite still-poignant thoughts of his wife, he was not suffering with more complicated guilt, grief, or depression. Eric's long-standing use of antihypertensives was also thought not to be the culprit, and his cardiovascular status was otherwise normal. An investigation of the potential physiological causes of erectile dysfunction revealed normal fasting glucose and thyroid function, but an abnormally low serum testosterone. A 3-month trial of testosterone replacement resulted in improved energy and more spontaneous sexual thoughts but only a minor improvement in erection quality, insufficient for intercourse. The doctor prescribed a PDE5 inhibitor and encouraged Eric to practice a bit with masturbation, including reacquainting himself with application of a condom. Eric was successful, and his sexual self-confidence improved. An opportunity for a romantic evening with Dolores finally arrived. Because the doctor had discussed age-related changes in sensation and response, Eric expected that both he and Dolores might need more direct genital touch for a longer period of time in order to optimize the body's sexual response. Dolores experienced some discomfort on attempts at vaginal penetration, but the use of a water-based lubricant resolved that issue. Eric continued to use testosterone and the PDE5 inhibitor, and he felt that his options for a full life had been entirely renewed.

PLISSIT: A Treatment Framework

Using a hierarchical scheme can be a helpful approach to treatment. One example is PLISSIT (Annon 1976): Permission, Limited Information, Specific Suggestion, and Intensive Therapy. This framework can be modified to suit various clinical skill levels.

Example: A clinician used PLISSIT as a treatment framework for a patient with depression and erectile dysfunction following myocardial infarction.

Permission

By asking questions about patients' sexual function, the clinician legitimizes and validates their concerns and gives them "permission" to pursue solutions—

a simple intervention that is already therapeutic. Going through the feedback model further normalizes the contributions of both psychological and physical aspects to the sexual problem(s).

Limited Information

By giving feedback about a patient's particular clinical picture, the clinician helps the patient to identify important present, proximate, and past elements (i.e., "light switches," ongoing life issues, and "circuit breakers"), as well as illness-related factors, both physical and psychiatric, that might be interfering with sexual response. Therapeutic targets might include, for example, the impact of mood or fatigability; concerns about parenting or economic implications of time off work; anxiety about a heart attack during sex; medication side effects; general vitality and physical comfort; partner needs, worries, or frustrations; the importance of patience, communication, trust, and respect during intimate encounters; and the value of a determination to work positively together on a problem important to the partners as a couple. The clinician can be very helpful by providing appropriate reassurance about the potential for "responsive" desire, even if the patient has no spontaneous sexual urges. Couples should know that there are various legitimate motivations for being sexual and that non-goal-oriented experiences can help rekindle feelings of closeness and sexual interest without adding performance pressures.

Specific Suggestion

The clinician should offer detailed guidance on the clinical evaluation. Suggestions might include

- Optimizing medications (e.g., exploring sex-friendlier antidepressants)
- Addressing modifiable risks, such as smoking, obesity, diet, and exercise
- Employing cognitive-behavioral treatments for mood or anxiety
- Suggesting a gentle return to sexual activity by deferring orgasm and intercourse, and focusing instead on sensual, nongenital pleasuring to rediscover intimacy and eroticism
- Discussing noncoital sexual options for achieving orgasm prior to resuming intercourse (including acceptability of helping partners reach orgasm even if the patient is not ready for that step)

- Discussing a couple's openness to alternative coital positions to reduce physical stress or discomfort
- Emphasizing avoidance of sex when fatigued or following heavy meals or alcohol
- Recommending a PDE5 inhibitor or other sexual aids as appropriate.

Intensive Therapy

Some patients require intensive therapy. This might include formal sexual therapy or various psychotherapy modalities for individuals or couples.

Special Clinical Considerations

Length and Termination of Therapy

Interventions for sexual problems depend on the nature of the dysfunction and the patient's or couple's expectations. On occasion, a single visit can be sufficient to provide information, reassurance, some basic suggestions, and possibly even treatment. More commonly, a series of visits, interweaving treatment with continuing assessment, is required. Patients with physical illnesses or disabilities may need to be encouraged to take the time to "relearn" their sexual capacities or to discover new potentials, through both genital and nongenital self-stimulation. Trained sexual rehabilitation clinicians can provide guidance. Therapy may 1) end when both the illness and the sexual problem resolve; 2) continue intermittently and indefinitely if the condition is chronic or deteriorating (as with interventions for other illness-related issues); 3) end when the residual sexual difficulties are accommodated into the relationship; or 4) end if the patient or couple decides to relegate sex to "a past part of life." Psychiatrists can help patients examine and adjust to all these outcomes.

Use of Sexual Aids

The clinician can help a patient or couple consider what types of sexual aids might be helpful to someone with a specific medical condition (e.g., loss of vaginal patency following cancer surgery; loss of genital sensation from multiple sclerosis or an injury). Ensuring that the options are presented in a professional, nonjudgmental, and respectful manner can be more important than the nature of the device itself. This rehabilitative approach should be practical and solution oriented.

Vacuum devices for erection enhancement are very helpful for men with serious illnesses or for those taking multiple medications, and are often better received by couples who have been together for a long time (vs. a young, single male). Vibrators, usually placed near a woman's clitoral area or around the glans area of men, may enhance the chance of orgasm (or ejaculation). Phallic or other devices for vaginal or anal insertion may allow an avenue of pleasure for some but not be acceptable to others. For some patients, self-stimulation may be the sole or preferred sexual activity. Various kinds of washable penile "sleeves" (e.g., the Fleshlight) can be used as masturbatory aids. Other sexual aids include modified support pillows (e.g., Love Bumper or Liberator Shapes) and chairs (e.g., Intimate Rider), as well as mounted ceiling bars and rails, which can substantially help with transfer, balance, strength, and relief from pain during sexual activities. The neutral presentation of any sexual aid is critical to helping patients make a fully informed decision about the use of a device as a temporary or permanent solution. The decision is also aided by reassurance that aids and devices are commonly used to good effect by other patients with similar conditions. Finally, the clinician should help a couple explore their capacity to recruit nongenital sensual or erotic areas into their sexual experience; to maximize their intimacy skills; to explore non-goal-oriented, non-coital-dependent methods of pleasure; and to nurture and strengthen their overall (nonsexual) relationship.

Obstacles to Identifying Sexual Problems

Despite their prevalence and importance, sexual concerns are possibly the most difficult area of health for patients and professionals to address. Sexual function is a subject that is uniquely private and sensitive, something that many individuals have never openly discussed with anyone, even a sexual partner. Meanwhile, North Americans are inundated with media images of people who are young, vibrant, mentally well, extroverted, and sometimes overtly erotic. These images propagate a mythical sexual standard suggesting that youth, beauty, and robust physical and mental health are all prerequisites to an active sexual life. This illusive and unrealistic stereotype is likely to be intimidating and unrealizable even for many healthy people. Individuals who are ill, injured, or elderly have little validation to see themselves as sexual beings whose concerns are legitimate and deserving of medical attention. Instead, the implication is that a disabled, infirm, psychiatrically unwell, or merely older person is unattractive, disinterested, incapable, or even unworthy of sexual thoughts, feelings, and needs. The combination of these insidious cultural myths and the intrinsically private nature of sexuality inhibits many patients from disclosing questions, concerns, or problems. Patients apparently expect little help from physicians in any event. Marwick (1999) reported on a public opinion poll in which 71% of respondents said they thought their doctor would dismiss any concerns about sexual problems, although 85% said they were inclined to broach the topic with their physician even if they might not get treatment for it. Still, embarrassment, misinformation, fear of stigma, or concerns about insurance coverage can all be factors that exacerbate nondisclosure. The clinician must therefore be proactive in evaluating and treating sexual problems.

Conclusion

Sexual problems are not distinctly organic or psychogenic, but instead are biopsychosocial phenomena with an extraordinarily high rate of comorbidity across the spectrum of physical and mental illness. Fortunately, some degree of resolution is achievable for many patients with sexual concerns. For that reason, and because loss of sexual function can have a significant effect on quality of life, psychiatrists, trained to deal with mind-body dysfunction, are well suited to include assessment of sexual issues as a routine part of their clinical work with most patients.

A sexual response feedback loop diagram can be used with patients to help elicit a full sexual history, and especially to identify specific elements in the present (including contextual, personal, interpersonal, medical, and psychiatric issues) and important experiences or themes from their psychosexual development that could be contributing to their problem. Specific details of a couple's sexual encounters, including thoughts, behaviors, and feelings, help to clarify areas of distraction, inhibition, or impairment, as well as areas for potential growth or recovery. In most cases, a patient's partner should be included in the assessment of all but the most private topics (e.g., affairs, self-stimulation), because this involvement usually fosters understanding, empathy, trust, and renewed commitment to problem solving as a couple. In working with patients with chronic illness, the clinician should utilize the rehabilitation principles and areas of inquiry to fully elucidate etiological factors. In addition to direct factors of the illness or treatments, the clinician should focus on coping skills and resilience, body image and self-esteem, mortality concerns, and functional issues such as pain or bowel and bladder control, among others listed earlier in the "Sexual Assessment Framework" section. Using a hierarchical intervention strategy such as PLISSIT allows every clinician to provide help at varying levels of sophistication.

Men and women who have previously experienced healthy, enjoyable sexual functioning have a positive mental and physical template on which to base recovery of sexual function after an acute injury or illness. However, when a condition becomes chronic or gradually debilitating, expectations of *recovery* must give way to pursuit of *adaptation*. For these reasons, especially for individuals with chronic medical conditions, the term *sexual rehabilitation* is sometimes a more accurate term than *treatment* (Stevenson and Elliott 2007). When the clinician provides a respectful, empathic, sincere, nonjudgmental, and compassionate exploration of the issues, and a holistic yet practical approach to the psychiatric and medical treatments, the majority of patients will be receptive and grateful.

Key Points

- Part of the psychiatrist's mandate is to help patients restore, maintain, or improve their quality of life, including sexual function.

- Sexual disorders have mixed biopsychosocial etiologies and frequently occur comorbidly with medical and psychiatric illness.

- Psychiatrists, trained in medicine and psychology, are well positioned to be clinical service, teaching, and research thought leaders regarding sexual disorders.

- Age, illness, and impairment do not signal an end to sexuality.

- Psychiatrists can approach the treatment of comorbid sexual dysfunctions by utilizing the following:
  - A comprehensive sexual framework for assessment (Table 3–1)
  - A sexual response model that engages patients in clarifying impairments and identifying specific targets for investigation or intervention (Figures 3–1 and 3–2)
  - Principles of rehabilitation: maximize remaining capacity, adapt to residual limitations, and persist with openness and optimism (Table 3–1)
- The clinician can help patients assume responsibility for meeting their sexual needs by encouraging a sense of control, exploring remaining potentials, and facilitating communication with partners.
- A hierarchical treatment scheme such as PLISSIT enables clinicians with various knowledge and skill levels to provide helpful guidance and important interventions.

References

Ambler N, Williams A, Hill P, et al: Sexual difficulties of chronic pain patients. Clin J Pain 17:138–145, 2001

Annon JS: The Behavioral Treatment of Sexual Problems: Brief Therapy. New York, Harper & Row, 1976

Aschka C, Himmel W, Ittner E, et al: Sexual problems of male patients in family practice. J Fam Pract 50:773–778, 2001

Bancroft J, Vukadinovic Z: Sexual addiction, sexual compulsivity, sexual impulsivity, or what? Toward a theoretical model. J Sex Res 41:224–234, 2004

Basson RJ: Human sex response cycles. J Sex Marital Ther 27:33–43, 2001

Blazer D: Depression in late life: review and commentary. J Gerontol A Biol Sci Med Sci 58:249–265, 2003

Blume SB: Alcoholism in women. Harv Ment Health Lett 14:5–7, 1998

Bronner G, Royter V, Korczyn A, et al: Sexual dysfunction in Parkinson's disease. J Sex Marital Ther 30:95–105, 2004

Bushnik T, Englander J, Wright J: The experience of fatigue in the first 2 years after moderate-to-severe traumatic brain injury: a preliminary report. J Head Trauma Rehabil 23:17–24, 2008

Chen Y, Chu S, Lin M, et al: Impact of renal transplantation on sexual function in female recipients. Transplant Proc 35:313–314, 2003

Colfax G, Coates TJ, Husnik MJ, et al: Longitudinal patterns of methamphetamine, popper (amyl nitrite), and cocaine use and high-risk sexual behavior among a cohort of San Francisco men who have sex with men. J Urban Health 82 (suppl 1):i62–i70, 2005

Cyranowski J, Frank E, Cherry C, et al: Prospective assessment of sexual function in women treated for recurrent major depression. J Psychiatr Res 38:267–273, 2004

Daniell HW: Hypogonadism in men consuming sustained-action oral opioids. J Pain 3:377–384, 2002

DasGupta R, Fowler CJ: Bladder, bowel and sexual dysfunction in multiple sclerosis. Drugs 63:153–166, 2003

de Groot M, Anderson R, Freedland KE, et al: Association of depression and diabetes complications: a meta-analysis. Psychosom Med 63:619–630, 2001

Ekland M, Krassioukov A, McBride K, et al: Incidence of autonomic dysreflexia and silent autonomic dysreflexia in men with SCI undergoing sperm retrieval: implications for clinical practice. J Spinal Cord Med 31:33–39, 2008

El-Bassel N, Gilbert L, Rajah V: The relationship between drug abuse and sexual performance among women on methadone: heightening the risk of sexual intimate violence and HIV. Addict Behav 28:1385–1403, 2003

Elliott S: Ejaculation and orgasm: sexuality in men with SCI. Top Spinal Cord Inj Rehabil 8:1–15, 2002

Elliott S: Sexual dysfunction and infertility in men with spinal cord disorders, in Spinal Cord Medicine: Principles and Practice. Edited by Vernon L. New York, Demos Medical Publishing, 2003

Elliott S: Sexuality after SCI, in Spinal Cord Injury Rehabilitation. Edited by Field-Fote E. Philadelphia, PA, FA Davis, 2009

Elliott SL: Sexual dysfunction in women with chronic medical illness, in Female Reproductive and Sexual Medicine. Edited by Kandel F. Totowa, NJ, Humana Press (in press)

Feldman HA, Goldstein I, Hatzichristou DG, et al: Impotence and its medical and psychosocial correlates: results of the Massachusetts Male Aging Study. J Urol 151:45–61, 1994

Figueira I, Possidente E, Marques C, et al: Sexual dysfunction: a neglected complication of panic disorder and social phobia. Arch Sex Behav 30:369–377, 2001

Fleischhacker WW, Cetkovich-Bakmas M, De Hert M, et al: Comorbid somatic illnesses in patients with severe mental disorders: clinical, policy, and research challenges. J Clin Psychiatry 69:514–519, 2008

Goldstein I: The mutually reinforcing triad of depressive symptoms, cardiovascular disease, and erectile dysfunction. Am J Cardiol 86(suppl):41f–45f, 2000

Gumus B, Yigitoglu MR, Lekili M, et al: Effect of long-term alcohol abuse on male sexual function and serum gonadal hormone levels. Int Urol Nephrol 30:755–759, 1998

Hallinan R, Byrne A, Agho K, et al: Erectile dysfunction in men receiving methadone and buprenorphine maintenance treatment. J Sex Med 5:684–692, 2008

Hibbard MR, Gordon WA, Flanagan S, et al: Sexual dysfunction after traumatic brain injury. Neurorehabilitation 15:107–120, 2000

Jackson G, Rosen R, Kloner R, et al: The Second Princeton Consensus on Sexual Dysfunction and Cardiac Risk: new guidelines for sexual medicine. J Sex Med 3:28–36, 2006

Kalpakjian CZ, Albright KJ: An examination of depression through the lens of spinal cord injury: comparative prevalence rates and severity in women and men. Womens Health Issues 16:380–388, 2006

Kaplan HS: The New Sex Therapy: Active Treatment of Sexual Dysfunctions. New York, Brunner/Mazel, 1974

Kennedy SH, Dickens SE, Eisfeld BS, et al: Sexual dysfunction before antidepressant therapy in major depression. J Affect Disord 56:201–208, 1999

Kettas E, Cayan F, Akbay E, et al: Sexual dysfunction and associated risk factors in women with end-stage renal disease. J Sex Med 5:872–877, 2008

Kumar RJ, Barqawi D, Crawford ED: Preventing and treating the complications of hormone therapy. Curr Urol Rep 6:217–223, 2005

La Pera G, Carderi A, Marianantoni Z, et al: Sexual dysfunction prior to first drug use among former drug addicts and its possible causal meaning on drug addiction: preliminary results. J Sex Med 5:164–172, 2008

Leavy S, Weitzel W: Endocrine abnormalities in chronic renal failure. Endocrinol Metab Clin North Am 31:107–119, 2002

Levine SB: More on the nature of sexual desire. J Sex Marital Ther 13:35–44, 1987

Marwick C: Survey says patients expect little physician help on sex. JAMA 281:2173–2174, 1999

McKee AL, Schover LR: Sexuality rehabilitation. Cancer 92:1008–1012, 2001

Morant S, Bloomfield G, Vats V, et al: Increased sexual dysfunction in men with storage and voiding lower urinary tract symptoms. J Sex Med 6:1103–1110, 2009

Muller JE: Sexual activity as a trigger for cardiovascular events: what is the risk? Am J Cardiol 84:2N–5N, 1999

O'Farrell TJ, Choquette KA, Cutter HSG, et al: Sexual satisfaction and dysfunction in marriages of male alcoholics: comparison with nonalcoholic maritally conflicted couples and nonconflicted couples. J Stud Alcohol 58:91–99, 1997

Parzeller M, Raschka C, Bratzke H: Sudden cardiovascular death in correlation with sexual activity: results of a medicolegal postmortem study from 1972–1998. Eur Heart J 22:610–616, 2001

Raja M, Azzoni A: Sexual behavior and sexual problems among patients with severe chronic psychoses. Eur Psychiatry 18:70–76, 2003

Romeo J, Seftel A, Madhun Z, et al: Sexual function in men with diabetes type 2. J Urol 163:788–791, 2000

Rybarczyk B, Nyenhuis DL, Nicholas JJ, et al: Body image, perceived social stigma, the prediction of psychosocial adjustment to leg amputation. Rehabil Psychol 40:95–110, 1995

Seidman SN, Roose SP, Menza MA, et al: Treatment of erectile dysfunction in men with depressive symptoms: results of a placebo-controlled trial with sildenafil citrate. Am J Psychiatry 158:1623–1630, 2001

Shabsigh R, Shah M, Sand M: Erectile dysfunction and men's health: developing a comorbidity risk calculator. J Sex Med 5:1237–1243, 2008

Smith GL, Christmas TJ: Potency preserving surgery, in Textbook of Erectile Dysfunction. Edited by Carson C, Kirby R, Goldstein I. Oxford, UK, ISIS Medical Media, 1999, pp 599–606

Son Y, Choi K, Park Y, et al: Depression, symptoms and the quality of life for end stage. Am J Nephrol 29:36–42, 2009

Stevenson RWD, Elliott SE: Sexuality and illness, in Principles and Practice of Sex Therapy, 4th Edition. Edited by Leiblum SR. New York, Guilford Press, 2007, pp 313–349

Szasz G: Sexual health care, in Management of Spinal Cord Injury, 2nd Edition. Edited by Zejdlik C. Boston, MA, Jones and Bartlett, 1992, pp 175–201

Taylor HA: Sexual activity and the cardiovascular patient: guidelines. Am J Cardiol 84:6n–10n, 1999

Teusch L, Scherbaum N, Bohme H, et al: Different patterns of sexual dysfunctions associated with psychiatric disorders and psychopharmacological treatment: results of an investigation by semistructured interview of schizophrenic and neurotic patients and methadone-substituted opiate addicts. Pharmacopsychiatry 28:84–92, 1995

Thomas DR: Medications and sexual function. Clin Geriatr Med 19:553–562, 2003

Tilton MC: Diabetes and amputation, in Sexual Function in People With Disability and Chronic Illness. Edited by Sipski M, Alexander C. Gaithersburg, MD, Aspen, 1997, pp 279–302

Tjandra BS, Janknegt RA: Neurogenic impotence and lower urinary tract symptoms due to Vitamin B$_1$ deficiency in chronic alcoholism. J Urol 157:954–955, 1997

Tsujimura A, Matsumiya K, Tsuboniwa N, et al: Effect of renal transplantation on sexual function. Arch Androl 48:467–474, 2002

Turvey C, Klein D: Remission from depression comorbid with chronic illness and physical impairment. Am J Psychiatry 165:569–574, 2008

Weizman R, Wiezman A, Levi J, et al: Sexual dysfunction associated with hyperprolactinemia in males and females undergoing hemodialysis. Psychosom Med 45:259–269, 1983

Whalen SR, Roth D: A cognitive approach, in Theories of Human Sexuality. Edited by Geer JH, O'Donohue T. New York, Plenum, 1987

Zanarini MC, Parachini EA, Frankenburg FR, et al: Sexual relationship difficulties among borderline patients and Axis II comparison subjects. J Nerv Ment Dis 191:479–482, 2003

4

Medications and Sexual Function and Dysfunction

Richard Balon, M.D.

The relationship between pharmacological agents (including herbal preparations and medications) and sexual functioning has been explored since the antiquities. For centuries, the main focus was on preparations or foods that could enhance one's sexual functioning or desire—that is, on aphrodisiacs (a word derived from the name of the Greek goddess of love, Aphrodite). Some of the aphrodisiacs may contain chemicals that potentially influence sexual desire or other aspects of sexual functioning. Some of them, such as rhinoceros horn or oysters, were considered to be aphrodisiacs mainly for their symbolic notion.

The human search for aphrodisiacs has continued to the present time. Chocolate has sometimes been promoted as a food that could enhance one's sexual functioning, and many so-called natural preparations have been touted the same way. Phosphodiesterase type 5 (PDE5) inhibitors and testosterone are not considered aphrodisiacs in a strict sense, yet their advertisements frequently border on promoting them as aphrodisiacs. The everlasting interest in pharmacological aids for sexual functioning has been demonstrated numerous times by the huge media attention to even the smallest findings of possible improvement or enhancement of sexual functioning via pharmacological agents.

During the last several decades, the complicated relationship between pharmaceutical agents and sexual functioning has also become a focus. The impairment of sexual functioning has been associated with various pharmacological agents, both psychotropic and nonpsychotropic. Numerous medications have been reported to be associated with impaired sexual functioning, affecting either the entire sexual response cycle or (less frequently) one phase of this cycle (although the phases are interconnected and cannot be clearly and unequivocally separated). Basically, the field of sexual pharmacology has gradually developed over the last few decades (see the books on sexual pharmacology by Crenshaw and Goldberg [1996] and Segraves and Balon [2003]). Impaired sexual functioning due to medications not only can significantly impact the patient's quality of life but also can lead to nonadherence to the medication regimen.

In this chapter, I focus on impaired sexual functioning due to various medications and its possible management, with the main focus on a prototypical group of medications associated with sexual dysfunction—antidepressants. In addition, I briefly mention pharmacological agents used for the treatment of various sexual dysfunctions and disorders, most of which are discussed in more detail in other chapters, and also some substances that may not help as much as previously believed or do not help at all. Importantly, this chapter serves as an overview and offers clinically oriented guidance for the assessment and management of sexual dysfunction associated with medications, not an exhaustive review of sexual pharmacology.

Definition of and Criteria for Sexual Dysfunction Associated With Medications

As noted in DSM-IV-TR (American Psychiatric Association 2000),

> A substance-induced sexual dysfunction due to a prescribed treatment for a mental disorder or general medical condition must have its onset while the

person is receiving the medication (e.g., antihypertensive medication). Once the treatment is discontinued, the sexual dysfunction will remit within days to several weeks (depending on the half-life of the substance). If the sexual dysfunction persists, other causes for the dysfunction should be considered. (p. 564)

The DSM-IV-TR criteria for sexual dysfunction associated with substances and medications are outlined in Table 4–1.

Some of the DSM-IV-TR criteria may not be perfectly clear (e.g., the etiological relationship, like many etiological relationships in psychiatry, is usually presumed) or may be a bit controversial (for recent case reports of persistent sexual dysfunction, see Bolton et al. 2006 and Csoka and Shipko 2006). However, these criteria succinctly summarize the issue in defining medication-induced sexual dysfunction.

Antidepressants

Depression is frequently associated with sexual dysfunction (e.g., Baldwin 1996), especially low sexual desire, but also other impairments, such as erectile dysfunction. The impairment of sexual functioning does not, however, mean that depressed and anxious patients consider sexual functioning unimportant, that they do not wish to have a good sexual life, or that they are contented to have their sexual functioning even more impaired due to medications. Therefore, the management of sexual dysfunction associated with antidepressants has emerged as an important clinical area.

Antidepressants have been the most studied group of medications with regard to sexual dysfunction, at least in psychiatry. Case reports and/or case series of sexual dysfunctions associated with antidepressants (tricyclic antidepressants [TCAs], monoamine oxidase inhibitors [MAOIs]) appeared not very long after the introduction of these agents (e.g., Beaumont 1977). However, like many other side effects, sexual dysfunctions associated with antidepressants have not been systematically studied for decades. Paradoxically, the development of newer, better tolerated antidepressants, such as the selective serotonin reuptake inhibitors (SSRIs), and their use in treating less severe conditions probably led to an increased awareness and focus on the impairment of sexual functioning associated with antidepressants.

Table 4–1. DSM-IV-TR diagnostic criteria for substance-induced sexual dysfunction

A. Clinically significant sexual dysfunction that results in marked distress or interpersonal difficulty predominates in the clinical picture.

B. There is evidence from the history, physical examination, or laboratory findings that the sexual dysfunction is fully explained by substance use as manifested by either (1) or (2):

   (1) the symptoms in Criterion A developed during, or within a month of, substance intoxication

   (2) medication use is etiologically related to the disturbance

C. The disturbance is not better accounted for by a sexual dysfunction that is not substance induced. Evidence that the symptoms are better accounted for by a sexual dysfunction that is not substance induced might include the following: the symptoms precede the onset of the substance use or dependence (or medication use); the symptoms persist for a substantial period of time (e.g., about a month) after the cessation of intoxication, or are substantially in excess of what would be expected given the type or amount of the substance used or the duration of use; or there is other evidence that suggests the existence of an independent non-substance-induced sexual dysfunction (e.g., a history of recurrent non-substance-related episodes).

Note: This diagnosis should be made instead of a diagnosis of substance intoxication only when the sexual dysfunction is in excess of that usually associated with the intoxication syndrome and when the dysfunction is sufficiently severe to warrant independent clinical attention.

   Code [Specific Substance]–Induced Sexual Dysfunction:

   (291.89 Alcohol; 292.89 Amphetamine [or Amphetamine-Like Substance]; 292.89 Cocaine; 292.89 Opioid; 292.89 Sedative, Hypnotic, or Anxiolytic; 292.89 Other [or Unknown] Substance)

   Specify if:

   With Impaired Desire

   With Impaired Arousal

Table 4–1. DSM-IV-TR diagnostic criteria for substance-induced sexual dysfunction *(continued)*

> With Impaired Orgasm
>
> With Sexual Pain

Specify if:

> **With Onset During Intoxication:** if the criteria are met for intoxication with the substance and the symptoms develop during the intoxication syndrome

Source. Reprinted from American Psychiatric Association: *Diagnostic and Statistical Manual of Mental Disorders,* 4th Edition, Text Revision. Washington, DC, American Psychiatric Association, 2000. Copyright 2000, American Psychiatric Association. Used with permission.

Since the early 1990s, numerous reports, studies, and review articles have addressed sexual dysfunction associated with antidepressants. Nobody questions the existence of sexual dysfunction associated with this group of medications. As Montgomery et al. (2002) pointed out,

> Sexual dysfunction is widespread in the healthy non-depressed population and is a recognized symptom of depression and/or anxiety disorders (some would add also others, such as eating disorders). Sexual dysfunction has been reported with all classes of antidepressants (MAOIs, TCAs, SSRIs, SNRIs [serotonin-norepinephrine reuptake inhibitors], and newer antidepressants) in patients with depression and various anxiety disorders. Numerous studies have been published, but only one used a validated sexual function rating scale and most lacked either a baseline or a placebo control or both. (p. 119)

These authors also felt that findings from the literature were not sufficiently robust to support claims of a difference in the incidence of drug-induced sexual dysfunction between existing antidepressant therapies. Nevertheless, most authors and clinicians would agree (based on some evidence) that various individual antidepressants (not groups), such as bupropion, mirtazapine, moclobemide, and nefazodone, are associated with sexual dysfunctions less frequently than the rest of antidepressants.

The estimates of incidence of sexual dysfunction associated with antidepressants are usually between 30% and 40% (some would claim up to 70%), but the numbers vary widely, from as low as 10% to as high as 90% with some medications (Monteiro et al. 1987). As pointed out by many researchers (e.g., Segraves and Balon 2003), the character and frequency of sexual dysfunction associated with different groups of antidepressants may vary somewhat. For instance, compared with other antidepressants, predominantly serotonergic antidepressants such as SSRIs and clomipramine seem to be more frequently associated with delayed orgasm or anorgasmia, and TCAs seem to be more frequently associated with erectile dysfunction. The reasons for the wide range of estimates include the imprecise definition of *sexual dysfunction*, the lack of using standard instruments, and the discrepancy between estimates obtained via self-reporting and via active questioning. For instance, in a study by Landen et al. (2005), more patients (41%) reported sexual dysfunction in response to direct questioning than through spontaneous reporting (6%).

The etiology of sexual dysfunction during antidepressant therapy is complicated and not well understood. The impact of antidepressants on various neurotransmitter systems, such as dopamine, norepinephrine, and serotonin systems, certainly plays a major role. Dopamine influences motivated sexual behavior, desire, and the ability to become involved in sexual activity (Clayton and Montejo 2006); norepinephrine stimulates sexual arousal and vasocongestion; and serotonin system activation may suspend vasocongestion, turning off arousal. Serotonin may also diminish nitric oxide function and decrease genital sensation (Clayton and Montejo 2006). As suggested in the study by Safarinejad (2008), some antidepressants (SSRIs) may decrease the levels of hormones involved in the regulation of sexual functioning, such as testosterone, luteinizing hormone, and others.

The complicated interaction of psychotropic medications, neurotransmitters, and the peripheral and central nervous systems was summarized by Segraves (1989). However, as Clayton and Montejo (2006) pointed out, many more potential causes of sexual dysfunction exist during antidepressant therapy, including, besides the mentioned ones, psychiatric illness; medical illness; interpersonal conflicts; substance abuse; developmental issues; sexual trauma; concerns about sexually transmitted diseases; psychological issues (self-esteem); cultural, religious, and environmental issues; pregnancy and childbearing issues; life cycle issues; neurological insult; and partner and/or sexual-specific issues. As pointed out in Chapter 2, "Clinical Evaluation of Sexual Dysfunctions," all these factors should be considered during the baseline evaluation of *any* sexual dysfunction, including sexual dysfunction associated with medications.

Other Psychotropic Medications

Antipsychotics

Sexual dysfunction has been linked to typical or traditional antipsychotics since the late 1960s (Kelly and Conley 2004). Kotin and Wilbert (1976) reported that among patients treated with thioridazine, 60% experienced sexual impairment, 44% had troubles with ejaculation, and 35% had difficulty maintaining an erection. The incidence of sexual dysfunction associated with antipsychotics has been estimated to be around 50% among patients with schizophrenia treated with these medications. However, some of the more recent studies reported rates as high as 80%–90% (Kelly and Conley 2004).

Determining the incidence of sexual dysfunction associated with antipsychotics is even more complicated than determining the incidence of sexual dysfunction associated with antidepressants. Although many newer antipsychotics have recently been approved by the U.S. Food and Drug Administration for wider indications, such as treatment of mood and anxiety disorders, most of the incidence reports are from samples of patients with schizophrenia treated with antipsychotics. Patients with schizophrenia are typically less engaged in sexual activities in general and have lower libido. These patients are also fairly unreliable when questioned about their sexual functioning, especially during a psychotic episode. In addition, psychiatrists may not feel comfortable speaking to these patients about their sexual problems or may not feel that this is an important area to address. Another problem is the lack of a reliable and valid instrument for estimating sexual dysfunction in this population. Additionally, most of the data on sexual dysfunction associated with antipsychotics has been obtained from studies and reports involving typical antipsychotics, yet these medications have been prescribed less frequently than the atypical antipsychotics in recent years. The incidence of sexual dysfunction associated with the newer antipsychotics is usually cited as fairly low, 10%–30%, and in some cases even in the single digits.

Sexual problems described as associated with antipsychotics (mostly the typical ones) include decreased libido, impaired erection, priapism, retrograde ejaculation, painful ejaculation, delayed orgasm, amenorrhea, and other disturbances of the menstrual cycle.

The mechanism of sexual dysfunction associated with antipsychotics is complex. Prolactin elevation has frequently been mentioned as the main culprit. Knegtering et al. (2008) reported that around 40% of emerging sexual side effects in patients with schizophrenia in their study were attributable to the prolactin-raising properties of antipsychotics. However, as Kelly and Conley (2004) pointed out, other factors, such as cholinergic antagonism, alpha-adrenergic blockade, serotonin activity, extrapyramidal side effects, tardive dyskinesia, and nonspecific effects such as sedation and weight gain (histamine receptors), may also play a significant role.

Mood Stabilizers

Evidence of sexual dysfunction associated with mood stabilizers is scarce. This scarcity of data has several possible explanations. First, with many antipsychotics being approved for various phases of bipolar disorder and claims of their mood-stabilizing properties, it is less clear what a "mood stabilizer" is and what drugs should be classified as mood stabilizers. Second, the incidence of sexual dysfunction with mood stabilizers seems to be low. Third, the available incidence data suffer from the fact that they were obtained mostly from case reports and series or from studies with poor methodology. Fourth, the estimate of sexual dysfunction associated with mood stabilizers is clouded by the changes of libido that typically occur during the course of bipolar disorder. During the manic phase, many patients report hypersexuality, but a few report diminished libido. As already mentioned, depression can be associated with diminished libido, erectile dysfunction, and other problems.

Unless combined with other medications, lithium appears to have limited adverse sexual side effects (Labbate 2008). Most of the data on sexual dysfunction associated with anticonvulsants that are used as mood stabilizers (e.g., carbamazepine, lamotrigine, oxcarbazepine, topiramate, valproic acid) comes from the epilepsy literature; the data on these drugs from bipolar disorder literature are either nonexistent or very limited. Sexual dysfunction associated with lamotrigine and valproic acid is considered to be rare. Carbamazepine induces metabolism of androgen and impacts other hormones, and thus is considered more prone to be associated with sexual dysfunction. Again, however, the evidence of this association is weak.

The mechanism of sexual dysfunction associated with mood stabilizers is probably multifactorial. These medications may combine effects on various neurotransmitters in the peripheral and central nervous systems, on metabolism of various hormones, and on sex hormone–binding globulin.

Antianxiety Medications

Medications usually used for treatment of anxiety and anxiety disorders include benzodiazepines, buspirone, various antidepressants, and more recently antipsychotics. All benzodiazepines have occasionally been reported as being associated with sexual dysfunction. However, the evidence is mostly anecdotal, and good studies are nonexistent. Decreased libido and impaired arousal and orgasm have been reported with benzodiazepines (Labbate 2008). Most benzodiazepines seem to have a dose-response relationship between the drug dose and sexual inhibition (Segraves and Balon 2003). Whether an association exists between benzodiazepines and sexual disinhibition is unclear. The estimate of frequency and the evaluation of sexual dysfunction associated with benzodiazepines are confounded by the association of sexual dysfunction with anxiety and anxiety disorders (Zemishlany and Weizman 2008). The mechanism of sexual dysfunction associated with benzodiazepines is not known but may involve gamma-aminobutyric acid receptors in the midbrain central gray or ventral tegmental area.

Buspirone is an anxiolytic that exerts its antianxiety effect through serotonin type 1A (5-HT$_{1A}$) presynaptic and postsynaptic receptors. It does not seem to have any effect on sexual functioning and has actually been used to reverse sexual dysfunction associated with SSRIs (Norden 1994).

Stimulants and Other Medications Used to Treat Attention-Deficit/Hyperactivity Disorder

Stimulants, such as various formulas of methylphenidate or amphetamine and its salts, are usually not associated with sexual dysfunction and are occasionally used for alleviation of sexual dysfunction associated with antidepressants. Treatment-emergent decreased libido and erectile dysfunction were described in one study with atomoxetine, a nonstimulant medication used to treat attention-deficit/hyperactivity disorder (Adler et al. 2006); in this study, the incidence of both these sexual side effects was low.

Other Medications Used to Treat Mental Disorders

Sexual dysfunction has not been reported to be associated with modafinil. The incidence of sexual dysfunction associated with guanfacine is low.

Nonpsychotropic Medications

Although the association between sexual functioning and psychotropic medications has received relatively more attention in the scientific and lay literature, nonpsychotropic medications are also frequently associated with impairment of sexual functioning. Frequently, sexual dysfunction is also associated with the physical illness treated by these medications, and the primary or secondary contributing roles of medications to sexual dysfunction are not fully appreciated. The focus in this chapter is on medications used for a longer period of time or chronically, rather than on agents used occasionally or for a brief period of time, such as antibiotics. For a full review of evidence regarding the latter medications, the interested reader is referred to books on sexual pharmacology by Crenshaw and Goldberg (1996) and Segraves and Balon (2003).

The following groups of medications are frequently mentioned as being associated with sexual dysfunction:

- *Cardiovascular medications* (e.g., antihypertensives, antiarrhythmics, beta-blockers, calcium channel blockers, diuretics, lipid-lowering medications, vasodilators, combination agents): These medications are most frequently associated with erectile dysfunction. However, decreased libido in both genders, impaired lubrication in women, and ejaculatory or orgasmic delay or inhibition may also occur.
- *Chemotherapeutic (antineoplastic, cytotoxic) agents* (e.g., antibiotics, antimetabolites, alkylating agents, hormones, immunomodulators, plant agents): These medications are frequently very toxic, and their impact on sexual organs and sexual functioning is not fully appreciated. Decreased libido is a frequent complication of chemotherapy, but impaired arousal (frequently due to vaginal dryness), dyspareunia, and difficulties in reaching orgasm also occur. Evaluation of sexual functioning associated with chemotherapeutic agents is complicated by other factors, such as nerve

damage by these agents, nerve and vascular damage by possible radiation, potential surgical damage (e.g., during prostate surgery), and associated medical symptoms (nausea) and psychological symptoms (anxiety, depression), as well as treatment of these symptoms with SSRIs.

- *Gastrointestinal agents* (e.g., antacids, antidiarrheals, antiemetics, antispasmodics, histamine receptor agonists, proton pump inhibitors): Physicians should remember that patients with severe nausea or frequent diarrhea are probably not involved in sexual activity, and therefore their sexual dysfunction may not be due to the gastrointestinal agents. The full scope and character of sexual dysfunction associated with these medications is not well known. Some of the gastrointestinal medications (e.g., cimetidine) may impact sexual functioning in a quite complex way (i.e., their impact on hormones and hormone receptors may result not only in various types of sexual impairment, such as erectile dysfunction, but also in gynecomastia). Because some of these medications are available over-the-counter (e.g., cimetidine), they may not be mentioned in the list of "prescribed" medications provided by patients.

- *Hormones and other medications used in obstetrics and gynecology* (antiandrogens—also used in urology, gonadotropin-releasing hormone agonists, selective estrogen receptor modulators): Sex hormones are usually thought (not always correctly) to be associated with positive changes in sexual functioning. Nevertheless, some of these medications, such as oral contraceptives, may be associated with sexual dysfunction (decreased libido), because exogenous estrogens and progesterones may lead to decreased levels of androgens.

- *Medications used in neurology* (antiepileptics, antiparkinsonian medications, migraine medications): As mentioned in the earlier section on mood stabilizers, medications used to treat epilepsy may be associated with sexual dysfunctions (e.g., decreased libido). However, the assessment of sexual dysfunction associated with these medications in patients with epilepsy is difficult due to known hyposexuality in these patients. Also, some of these medications (e.g., carbamazepine) affect the levels of sex hormones and sex hormone–binding globulin. Medications used to treat Parkinson's disease usually do not have a negative impact on sexual functioning and actually may be associated with hypersexuality (Klos et al. 2005). Migraine medications have not been reported to cause sexual dysfunction.

- *Medications used in urology* (drugs used for incontinence, drugs used for benign prostatic hypertrophy and/or prostatic cancer): Finasteride, used in benign prostatic hypertrophy, may be associated with erectile dysfunction or delayed ejaculation. The TCA imipramine, used in enuresis and occasionally in incontinence, is associated with erectile dysfunction and other impairment of sexual functioning.

Other medications, such as nonsteroidal anti-inflammatory drugs or even topical glaucoma medication (timolol, a beta-blocker), may occasionally be associated with various sexual dysfunctions. Some of the medications used for treatment of substance abuse have been reported to be associated with sexual dysfunction (e.g., methadone has been associated with erectile dysfunction; Hallinan et al. 2008), but others have not (e.g., buprenorphine; naltrexone, which has been actually tested for treating erectile dysfunction).

Substance Abuse and Toxins

Although the focus of this chapter is on sexual dysfunction associated with medications, sexual dysfunctions also may be associated with recreational drugs (alcohol, cocaine, heroin, marijuana, nicotine), especially when used chronically (Palha and Esteves 2008). Similarly, numerous workplace toxins (e.g., carbon disulfide, chlordecone, manganese, nitrous oxide, stilbene, trinitrotoluene) may be associated with sexual dysfunctions (Segraves and Balon 2003).

Management of Sexual Dysfunction Associated With Medications

The management of sexual dysfunction associated with medications starts with the initial evaluation of the patient. The clinician has to carefully evaluate the patient's sexual functioning at baseline, prior to starting any medication (for discussion of evaluation, see Chapter 2). Nothing can replace a thorough baseline evaluation. The clinician cannot rely on patient memory in making sure that the sexual dysfunction definitely started after the onset of treatment. Also, because the "cause" of sexual dysfunction can be quite complicated, considerations should include the presenting disorder, the possibility of one or more comorbid disorders (mental and/or physical), more than one medication, interpersonal problems, and even primary sexual dysfunction.

An important part of the baseline evaluation is proactive, pointed questioning. The clinician should ask very specific questions, not general, vague ones. Proactive and specific questioning should continue during follow-up visits and should become part of the clinician's routine, not occurring just in response to a patient's spontaneous reporting of sexual dysfunction (as mentioned earlier, spontaneous reporting and active questioning lead to differences in the numbers of reports of sexual dysfunction associated with medication; see Landen et al. 2005). Some clinicians may decide to use questionnaires completed by patients or by clinicians (see Chapter 2). Patients' self-reports should always be followed by a clinical interview, including going over the questions and possibly asking additional ones (for examples of questions about sexual functioning, see Table 2–2 in Chapter 2). Laboratory testing is almost never necessary in evaluating medication-associated sexual dysfunction (an exception may be measuring prolactin levels in antipsychotic-associated sexual dysfunction).

The clinician should also obtain information about the patient's use of over-the-counter medications, herbal preparations, and contraceptives, and about possible substance abuse (including nicotine and alcohol). The effect of a treated illness (e.g., depression, anxiety, cancer, hypertension, coronary artery disease) on sexual functioning should also be considered. Some preventable and/or treatable risks or factors, such as diabetes mellitus, hypertension, obesity, sleep apnea, or smoking, may be contributing to the sexual dysfunction. Addressing these risks or factors may either decrease the need for the medication that is causing sexual dysfunction or improve the patient's general physical well-being and possibly sexual functioning.

The clinician should also actively discuss the possibility of medication-associated sexual dysfunction with the patient. Patients appreciate being informed by the physician and being part of the clinical decision making, and some patients may have heard that sexual dysfunction may be associated with their medication. Inviting the partner to discuss sexual activity may also be helpful.

For patients with certain diseases, the discussion of sexual activity prior to treatment may include some practical tips (Segraves and Balon 2003). For example, for patients with cardiovascular disease, especially during the post-myocardial infarction period, these tips may include suggestions of avoiding sex after meals (wait 3 hours) or after alcohol consumption; avoiding sex in extreme temperatures; avoiding sex when tired or fatigued; avoiding sex during periods of extreme stress; and reporting to the treating physician any unusual symptoms (e.g., chest pain, long palpitations, marked fatigue, sleeplessness) that occur during or after sexual activity.

Several strategies have been used in the management of sexual dysfunction associated with medications, most of which were used originally for the management of antidepressant-associated sexual dysfunction. Most of these strategies have not been properly evaluated in a gold-standard, double-blind placebo fashion and probably never will be evaluated in this fashion. As Taylor et al. (2005) pointed out in their analysis of management strategies for antidepressant-associated sexual dysfunction, only the addition of sildenafil or tadalafil and possibly bupropion seem to be effective strategies, supported by relatively solid evidence. Thus, the use of management strategies remains a clinical art rather than a science. Again, a complete review of evidence is beyond the scope of this chapter, and the interested reader is referred to the book by Segraves and Balon (2003).

Management strategies for medication-associated sexual dysfunction are discussed below and are summarized in Table 4–2. Importantly, none of the medications mentioned in the management strategies of medication-associated sexual dysfunction has been approved by the U.S. Food and Drug Administration for these indications.

1. *Select a medication with a low incidence of sexual dysfunction, especially for sexually active patients.* This proactive strategy may be quite helpful for sexually active patients. In the case of antidepressants, one may choose bupropion, mirtazapine, moclobemide, or nefazodone as the initial treatment of depression or some of the anxiety disorders. Similarly, in the case of antipsychotics, one may choose either any of the atypical antipsychotics, or some of the older antipsychotics, such as loxapine or molindone, that are reportedly associated with a lower incidence of sexual dysfunction. Among antihypertensives, one may choose captopril, which reportedly has been associated with a lower incidence of sexual dysfunction.

2. *Wait for spontaneous remission of the dysfunction or accommodation to it.* This strategy is rarely used because "remission" rates are quite low and the

Table 4–2.   Management strategies for medication-associated sexual dysfunction

1. Select a medication with a low incidence of sexual dysfunction, especially for sexually active patients.

2. Wait for spontaneous remission of the dysfunction or accommodation to it.

3. Make lifestyle adjustments or changes.

4. Schedule sexual activity around the dose of medication.

5. Reduce to minimal effective dose.

6. Switch to another medication from the same class (or one that exerts a similar effect) with a lower incidence of sexual dysfunction.

7. Use drug holidays.

8. Use "antidotes" or other agents to counteract sexual dysfunction or alleviate its symptoms.

9. Use psychotherapy and sex therapy.

time to achieve remission could be quite long (6 months), and even waiting for that long may not work. In addition, this strategy may be acceptable only to patients with a low frequency of sexual activity.

3. *Make lifestyle adjustments or changes.* Some lifestyle changes, such as smoking and substance abuse cessation, exercise, and weight loss, may contribute to the improvement of sexual functioning. However, no matter whether intuitively correct and recommended by some clinicians, the efficacy of lifestyle changes has not been demonstrated in the management of medication-associated sexual dysfunction.

4. *Schedule sexual activity around the dose of medication.* The patient may be advised to get involved in sexual activity prior to taking the entire daily dose of medication suspected of causing the sexual dysfunction. Although this strategy has been suggested by some clinicians, it has not been properly tested.

5. *Reduce to minimal effective dose.* This strategy seems logical, and evidence indicates that sexual dysfunction in some cases may be dose dependent. This strategy has been frequently suggested in the management of erectile dysfunction, and it may be helpful for patients who are bothered also by

other side effects. However, this strategy may be clinically problematic, because the likelihood of relapse or medication discontinuation symptoms may increase with a decreased dose.

6. *Switch to another medication from the same class (or one that exerts a similar effect) with a lower incidence of sexual dysfunction.* This strategy is basically the same as the first discussed strategy—selection of a medication with a lower incidence of sexual dysfunction—but after the sexual dysfunction has developed. The clinician may decide to switch to a medication within the class (the evidence is weak) or out of the class. Examples in the case of antidepressants may include switching from one MAOI to another, such as from phenelzine to moclobemide (within-class switch), or from an SSRI to either bupropion, nefazodone, or mirtazapine (out-of-class switch). Other examples include switching to antipsychotics mentioned earlier (atypical antipsychotics, loxapine, molindone) or switching from a benzodiazepine to bupropion.

7. *Use drug holidays.* This strategy is based on one small study (Rothschild 1995) in which paroxetine, sertraline, and fluoxetine were stopped for a few days in patients with sexual dysfunction associated with these antidepressants, and sexual activity was recommended at the end of this "holiday," just prior to restarting the antidepressant. The strategy did not work for fluoxetine-associated sexual dysfunction, probably due to this drug's long half-life. This strategy seems to be problematic, because it may reinforce nonadherence and because discontinuation symptoms may occur when taking a break from medications with a short half-life. The strategy has not been tested in any other class of medications.

8. *Use "antidotes" or other agents to counteract sexual dysfunction or alleviate its symptoms.* Although numerous "antidotes" or drugs that counteract sexual dysfunction associated with medications have been described in the literature, the evidence from double-blind, placebo-controlled trials, as pointed out by Taylor et al. (2005), is mostly nonexistent or weak. Most of the evidence comes from case reports, case series, or open trials. Some antidotes have been tried based on consideration of their mechanism of action (e.g., dopaminergic drugs for medication-associated low libido), and others have been tried based on an accidental finding (buspirone improving sexual functioning of anxious patients; Othmer and Othmer 1987). The antidotes used in antidepressant-associated sexual dysfunction include

amantadine, bethanechol, bromocriptine, bupropion, cyproheptadine, dextroamphetamine, ginkgo biloba, granisetron, loratadine, methylphenidate, mirtazapine, nefazodone, neostigmine, sildenafil, tadalafil, trazodone, vardenafil, and yohimbine. Many of these have side effects of their own (e.g., sedation with cyproheptadine, anxiety with yohimbine), and the efficacy of some (e.g., ginkgo biloba) has been questioned. As mentioned before, the best evidence (Taylor et al. 2005) exists for using sildenafil and tadalafil for antidepressant-associated erectile dysfunction and for using bupropion for antidepressant-associated low libido. A recent small study suggested the possible usefulness of sildenafil in female sexual dysfunction associated with antidepressants (Nurnberg et al. 2008). PDE5 inhibitors (sildenafil, tadalafil, vardenafil) have been attempted in other medication-associated sexual dysfunctions (e.g., antipsychotic-associated ones). The use of PDE5 inhibitors requires a bit of caution: these drugs are contraindicated in patients taking nitrates, because fatal hypotension may develop, and PDE5 inhibitors should be used carefully in patients with recent (within 6 months) cardiovascular disease (e.g., myocardial infarction, stroke, unstable angina), resting hypotension (blood pressure<90/50) or hypertension (blood pressure>170/110), or retinitis pigmentosa. PDE5 inhibitors have usually been used prior to planned sexual activity, although a recent report suggests that a low dose of tadalafil (5 mg/day) may be useful in treating erectile dysfunction (Forst et al. 2008). It may be only a matter of time before this approach will be suggested for medication-associated sexual dysfunction.

Various gels and lubricants could possibly be used for impaired female arousal associated with medication, but solid evidence is lacking.

9. *Use psychotherapy and sex therapy.* This approach has not been formally tested. The use of cognitive-behavioral therapy and other therapy modalities to decrease anxiety associated with medication use or sexual performance could theoretically be useful. Similarly, sex therapy and sex education may be helpful in general but remains untested in this indication.

Final Remark Regarding the Management of Medication-Associated Sexual Dysfunction

The management of medication-associated sexual dysfunction should be tailored to the type of dysfunction (e.g., dopaminergic drugs or stimulants for decreased libido, PDE5 inhibitors for erectile dysfunction), the type of medication "causing" the sexual dysfunction, the type of underlying illness (e.g., avoiding use of yohimbine in anxious patients), the patient's comfort, and the physician's expertise and skills.

Medications Used for Primary Sexual Dysfunction

Many medications have been used for the treatment of primary sexual dysfunctions in recent years, as discussed throughout this book. These medications include hormones (e.g., testosterone) and bupropion for low libido (see Chapter 5, "Disorders of Sexual Desire and Subjective Arousal in Women," and Chapter 6, "Male Hypoactive Sexual Desire Disorder"); PDE5 inhibitors, apomorphine, phentolamine, yohimbine, intraurethral or intracorporeal alprostadil, and other medications for male erectile disorder (see Chapter 8, "Male Erectile Disorder"); using these agents, arginine, and lubricants for female arousal disorder (see Chapter 7, "Female Sexual Arousal Disorders"); and SSRIs, clomipramine, and anesthetizing creams (used locally) for premature ejaculation (see Chapter 10, "Delayed and Premature Ejaculation"). On the other hand, many pharmacological agents, substances of abuse, and herbal remedies (e.g., ginkgo biloba) touted for these indications do not work or lack solid evidence beyond case reports.

Case Example

A 40-year-old divorced female started taking fluoxetine 20 mg/day for depression, low energy, poor sleep, and low appetite. At the time of her initial evaluation, she confided that she was sexually active with her boyfriend and had no problems achieving orgasm. During her follow-up visit a month later, she felt a bit more depressed because "I had some arguments with my boyfriend regarding his and my kids." When asked about her sexual functioning, she hesitantly responded that her "sex life was OK." However, when asked specifically about her ability to reach orgasm, she reported that it "takes me much longer to come than before, and it happened that I was not able to come at all. You know, we have had some problems with kids, and I don't feel very excited about sex." Because the sexual dysfunction 1) might have been causing some problems in her relationship with her boyfriend and 2) might have been related to fluoxetine, she agreed to the clinician's suggestion that she switch to bupropion. She reported improved mood and a return to pre-morbid (i.e., prefluoxetine) sexual functioning a month later.

This case illustrates several points made in this chapter: 1) the importance of baseline evaluation, 2) the importance of active questioning at baseline and during follow-up visits, and 3) the fact that patients may interpret their sexual dysfunction as a consequence of interpersonal and other problems when it could be associated with medication.

Key Points

- Sexual dysfunction may occur with almost any medication, may be dose dependent, and is fairly frequent with some psychotropic medications, such as antidepressants.

- Physicians should not rely on a patient's spontaneous reporting of sexual dysfunction associated with medication. They should take a proactive stance and ask specifically about sexual dysfunction, the type and duration, and so forth. They should also monitor for possible sexual dysfunction during the administration of medication.

- Baseline evaluation of sexual function—that is, evaluation prior to starting a medication—is absolutely necessary for detecting, assessing, and managing sexual dysfunction associated with medications.

- The contribution of other factors, such as the treated illness, co-morbid illness, substance abuse, and interpersonal problems, should not be underestimated in the evaluation and management of medication-associated sexual dysfunction.

- Management of medication-associated sexual dysfunction should be tailored to the type of sexual dysfunction, medication used, underlying treated illness, patient comfort, and physician skills.

- Several strategies are useful in managing medication-associated sexual dysfunction, as summarized in Table 4–2. Solid evidence beyond case reports or case series for using these strategies is usually weak or nonexistent. The best existing evidence supports use of PDE5 inhibitors for erectile dysfunction and bupropion for low libido.

References

Adler L, Dietrich A, Reimherr FW, et al: Safety and tolerability of once versus twice daily atomoxetine in adults with ADHD. Ann Clin Psychiatry 18:107–113, 2006

American Psychiatric Association: Diagnostic and Statistical Manual of Mental Disorders, 4th Edition, Text Revision. Washington, DC: American Psychiatric Association, 2000

Baldwin DS: Depression and sexual function. J Psychopharmacol 10 (suppl 1):30–34, 1996

Beaumont G: Sexual side effects of clomipramine. J Int Med Res 51:37–44, 1977

Bolton JM, Sareen J, Reiss JP: Genital anesthesia persisting six years after sertraline discontinuation. J Sex Marital Ther 32:327–330, 2006

Clayton AH, Montejo AL: Major depressive disorder, antidepressants, and sexual dysfunction. J Clin Psychiatry 67 (suppl 6):33–37, 2006

Crenshaw TL, Goldberg JP: Sexual Pharmacology: Drugs That Affect Sexual Function. New York, WW Norton, 1996

Csoka AN, Shipko S: Persistent sexual side effects after SSRI discontinuation. Psychother Psychosom 75:187–188, 2006

Forst H, Rajfer J, Casabe A, et al: Long-term safety and efficacy of tadalafil 5 mg dosed once daily in men with erectile dysfunction. J Sex Med 5:2160–2169, 2008

Hallinan R, Byrne A, Agho K, et al: Erectile dysfunction in men receiving methadone and buprenorphine maintenance treatment. J Sex Med 5:684–692, 2008

Kelly DL, Conley RR: Sexuality and schizophrenia: a review. Schizophr Bull 30:767–779, 2004

Klos KJ, Bower JH, Josephs KA, et al: Pathological hypersexuality predominantly linked to adjuvant dopamine agonist therapy in Parkinson's disease and multiple system atrophy. Parkinsonism Relat Disord 11:381–386, 2005

Knegtering H, van den Bosch R, Castelein S, et al: Are sexual side effects of prolactin-raising antipsychotics reducible to serum prolactin? Psychoneuroendocrinology 33:711–717, 2008

Kotin J, Wilbert D: Thioridazine and sexual dysfunction. Am J Psychiatry 133:82–85, 1976

Labbate LA: Psychotropics and sexual dysfunction: the evidence and treatment. Adv Psychosom Med 29:107–130, 2008

Landen M, Hogberg P, Thase ME: Incidence of sexual side effects in refractory depression during treatment with citalopram or paroxetine. J Clin Psychiatry 66:100–106, 2005

Monteiro WO, Noshirvani HF, Marks IM, et al: Anorgasmia from clomipramine in obsessive-compulsive disorder: a controlled trial. Br J Psychiatry 151:107–112, 1987

Montgomery SA, Baldwin DS, Riley A: Antidepressant medications: a review of the evidence for drug-induced sexual dysfunction. J Affect Disord 69:119–140, 2002

Norden M: Buspirone treatment of sexual dysfunction associated with selective serotonin re-uptake inhibitors. Depression 2:109–112, 1994

Nurnberg HG, Hensley PL, Heiman JR, et al: Sildenafil treatment of women with antidepressant-associated sexual dysfunction: a randomized controlled trial. JAMA 300:395–404, 2008

Othmer E, Othmer SC: Effect of buspirone on sexual function in patients with generalized anxiety disorder. J Clin Psychiatry 48:201–203, 1987

Palha AP, Esteves M: Drugs of abuse and sexual functioning. Adv Psychosom Med 29:131–149, 2008

Rothschild AJ: Selective serotonin reuptake inhibitor-induced sexual dysfunction: efficacy of a drug holiday. Am J Psychiatry 152:1514–1516, 1995

Safarinejad MR: Evaluation of endocrine profile and hypothalamic-pituitary-testis axis in selective serotonin reuptake inhibitor-induced male sexual dysfunction. J Clin Psychopharmacol 28:418–423, 2008

Segraves RT: Effects of psychotropic medication on human erection and ejaculation. Arch Gen Psychiatry 46:275–284, 1989

Segraves RT, Balon R: Sexual Pharmacology: Fast Facts. New York, WW Norton, 2003

Taylor MJ, Rudkin L, Hawton K: Strategies for managing antidepressant-induced sexual dysfunction: systematic review of randomized controlled trials. J Affect Disord 88:241–254, 2005

Zemishlany Z, Weizman A: The impact of mental illness on sexual dysfunction. Adv Psychosom Med 29:89–106, 2008

PART II

Management of Sexual Disorders

5

Disorders of Sexual Desire and Subjective Arousal in Women

Rosemary Basson, M.D., FRCP

Lori A. Brotto, Ph.D.

Having too little sexual desire is the most common sexual complaint in clinical settings and identified on questionnaires or interviews in epidemiological surveys of women. However, exactly what women mean when they speak of low sexual desire may vary considerably, even among women of similar ages, cultures, and relationship duration. Qualitative, empirical, and clinical research confirms the overlap of women's concepts of sexual desire and sexual arousal, in keeping with the well-documented comorbidity of arousal and desire disorders. Therefore, problematic low desire and problematic low arousal should be addressed together.

To understand a patient's complaint of lack of desire to engage sexually, one needs to know the variety of reasons women *do* choose to have sex. Recent empirical data confirm the clinical experience that so-called desire, as in having a hunger, drive, or need for sex, is but one motivation for sexual activity. In a study of 750 mostly younger women, researchers divided the 237 separate reasons the women identified for having sex into four domains: 1) emotional reasons, including love and commitment; 2) physical reasons, including pleasure; 3) goal attainment reasons, such as resources and social status; and 4) insecurity reasons, such as boosting self-esteem, duty/pressure, and "mate guarding" (Meston and Buss 2007). That compatibility with the partner is a major influence on desire and sexual distress received empirical support in recent study (Witting et al. 2008). Baseline data from the Study of Women's Health Across the Nation confirm that absence of sexual desire does not preclude women's satisfaction with their sexual lives (Cain et al. 2003). The data from 3,250 multiethnic middle-aged women in North America indicated that the vast majority were satisfied with their physical sexual pleasure, although 42% never or very infrequently sensed desire between sexual experiences or at the outset (frequently referred to as "spontaneous" sexual desire), with even higher figures for Chinese and Japanese women in this sample (61.4% and 67.8%, respectively) (Cain et al. 2003).

Women's Sexual Response Cycle

Although various models of sexual response have been proposed, we consider the sexual response cycle described by Basson (2000) to be most applicable to the majority of women. In this model, the sexual response cycle of women is conceptualized as circular, comprising overlapping phases of variable order: desire may not be present initially (Basson 2006).

Figure 5–1 shows that even when a woman begins from sexual neutrality, her deliberate attention to appropriate sexual stimulation and ability to stay focused allows reflexive, prompt genital congestion, potentially followed by subjective arousal (i.e., mental/sexual excitement). Providing that this complex state of arousal is accompanied by positive emotions and thoughts, then the arousal increases in intensity and triggers sexual desire; the arousal and desire then coexist and reinforce each other. Recent functional brain imaging performed while women were aroused from visual erotica (Arnow et al. 2009), plus genital imaging under the same conditions, as well as psychophysiological assessment using vaginal photoplethysmography over the past sev-

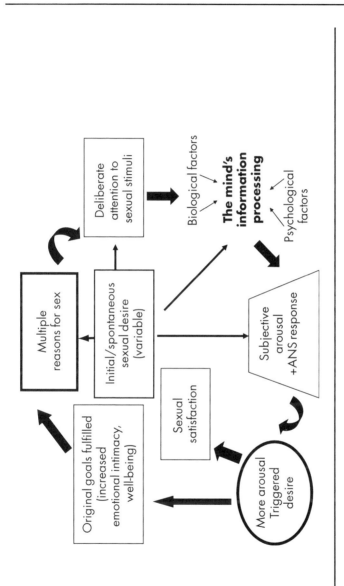

Figure 5–1.   Sexual response cycle.

Note.   Phases overlap and are in variable order. Initial desire may be present to augment motivation and arousability. ANS=autonomic nervous system.

Source.   Reprinted from Basson R: "Female Sex Response: The Role of Drugs in the Management of Sexual Dysfunction." *American College of Obstetrics and Gynecology* 98:350–352, 2001. Used with permission of Lippincott Williams & Wilkins.

eral decades, confirms the complexity of arousal and the usual poor correlation between subjective excitement and congenital congestion (Basson 2008). Once the woman is experiencing high arousal, she is more receptive to more erotic types of stimulation that she may have previously declined, and thus arousal can be even more intense. The circular response shown in Figure 5–1 may be cycled many times during one sexual encounter. Although positive experiences provide further motivation for sex in the future, negative outcomes will efficiently do the opposite. Any initial (i.e., spontaneous) desire can augment the cycle at any or all points, as shown in the figure.

The conceptualization shown in Figure 5–1 includes and expands the work of many others. Masters and Johnson (1966) described a linear sequence of arousal, plateau of excitement, orgasm, and resolution. Although after the publication of *Human Sexual Response* by Masters and Johnson, the arousal phase in women often became equated to genital events (lubrication and swelling), the original description included both genital and subjective arousal (Masters and Johnson 1966). Helen Singer Kaplan (1979) noted that desire could be triggered during the sexual experience and/or it could be present at the outset. She called the former "extrinsic/responsive" and the latter "intrinsic/biological." No simple drawing was used to emphasize the extrinsic/responsive component, and, therefore, the accepted model of human sex response for three decades was linear: desire, arousal, orgasm, and resolution.

Clinicians involved with patients with disabilities and chronic illness emphasized the importance of a positive outcome, which would allow "reflection," which in turn would subsequently fuel a "seduction phase" that encompassed desire (Whipple and Brash-McGreer 1997). Thus, a more circular response was envisioned. Levine (2003), in his tripartite model of sexual desire, identified drive, motivation, and wish components. That there are many motives for men and women to be sexual, only one of which is an awareness of an intrinsic urge for sexual activity, had already been discussed by other authors, including Regan and Berscheid (1996), Singer and Toates (1987), and Whalen (1966). These "nondesire" motivations awaited incorporation into a composite model. The importance of the mind's processing of sexual stimuli has been integral to Janssen et al.'s (2000) information processing model of sexual arousal: both unconscious processing leading to an automatic genital response and conscious cognitive processing appraising the sexual content of the stimulus to allow subjective arousal are involved. This model and that of Basson (2001) emphasize that the genital activation and the awareness of excitement can then become further sexual stimuli, adding to the original sexual stimulus. Divergence between automatic genital response and the more slowly developed conscious appraisal of arousal underlies dysfunctional arousal in men and women. More recent work by Sanders et al. (2008) has begun to identify themes commonly underlying women's propensity to become aroused from sexual stimulation and factors that tend to preclude or inhibit arousal. None of the models discussed previously were meant to represent the sexual response cycle of only one gender. Possibly one major difference between the sexual experiences of a majority of women compared with a majority of men is that the initial desire leading up to a sexual experience and present at its outset is less frequent in women. Indeed, data are numerous documenting reduction of this type of desire in women compared with men (Baumeister et al. 2001).

Empirical support for the triggering of desire, first mentioned by Kaplan (1979), includes the recent work by McCall and Meston (2007). Studying 65 premenopausal women, 30 diagnosed with hypoactive sexual desire disorder, and 50 postmenopausal women, 39 diagnosed with hypoactive sexual desire disorder, these researchers found that all women acknowledged triggers or cues for desire. Triggers include those involving love and emotional bonding, those involving erotica, those that are visual, and those that are romantic. They found no significant difference in the reporting of cues by premenopausal women and postmenopausal women. Not surprisingly, the sexually healthy women recognized somewhat higher numbers of triggers than women diagnosed with hypoactive sexual desire disorder. This recent research confirms that triggered desire is not limited to dysfunctional women.

The Basson model is a composite of other models, but it also allows for the marked flexibility and variability of response among women who consider their sexual lives as rewarding and functional. By focusing on context, the model echoes themes from "the new view" of women's sexual function (Tiefer et al. 2002). This view maintains that there is no one "normal" sexual response or experience, and that any of four major aspects of women's sexual lives could potentially cause sexual difficulty. These are sociocultural/political/economic, relationship, medical, and psychological aspects. This view is very much in keeping with our view that women with so-called sexual disorder often do not have innate dysfunction of sexual response; instead, their reported problematic sexual encounters result from 1) a paucity of reasons to begin engaging in sex or 2) problematic stimuli and/or context.

Assessment

Patient History

Assessment not only is a guide to therapy but in itself can be therapeutic. Preferably, both partners are seen alone and together. A number of published self-administered screening questionnaires have been designed to identify progress with treatment, but these cannot replace the diagnostic interview. For a thorough assessment, the clinician should do the following.

1. *Assess mood, anxiety, self-esteem, and sexual self-image.* Results from both longitudinal and cross-sectional studies have indicated that a robust correlation exists between women's mental health and their sexual desire (Bancroft et al. 2003; Dennerstein et al. 2001). The majority of women with concerns about low desire and arousal have either clinical depression or symptoms of low self-esteem, mood lability, and more anxious and depressed thoughts than control women (Hartmann et al. 2004). Of 445 women with major depressive disorder, close to 80% had endorsed sexual dysfunction on a validated self-report questionnaire. Their dysfunction improved with successful antidepressant therapy but worsened if the depression continued (Clayton et al. 2007). For women with diabetes, renal failure, or multiple sclerosis, it is the comorbid depression, and not the medical disease itself, that is associated with a higher prevalence of sexual dysfunction compared with control women (Basson and Weijmar Schultz 2007). Depression accompanied by negative thoughts, especially about the future of the woman's relationship, emerges as a risk factor for every sexual dysfunction in women ages 40–80 years (Laumann et al. 2005). Anxiety disorders can preclude women's ability to attend to sexual stimuli and to be (positively) lost in the moment. In cognitive models of sexual dysfunction, anxiety is purported to reduce the effectiveness of sexual stimuli and enhance attention to nonsexual stimuli (Barlow 1986). Also, assess for schizophrenia, eating dis-

orders, personality disorders (especially borderline personality disorder), and obsessive-compulsive disorder, because these may occur comorbidly with disorders of desire and arousal. Treatment of the underlying mental health issue is needed before specific sexual therapy is begun.

2. *Assess the patient's present and former reasons for sex and the reasons she now gives for declining or avoiding sexual activity.*

Practice Point

After explaining the variety of reasons women decide to have sexual activity, ask the patient to list reasons she previously agreed to sex or initiated sex with her partner. Next, have the patient list reasons she now declines her partner's sexual invitation or suggestion, or decides not to initiate sex herself.

---

3. *Assess any apparent internally triggered (i.e., spontaneous) desire, possibly at a particular time in the patient's menstrual cycle or after a period of abstinence or separation from her partner.* Assess any sexual fantasizing or self-stimulation. Of note, many women self-stimulate to feel more relaxed and even more commonly to promote sleep (in other words, self-stimulation may not signify sexual desire). Consider any medical factors impacting on loss of apparently spontaneous desire. Although gradual loss of this type of desire with age and with relationship duration may be within normal limits, sudden loss may indicate important psychological issues (intrapersonal or interpersonal) or medical entities such as hyperprolactinemia; medication effects, particularly those due to selective serotonin reuptake inhibitors (SSRIs), beta-blockers, narcotics, antiandrogens, or combined hormonal contraceptives; or, in younger women, unwanted loss of ovarian function from surgery, chemotherapy, or some types of primary ovarian insufficiency. Other chronic illness, such as hypothyroidism or diabetes, may contribute to low desire. Current and past alcohol intake should be checked. Current high alcohol intake reduces sexual desire, but so may a past high intake with current sobriety. Also screen for other substance abuse.

4. *Assess emotional intimacy between the partners.* Explain that many women choose to have sex because of the associated emotional closeness both during sexual engagement and subsequently. Ask about the degree of trust, consideration, and respect. Does the couple have interpersonal difficulties such that the woman's withholding sex has some value? Are secrets being held (e.g., a prior affair, or her feigning sexual arousal or orgasm)?

5. *Assess the sexual context.* Is the immediate environment erotic and safe (e.g., from sexually transmitted disease and from unwanted pregnancy)? Is the environment private (e.g., so that no members of the family can enter the bedroom door or overhear)? Is the couple attempting sexual activity at the end of the day when fatigue is a genuine obstacle? Assess also the cultural context. Sexual desire has been found in recent research to be significantly lower in East Asian than in Euro-Canadian/American samples, and increasing acculturation to the mainstream culture is associated with increasing levels of sexual desire (Woo et al. 2009). This relationship between culture and sexual desire appears to be mediated, in large part, by sexual guilt. For example, the association between East Asian culture and lower sexual desire is mediated by increasing levels of sex guilt. Moreover, the acculturation-associated increase in desire seen in East Asian women is also mediated by a significant decline in sex guilt. The extent to which these findings apply to other ethnic and cultural groups remains to be determined.

6. *Assess the sexual stimuli.* Often, a necessary first step is simply being together, emotionally close, with no specific sexual touching occurring. Does the couple engage in sexual talking or any activity that encourages sexual feelings (e.g., showering together, dancing), sufficient nongenital physical pleasuring, and sufficient nonpenetrative genital stimulation? Does the woman find any forms of stimulation (either to herself or to her partner) offensive or anxiety provoking? How aware is she of the physical stimuli that will reliably excite her, and how comfortable is she communicating this information to her partner? How well can he or she follow her guidance?

7. *Assess how able the woman is to attend to the stimuli or to stay focused.* Are there distractions? Recent research supports the clinical observation that distractions commonly inhibit women's arousal (Sanders et al. 2008). Also, the degree of attention that a person can give to sexual stimuli cor-

relates with the person's reported level of desire (Prause et al. 2008). Does the woman self-monitor? A term coined by Masters and Johnson to describe this phenomenon is "spectatoring" (Masters and Johnson 1966); this has been confirmed to decrease women's genital arousal (Meston 2006). Moreover, recent functional magnetic resonance imaging suggests that women with hypoactive sexual desire disorder focus more on their own physical response than do control women (Arnow et al. 2009). Do the partners try and mutually stimulate each other, or do they take turns so she can have time to focus on her own pleasure? When she states that she is not feeling aroused, inquire as to what she is feeling and thinking. Feeling anxious and having critical thoughts is common.

8. *Assess the patient's arousal in some detail by questioning her about any mental sexual excitement; increase in body temperature; increase in muscle tension; changes in breathing pattern; increase in breast and nipple sensitivity; and perception of genital engorgement from tingling, throbbing, or extra lubrication.*

9. *If intercourse is part of the couple's activities, inquire as to who moves the process on from nonpenetrative sex to intercourse.* Does thrusting continue once a male partner has ejaculated to maintain pubis-to-pubis stimulation while the penis is still inside? (For some women, this contact is necessary for satisfaction and orgasm.) Does the couple continue with nonpenetrative genital stimulation if necessary after intercourse?

10. *Assess the outcome in terms of emotional closeness as well as physical satisfaction.* Does either partner feel any pain or discomfort? Does either experience any sexual dysfunction (e.g., erectile difficulties, premature or delayed ejaculation, lack of wanted orgasm)?

Physical Examination

Although a physical examination may be done simply as a component of good medical care, it is necessary for assessment of certain sexual dysfunctions. A pelvic and genital exam is of major importance when there is comorbid dyspareunia. Also, a physical examination is important for patients with chronic medical disease (e.g., neurological disease may be accompanied by sensory loss in the genitalia; renal disease may be accompanied by anemia and vulvovaginal atrophy; hyperprolactinemia may be accompanied by galactorrhea; hypoadrenal states may cause a loss of pubic hair). When the patient complains of a loss of genital sexual sensitivity, a genital examination is necessary to exclude conditions such as lichen sclerosis. Also, genital and pelvic examinations are often performed for reasons of reassurance and as a means to encourage the woman to consider what is going on in her mind when she is sexual rather than believing the etiology of her arousal dysfunction is confined to her genitalia.

Diagnoses

Table 5–1 lists the definitions of sexual disorders given in DSM-IV-TR (American Psychiatric Association 2000); revised definitions published in 2003 following the 2-year deliberation of an American Foundation for Urologic Disease/American Urological Association Foundation (AFUD/AUAF) International Consensus Committee (Basson et al. 2003); and further recommendations published in 2007 (Segraves et al. 2007). The following were major recommended changes to the sexual desire and arousal disorders:

1. Reliable triggered (or responsive) desire, in the absence of apparently spontaneous desire, is acknowledged as a normal variant.
2. The importance of women's subjective arousal is acknowledged.
3. The degree of personal distress is to be noted (Basson et al. 2008) (rather than giving or withholding a diagnosis based on personal or interpersonal distress as in DSM-IV-TR).

Dysfunction can be present even though the cause is external to the woman herself. For example, the issue may be simply an unsuitable sexual context. To avoid overpathologizing such an experience, the AFUD/AUAF committee (Basson et al. 2003) recommended that clinicians note, alongside a diagnosis of sexual disorder, if any of the following three descriptors apply:

1. Past psychosexual developmental factors
2. External factors in current life and/or sexual context
3. Medical factors, including comorbid illness, use of prescription or illicit drugs, or previous surgery

A DSM-V work group has been convened by the American Psychiatric Association to consider revising the official definitions of sexual disorders in men and women, and the revision is due to be published in 2012. Despite increasing clinical usage internationally, the revisions recommended by the AFUD/AUAF committee (Basson et al. 2003) and those of Segraves et al. (2007) remain unofficial.

Formulation

From the in-depth biopsychosocial assessment, the clinician can make a formulation of the patient's problem(s). The formulation is a concise summary of the etiological factors considered most important, and this understanding becomes the basis for treatment. Rapport is increased by sharing this formulation with the patient. In addition to the historical details, information from direct observation of the couple—including their behaviors and interactions, their attitude toward any homework assignments, and their response to initial treatments—frequently modulates the original formulation. In other words, the initial formulation may well change as patient visits continue.

Some clinicians recommend using the "four P's" model of formulation (see Table 5–2). An alternative model for the formulation is a "pie chart." The various sections of the pie are for the various etiological factors that make up the formulation (see Figure 5–2).

Therapy

For some women, improving general well-being, such as by eating a healthier diet, exercising more, limiting use of alcohol, and discontinuing substance abuse, may benefit problematically low desire. For other women, specific therapy is needed depending on the reason for the disrupted response cycle. When medications are suspected of contributing to the dysfunction, they are addressed first (see Chapter 4, "Medications and Sexual Function and Dysfunction").

Behavioral, Cognitive, and Sexual Therapies

Behavioral, cognitive, and sexual therapies have been the mainstay of management of desire disorders and subjective sexual arousal disorders. Figure 5–3

Table 5–1. Changing definitions of women's sexual dysfunctions

Sexual symptom category	DSM-IV-TR (American Psychiatric Association 2000)	Revised definition from AFUD/AUAF International-al Consensus Committee (Basson et al. 2003)	Revisions suggested by Segraves et al. (2007)	Comments
Lack of sexual desire	Hypoactive sexual desire disorder: Persistently or recurrently deficient (or absent) sexual fantasies and desire for sexual activity. The judgment of deficiency or absence is made by the clinician, taking into account factors that affect sexual functioning, such as age and context of the person's life.	Sexual desire/interest disorder: Absent or diminished feelings of sexual interest or desire, absent sexual thoughts or fantasies, and a lack of responsive desire. Motivations (here defined as reasons/ incentives) for attempting to become sexually aroused are scarce or absent. The lack of interest is beyond a normative lessening with life cycle and relationship duration.	Hypoactive sexual desire disorder: Persistent lack of desire for sexual activity and/or lack of responsive desire. This is beyond normative lessening due to relationship duration or aging.	Data on women in sexually satisfactory established relationships confirm that minimal spontaneous desire of sex ahead of sexual experiences does not necessarily constitute disorder. *Lack of desire triggered during the sexual encounter (i.e., "responsive" desire) is integral to the revised diagnosis.* Segraves et al. noted, "many women do not report presence of spontaneous desire." Thus *"or lack of responsive desire"* seems incorrect.

Table 5–1.   Changing definitions of women's sexual dysfunctions (continued)

Sexual symptom category	DSM-IV-TR (American Psychiatric Association 2000)	Revised definition from AFUD/AUAF International Consensus Committee (Basson et al. 2003)	Revisions suggested by Segraves et al. (2007)	Comments
Lack of subjective and genital sexual arousal	No DSM-IV-TR definition addresses lack of subjective arousal.	**Combined arousal disorder:** Absent or markedly reduced feelings of sexual arousal (sexual excitement and sexual pleasure) from any type of stimulation and absent or impaired genital sexual arousal (vulval swelling and lubrication).	**Female sexual arousal disorder:** Persistent or recurrent lack of sense of building sexual excitement and pleasure during sexual activity and/or inability to attain and maintain the lubrication/swelling response until completion of sexual activity.	The two revised versions identify the lack of sexual excitement (in the mind) and no *awareness* of reflexive genital vasocongestion.
Lack of subjective sexual arousal	No DSM-IV-TR definition addresses lack of subjective arousal.	**Subjective arousal disorder:** Absent or markedly reduced feelings of sexual arousal (sexual excitement and sexual pleasure) from any type of stimulation. Vaginal lubrication and other signs of physical response still occur.	There was no recommendation to separate different types of arousal that might be lost.	In the AFUD/AUAF definition, there is no sexual excitement (in the mind) but there is awareness of adequate lubrication.

Table 5–1. Changing definitions of women's sexual dysfunctions *(continued)*

Sexual symptom category	DSM-IV-TR (American Psychiatric Association 2000)	Revised definition from AFUD/AUAF International Consensus Committee (Basson et al. 2003)	Revisions suggested by Segraves et al. (2007)	Comments
Lack of genital sexual arousal	**Female sexual arousal disorder:** Persistent or recurrent inability to attain, or to maintain until completion of the sexual activity, an adequate lubrication-swelling response of sexual excitement.	**Genital arousal disorder:** Absent or impaired genital sexual arousal—minimal vulvar swelling or vaginal lubrication from any type of sexual stimulation and reduced sexual sensations from caressing genitalia. Subjective sexual excitement still occurs from nongenital sexual stimuli.	There was no recommendation to separate different types of arousal that may be lost.	The presence of subjective arousal (sexual excitement) from nongenital stimuli (e.g., erotica, stimulating the partner, receiving breast stimulation, kissing) is key to the revised AFUD/AUAF diagnosis. Women describe "genital deadness."

Table 5–1. Changing definitions of women's sexual dysfunctions (*continued*)

Sexual symptom category	DSM-IV-TR (American Psychiatric Association 2000)	Revised definition from AFUD/AUAF International Consensus Committee (Basson et al. 2003)	Revisions suggested by Segraves et al. (2007)	Comments
Persistent genital arousal	No DSM-IV-TR definition addresses persistent genital arousal.	Persistent genital arousal disorder: Spontaneous, intrusive, and unwanted genital arousal (tingling, throbbing) when sexual interest or desire is absent. Awareness of subjective arousal is infrequent but mostly unpleasant. The arousal is unrelieved by orgasms, and the feelings persist for hours or days.	There was a recommendation to address persistent genital arousal.	This condition is poorly understood, and prevalence is unknown. Hypervigilance toward genital sensations and increasing anxiety that the symptoms are highly abnormal are clinical findings. Reliable treatment has not been found.

Note.   AFUD/AUAF=American Urological Association Foundation, formerly American Foundation for Urologic Disease.
Source.   Adapted from Basson R: "Sexual Desire and Arousal Disorders in Women." *New England Journal of Medicine* 354:1497–1506, 2006.

Table 5–2. The "four P's" model of formulation

Factor	Comments
Predisposing	Factors setting the stage for later sexuality, including early sex education, in-home and sociocultural messages/taboos around sexuality, first sexual experiences, past history of sexual assault, dynamics of family of origin, family history of mental illness, important early experiences or losses, personality and temperament, sociocultural background
Precipitating	Factors linked to the onset of the sexual complaint, including medical illness, surgery, medical interventions, medication, trauma, substance abuse, stresses, losses (e.g., of relationship, of person, of job)
Perpetuating	Factors in the present that maintain a sexual complaint, such as ongoing illness or medication or substance abuse, nonadaptive coping, defenses, lack of social support, ongoing interpersonal difficulties in relationship, ongoing external stresses (e.g., unemployment or difficult work or social environment)
Protective	Protective factors in the patient's current and past history that buffer against negative influences on her sexuality; these factors include absence of history of family mental illness, ongoing positive feelings for sexual partner, compliance with therapy, adaptive coping, absence of substance abuse, insight, psychological mindedness, history of previous rewarding sex, history of rewarding nonsexual relationships

shows a treatment algorithm that indicates the priority and options of treatment. Any symptoms of a mood disorder or low self-image and any relationship difficulties must be addressed first.

Using Figure 5–1 as an illustrative guide with a patient, we find that explaining the women's sex response cycle and identifying interruptions in this patient's own cycle is often itself therapeutic. Following such an explanation, some women state that they now understand why they are not motivated to

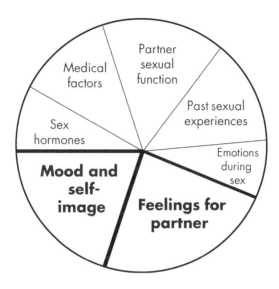

Figure 5–2.   "Pie chart" model of formulation.

Source.   Reprinted from Basson R: "Recent Conceptualization of Women's Sexual Response." *Menopause Management* 16(3):16–28, 2007. Used with permission of HealthCom Media.

be sexual or why they are not getting aroused and having pleasure, and they can see what changes need to be made (e.g., by getting help with the emotional intimacy or by attending to the currently unsatisfactory sexual stimuli and context). For women with a diagnosis of hypoactive sexual desire disorder (as defined by DSM-IV-TR) but no loss of arousal or pleasure when they do engage, the detailed assessment of women's reasons for sex can be very therapeutic. When they learn that they do not have a disorder according to more recently recommended definitions, patients' self-image improves, and they often experience more arousability on subsequent occasions. For many women, the normalization of the lack of spontaneous desire may be sufficient to motivate them to initiate sexual activity themselves (for all the other benefits that sex brings). Their awareness of a normal need to notice sexual cues during the day can even foster that apparently "spontaneous" or initial desire.

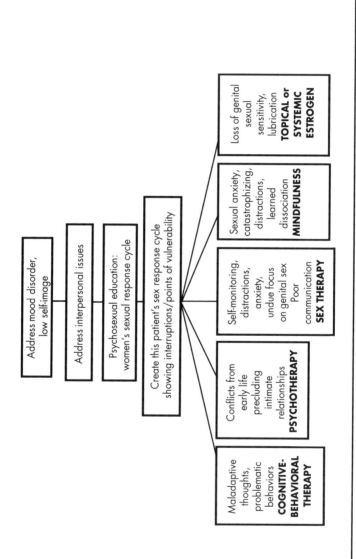

Figure 5–3.   Treatment algorithm for management of desire disorders and subjective sexual arousal disorders.

Source.   Reprinted from BMJ Point of Care with permission from BMJ Publishing Group.

Practice Point

Explain women's sex response cycle (Figure 5–1) to patient and partner. Adapt the cycle to this particular patient's response, showing the areas of interruption that have caused her dysfunction. (Figure 5–4, later in this chapter, shows an example of how disruptions to the sexual response cycle can lead to desire and/or arousal impairment.) Table 5–3 details the various standard psychological approaches to treatment of women's disordered desire and subjective arousal.

Medical Components of Therapy

Addressing Medication-Induced Dysfunction

Drugs with sexually negative effects include antidepressants (most typically the SSRIs), narcotics, gonadotropin-releasing hormone agonists, combined contraceptives, depot progesterone, aromatase inhibitors, antiandrogens, and beta-blockers (see Table 5–4 for a more complete list). If a patient is unable to discontinue or switch a drug, the clinician discusses with the couple the etiology of dysfunction and explains that although the problem is the medication, understanding the woman's sex response cycle will help them cope with the drug's effects. The couple is advised that the more erotic the context, the more attention to her stimulation, and the more she can learn to focus, the less detrimental the drug effect will be. Psychological strategies, including sensate focus therapy and mindfulness training, can help the woman learn to begin a sexual encounter despite lack of initial desire and a muted response.

In addition to psychological interventions, the clinician may suggest adjustments in medication dosage or formulation. Results from open-label trials and case series have indicated that a number of pharmacological agents might improve or reverse the loss of arousal, desire, and orgasm commonly associated with serotonergic antidepressants. Authors of a Cochrane Review (Taylor et al. 2005) could make no recommendations for women but did note that bupropion is of interest according to one of two randomized clinical trials (Clayton et al. 2004). Recently, sildenafil 50–100 mg taken 1–2 hours before sex proved beneficial over an 8-week period for women with orgasmic dys-

Table 5–3.   Psychological therapies for women's desire and arousal disorders

Therapy	Explanation	Outcome
Psychoeducation	Psychoeducation is given to all women treated for sexual concerns.	Women whose response is within the normal range, even though changed from their past sexual function, are reassured. Others become aware of the complexity of sexual function. Recently, incorporating mindfulness techniques with psychoeducation has shown benefit for women with sexual desire/interest disorder (Brotto et al. 2008).
Cognitive-behavioral therapy (CBT)	The model of women's sex response cycle is used to identify problematic areas. Behavioral changes include attending to inappropriate sexual context or behaviors in either partner that reduce attractiveness or trust and the ability to focus on the sexual stimuli and feelings. Unhelpful thoughts that can change include distractions, believing she is unattractive, and idealizing an unrealistic mode of sexual response portrayed by media.	Group CBT improved sexual desire disorder in 74% of couples, which was maintained in 64% of them at 1 year (Trudel et al. 2001). Modified Masters and Johnson sex therapy improved sexual response in 57% of women with loss of desire (Hawton et al. 1991).

Table 5–3. Psychological therapies for women's desire and arousal disorders (*continued*)

Therapy	Explanation	Outcome
Short-term psychotherapy	This approach may be needed to address more distant factors (e.g., when sexual symptoms are thought to result from themes from childhood, including abuse or neglect, control issues, low sexual self-image).	Benefit has been reported in the clinical literature (Pridal and LoPiccolo 2000), but minimal empirical study has been reported.
Sex therapy	This therapy focuses on the interpersonal relationship plus sexual details. It includes sensate focus therapy consisting of exchanging physical touch, moving from nonsexual to sexual areas of the body, and the partners' taking turns and giving feedback.	Outcome studies are limited. One study showed that 65% of 365 married couples were improved by clinical judgment at the end of therapy (Sarwer and Durlak 1997).
Mindfulness	Variously defined as nonjudgmental, present moment awareness or relaxed wakefulness, this practice originated in Buddhist meditation and is increasingly incorporated into Western medical and mental health.	Alongside psychoeducation, mindfulness is especially beneficial for women with sexual desire and arousal disorders who had past sexual abuse (Brotto et al. 2008). Relationship happiness, relationship stress, and stress coping efficacy has also been reported (Carson et al. 2004).

Table 5–4. Medications affecting sexual response

Drugs with negative sexual effects

Antihypertensives: beta-blockers, thiazides

Serotonergic antidepressants

Anticonvulsants

Antipsychotics

Benzodiazepines

Lithium

Narcotics

Oral contraceptives and oral estrogen therapy

Gonadotropin-releasing hormone agonists

Depot progesterone

Aromatase inhibitors

Antiandrogens

Spironolactone

Alcohol

Cocaine

Drugs that appear to be prosexual

Amphetamines

Bupropion

Danazol

Levodopa

function associated with SSRI use for major depression. Recruitment over 4 years at seven U.S. medical outpatient centers led to enrollment of 98 premenopausal women (Nurnberg et al. 2008). Exclusion criteria were extensive. Inclusion criteria included SSRI-associated impairment of orgasm and/or impairment of genital congestion. Sexual function questionnaires confirmed overall benefit with active drug—and specifically in the domain of orgasm—but not in the domains of arousal, lubrication, and desire.

Estrogen Therapy for Sexual Desire and Arousal Disorders

Estrogen activity has been found to correlate directly only with dryness dyspareunia of vulvovaginal atrophy and with loss of sexual sensitivity of genital structures. However, motivation for sexual activity can markedly decrease as a result. Lubrication, elasticity, and genital sensitivity are usually improved by the use of local estrogen (e.g., vaginal estradiol 25 μg as a vaginal pill twice weekly or use of a Silastic ring releasing 7.5 μg/day). Systemic estrogen is indicated only if the woman has other menopausal health considerations, including ongoing severe vasomotor symptoms. The nonoral route is preferred to avoid increasing sex hormone–binding globulin and reduction of testosterone availability.

Testosterone Therapy for Sexual Desire and Arousal Disorders

Although testosterone supplementation has been prescribed for complaints of low sexual desire since the 1930s, only recently has scientific evaluation been done. At the present time, the U.S. Food and Drug Administration has not approved any formulation of systemic testosterone for women's sexual disorders, and the American Endocrine Society recommends against generalized use of testosterone in women because the indications are inadequate and evidence of long-term safety is lacking (Wierman et al. 2006). This recommendation came about in the knowledge that there is evidence for short-term efficacy of testosterone in selective populations such as surgically menopausal women. Nevertheless, many clinicians are prescribing testosterone off-label by adapting formulations created for men or by using compounded creams or gels. The clinician should be well informed about what is known and what is not known before embarking on any investigational treatment with systemic testosterone.

What is known regarding testosterone therapy.

1. *Randomized trials in surgically menopausal estrogen-replete women.* In surgically menopausal estrogen-replete women who reported a bothersome reduction of their level of desire for sex and a decrease in sexual activity since the loss of both ovaries, supplementing testosterone to levels that are high normal for young women increases the number of sexually satisfactory events per month. Pooling the data from recent randomized controlled trials showed that surgically menopausal women receiving 300 μg/day of transdermal testosterone reported 1.9 more sexually satisfying events per month than at baseline, compared with 0.9 more in women receiving placebo. All studies showed that women taking active drug had increased scores in the desire and response domains of the questionnaire, and their distress was reduced in three of the four trials. Whereas 350 μg/day of transdermal testosterone allowed sexual benefit,

150 μg/day and 450 μg/day did not provide benefit (Basson 2006; Braunstein et al. 2005). Of note, recruited women already reported 2–3 sexually satisfying events per month at baseline.

2. *Randomized trials in naturally menopausal estrogen-repleted women.* Naturally menopausal estrogen-replete women in one randomized controlled trial that used the same protocol as for the surgically menopausal women reported similar benefit from the active drug and lower response to the placebo (Shifren et al. 2006).

3. *Randomized trials in premenopausal women.* A recent randomized controlled trial to ameliorate premenopausal women's sexual dissatisfaction using transdermal testosterone showed only marginal benefit (Davis et al. 2008b). Exclusion criteria included serum testosterone levels >1.1 pg/mL. The highest of three doses increased the free testosterone levels to high normal (in 65% of women) or slightly above normal (in 35% of women) and failed to show benefit beyond placebo, as did the smallest (one-third) dose. The medium (one-half) dose allowed 0.8 more "sexually satisfactory events" per month, but outcome as measured by the Sabbatsberg Sexual Rating Scale was similar to that of placebo.

4. *Safety data in recent randomized trials.* In five recently published randomized controlled trials by Procter & Gamble using the same protocol, treatment was safe for the duration of the trial (i.e., 6 months) (see Basson 2008 for review).

5. *Testosterone supplementation in estrogen-depleted women.* Testosterone supplementation in estrogen-depleted women would be nonphysiological; the already high androgen:estrogen ratio would be further increased. Furthermore, no benefit was seen in a study of postmenopausal, estrogen-depleted women with past history of cancer, which included breast cancers (Barton et al. 2007). Modest benefit has recently been shown in naturally but not surgically menopausal women. Again, recruited women already reported 2–3 sexually satisfying events per month at baseline (Davis et al. 2008a).

6. *Relation of testosterone serum levels to women's sexual function.* In large population studies, serum levels of testosterone do not correlate with any measure of women's sexual function (Wierman et al. 2006).

7. *Loss of ovarian androgen.* Cross-sectional epidemiological surveys of convenience samples of women have reported lower sexual desire in women

with surgical menopause (Dennerstein et al. 2006; Leiblum et al. 2006), but a recent, larger national survey of 2,207 American women using the same validated questionnaire as the previous surveys did not (West et al. 2008). Rather, the results confirmed an increased prevalence of distress about low desire in women with relatively recent bilateral salpingo-oophorectomy (BSO). Both older and younger women with relatively recent BSO reported the presence of low sexual desire as frequently as did age-matched women with intact ovaries. Of interest, despite their continued hormone deficit, women older than 45 years who had undergone oophorectomy prior to menopause had fewer complaints of low desire than women of similar age with intact ovaries. Three prospective studies involving perimenopausal hysterectomy combined with elective bilateral oophorectomy for benign disease showed no loss of sexual function afterward (Ariz et al. 2006; Farquar et al. 2006; Teplin et al. 2007).

8. *Relation of androgen metabolites to sexual function.* Measures of androgen metabolites have not been shown to correlate with sexual function. The majority of testosterone produced in midlife and older women is intracellular; however, a test of intracellular testosterone is not currently available except on a research basis. Androgen metabolites are being evaluated as a useful measure of total androgen activity (Labrie et al. 2006) and may replace serum measurement of testosterone in the future.

9. *Serum levels of precursor sex hormones.* Precursor sex hormones—that is, hormones that can be converted into either testosterone or estrogen, such as dehydroepiandrosterone—do not correlate consistently with sexual function (Wierman et al. 2006).

10. *Relationship of estrogen treatment to risk of cardiovascular disease and breast cancer.* If systemic estrogen (needed with systemic testosterone) is not initiated within a few years of menopause, the risk of cardiovascular disease is increased. After 10 years, regardless of onset of therapy, the patient has a small increase in breast cancer risk (as reviewed by Schover 2008).

What remains unknown about testosterone therapy.

1. *Usefulness for sexual desire/interest disorder.* Research has not yet definitively indicated whether testosterone therapy would be beneficial for women

with sexual desire/interest disorder, which is typically comorbid with an arousal disorder. Benefit is expected given the improvement in arousal and response domains in the questionnaires used in the recent randomized controlled trials (Basson 2008; Braunstein et al. 2005). However, participants from those studies were not recruited on the basis of problematic responsive desire and arousal. In all the randomized controlled trials of transdermal testosterone, subjects were reporting 2–3 sexually satisfying events per month at baseline. Such women would be unlikely to be given a diagnosis of sexual desire/interest disorder or of arousal disorder (although distress about lack of spontaneous desire may have merited a DSM-IV-TR diagnosis of hypoactive sexual desire disorder).

2. *Long-term efficacy of testosterone.* Long-term efficacy (i.e., beyond 2 years) is unknown (Braunstein 2007).

3. *Long-term effects on cardiovascular disease.* A link between higher androgens and cardiovascular disease continues to be debated. Cross-sectional studies have given conflicting results, but a prospective study—a nested case controlled study—showed weak trends toward increased risk of cardiovascular disease among women having higher androgen:estrogen ratios: among postmenopausal women not taking hormone therapy, those women with lower sex hormone–binding globulin or with higher free androgen indexes were at increased risk of cardiovascular events (Wild 2007).

4. *Long-term safety regarding risk of breast cancer.* The long-term safety regarding risk of breast cancer in women taking testosterone is not known. In vitro and in vivo studies have reported both proliferative and antiproliferative effects on growth of breast cancer cells brought about by testosterone. Results from an epidemiological review suggest that endogenous androgen levels are positively correlated with breast cancer risk (Tamimi et al. 2006). However, recent research has shown testosterone's reduction of the typical proliferative effects of postmenopausal estrogen and progesterone therapy (Hofling et al. 2007).

5. *Effect of age on sensitivity of androgen receptors.* Whether older women may have a degree of loss of sensitivity of androgen receptors is not yet known. Note that little sexual benefit has been documented from supplementing testosterone in older as opposed to younger hypogonadal men (Bhasin et al. 2007). This lack of benefit may be due to the relative resistance of the androgen receptor. Whether genetic polymorphism of the androgen re-

ceptor will prove to be relevant to the efficacy and safety of supplemental testosterone in women (or men) is unknown.

6. *Effect of exogenous testosterone on production of neurosteroids postmenopause.* Research has not yet determined whether the recently identified increased production of neurosteroids postmenopause would be negatively affected by exogenous testosterone. Adaptive changes in the brain to the drop in systemic sex hormones have been documented: upregulation of steroid-ogenic enzymes and of sex receptors occurs (Ishunina and Swaab 2007). Sex steroids are produced de novo (from cholesterol) in the human brain. A theoretical concern is that peripheral supplementation could impair this adaptation.

Investigational Nonhormonal Pharmacological Therapies

Both basic science and the unwanted sexually negative effects of antidepressants have indicated that some molecules having actions on certain dopamine, serotonin, melanocortin, and noradrenaline receptors are likely to be prosexual. Table 5–5 lists investigational therapies and their current status in terms of industry-sponsored research. Various drugs, including phosphodiesterase inhibitors, alpha-blockers, selective estrogen receptor modulators, and peptidase inhibitors, have been studied to treat deficient genital congestion. However, the documented lack of correlation between women's sexual symptoms and any measurable deficit in genital congestion limits this research approach.

Holistic Therapy

Although limited research is available on combined medical and psychological approaches, clinical practice is generally based on the psychological methods, and any investigational medication is adjunctive.

Case Example

Mia, age 32 years, has been in a relationship with Bob, also age 32, for 7 years. The sexual complaint is that for the past 5–6 years, Mia has had difficulty becoming aroused and has minimal sexual desire. Mia and Bob were seen both together and separately. When seen together, both partners stated that their relationship is sound, caring, and respectful, and that they have many common interests and goals. They recalled that Mia had sexual desire and reliable

Table 5–5.   Investigational drugs for low sexual desire and arousal disorders in women

Drug type/name	Rationale/comments	Published trials
Systemic testosterone	Clinical benefit noted since the 1930s. Serum levels of testosterone or its precursors do not correlate with sexual function. Precursors of intracellular testosterone decrease in women by some 60% from mid-30s to early 60s, and postmenopausal ovarian production of testosterone varies. Thus, intracellular testosterone production may decline with age, but prevalence of excessive loss or deficiency is unknown. Moreover, changes in androgen receptors, coregulators, and the brain's own production of testosterone (and estrogen) from cholesterol with age are largely unknown. Testosterone is not approved in the United States or Canada, and the American Endocrine Society recommends against its use. However, currently some physicians adapt off-label formulations approved for men.	Modest sexual benefit beyond placebo from 300-µg (but not 450-µg) transdermal testosterone has been shown in four studies of surgically postmenopausal and one study of naturally menopausal women (Basson 2006). Frequency of "sexually satisfying events" increased from approximately 2–3 to 5 per month (from 3 to 4 with placebo). Scores in desire domain of validated unpublished questionnaire increased in all trials. Scores in arousal, pleasure, and orgasm domains increased and distress scores decreased in some, but not all, studies. A recent RCT to ameliorate premenopausal women's sexual dissatisfaction using transdermal testosterone showed minimal benefit (Davis et al. 2008b). No RCTs to date have recruited women unable to have any sexually satisfying events. No long-term safety data are available. Major concerns are possible increased risk of breast cancer, cardiovascular disease, insulin resistance, and metabolic syndrome. Also, concerns remain with long-term systemic estrogen. Supplemental testosterone in estrogen-depleted women is nonphysiological and has been shown to be of no benefit in women with a past history of cancer (Barton et al. 2007).

Table 5–5. Investigational drugs for low sexual desire and arousal disorders in women *(continued)*

Drug type/name	Rationale/comments	Published trials
Tibolone	Androgenic, progestogenic, and estrogenic effects have been shown. The drug has been available in Europe for more than a decade for menopausal symptoms.	Sexual benefits are comparable to transdermal norethisterone acetate plus estradiol in women with sexual dysfunction (Nijland et al. 2008). Vulvar atrophy improved in women recruited for reasons other than sexual dysfunction. The U.S. Food and Drug Administration determined, in June 2006, that the drug was not approvable for indication applied for (female sexual function postmenopause). Concerns include possible higher risk of breast cancer than from estrogen only (found in Million Women Study) and doubled incidence of stroke, compared with placebo (found in Long-Term Intervention on Fractures With Tibolone trial).
Bremelanotide (synthetic peptide): alpha-melanocyte-stimulating hormone (MSH) analogue-agonist at MC3R and MC4R receptors	Alpha-MSH has been implicated in male and female sexual responses in rodents. Of note, MC4R is also involved in satiety for food, stress response, and nociception. Safety concerns have suspended further trials.	No significant differences in psychophysiological or questionnaire responses to viewing erotic videos 15 minutes after intranasal drug but increased arousal during subsequent activity found in eight women given alpha-MSH compared with seven women given placebo (Diamond et al. 2006). Recent small RCT showed benefit for women's arousal disorder with in-home use of nasal drug 45 minutes before sex (Safarinejad 2008). Pharmaceutical company discontinued trials in June 2008.
Flibanserin: 5-HT_{1A} agonist and 5-HT_{2A} antagonist	Serotonin acting on 5-HT_{1A} receptors has prosexual effects in rodents.	None.

Table 5–5. Investigational drugs for low sexual desire and arousal disorders in women (*continued*)

Drug type/name	Rationale/comments	Published trials
Bupropion	Bupropion blocks noradrenaline and dopamine reuptake and is less likely to cause medication-associated dysfunction when used as an antidepressant and may ameliorate SSRI-induced dysfunction.	One small 4-month study of nondepressed premenopausal women showed increased arousability and sexual response but no increase in initial (spontaneous) desire (Segraves 2004).
Phosphodiesterase inhibitors: sildenafil	Nitric oxide is a major neurotransmitter involved in vasodilation of clitoral structures and is also present in vagina. However, most women with arousal disorders have normal genital congestion.	Increased genital congestion benefited women with diabetes and multiple sclerosis in small RCTs. One RCT showed an improvement in women with genital arousal disorder who had an impaired physiological response on the vaginal photoplethysmograph. Large multisite RCTs of women with arousal and desire disorders showed no benefit (Basson et al. 2002). Pharmaceutical company discontinued support for trials of sildenafil in women in 2004.
L-Arginine	Arginine is a substrate for nitric oxide. However, most women with arousal disorders have normal genital vasocongestion.	One RCT has shown some benefit in sexual dysfunction in premenopausal and perimenopausal women but not postmenopausal women (Ito et al. 2006).

Note.   RCT = randomized controlled trial; SSRI = selective serotonin reuptake inhibitor.

arousal and enjoyment, with orgasms from direct genital stimulation and occasionally from intercourse, in their first approximately 18 months together.

Mia's sexual response changed in the context of medical illness. Mia had a second episode of ulcerative colitis 18 months into the relationship with Bob. She was hospitalized, and her medications over the next 20 months included intermittent high-dosage prednisone and some immunosuppressive drugs. Mia had three hospital admissions of a few weeks each during that time period. At that time, Mia had been studying to complete an undergraduate degree in general sciences and working as a bank teller. She has not continued with the studies but has continued working at the bank.

Mia rarely has any spontaneous sexual desire. Every 1–2 months, she agrees to Bob's initiation of sexual activity, mostly out of obligation and guilt. Although Bob repeatedly asks what kind of pleasuring he can do for her, typically Mia hurries them on to the act of intercourse "to get it over with." Her pleasure is minimal, other than feeling better about herself after intercourse, less guilty, and relieved that they will not be sexual for the next many days. Mia still enjoys affectionate hugging, cuddling, and holding hands and is grateful that Bob does not see these interactions as preludes to sexual activity.

Mia is not content with the current situation. She explained that even though "it will be fine for me never to have sex again," she knows this is not fair to Bob, and their infrequency of sexual activity also makes her feel unworthy and unattractive. When seen alone, Bob explained that his frustration with the situation is now far less than before. Initially, he was confused, thinking that Mia's reluctance to be sexual was about him. The more they have spoken and Mia has reassured him that this is not so, he has come to believe that her illness or the medications or her childhood history may be relevant.

Mia's developmental history includes being brought up by two rather distant parents. Most of the parenting was done by her mother who, although caring and involved in Mia's life, was described as cold and critical. Mia has a younger sister, Angelina, but Mia suggests that she was not close to Angelina and felt inferior to her. When seen alone, each partner referred to Mia's history of sexual abuse by an uncle. Mia was about 9 or 10, and the uncle would call by phone for Mia to come and help him with various jobs around the house. Genital touching of both Mia and himself occurred. Mia recalls knowing this behavior was wrong, does not recall being frightened, and does not recall trying to tell her parents. One day, after a number of occurrences, perhaps a dozen, Mia decided to send her younger sister instead. Angelina returned home and immediately told her mother about the sexual abuse and that Mia had told her to go and that the uncle had said it was his and Mia's secret. Mia recalls feeling responsible, blamed, dirty, and very confused. She has no recall of how things went in the family regarding this subject after that incident but does know that neither of the girls again visited the uncle, who subsequently moved away. Home life was described as not particularly happy, even though no abuse or conflict occurred. Mia was much happier from age 14 to age 17 years, when she spent as much time as possible with her boyfriend's family. She felt accepted and loved by them. She recalled sex with the boyfriend as being fun and problem free. The couple used condoms and then the pill, and Mia recalled having been aroused and orgasmic consistently.

Mia was distressed at the breakup with her first boyfriend, had a couple of short-term monogamous heterosexual relationships, and then became ill with her first episode of ulcerative colitis between the ages of 22 and 24 and did not have sexual partners during that time. She met Bob when she was 25 and recalled that she had rewarding sexual times during the first 18 months with him, as well as having sexual desire preceding sexual activity.

Regarding Mia's mental health, she explained that she has always been a "worrier"; she said that frequently she anticipates the worst scenario and has catastrophic thoughts. She agreed that these thoughts interfere when she is trying to be sexual. She has had no psychological intervention, but for the past 6 months she has used citalopram (Celexa) 10 mg with only modest benefit. Depressive symptoms were present at the breakup with her first boyfriend for a few months and during each bout of ulcerative colitis. No therapy was given. Mia's mother and grandmother both have histories of depression.

Mia rarely has sexual fantasies—she says this is long term as far as she can remember. She self-stimulated as a teenager, mostly out of curiosity and never frequently. Her family members provided no advice regarding sexuality. Mia recalled some sex education classes at school, but no one spoke of sexual response or feelings. Religion has not been part of her life and is therefore not likely to have influenced her sexuality. When the couple is sexual, Mia has no discomfort or dyspareunia. She feels that lubrication is adequate. Her genital structures seem appropriately sexually sensitive, but she declines to have much in the way of direct stimulation. Occasionally, erotic movies or books can cause some sexual arousal, but mostly Mia does not choose to read or view erotic materials.

Mia's general health is currently good. She is taking no other medications. Switching from oral contraceptives to condoms 2 years ago made little change to her sexual symptoms.

Diagnosis

Mia's diagnoses were acquired sexual desire/interest disorder and subjective sexual arousal disorder.

Formulation

Predisposing factors include Mia's low self-esteem associated with her mother's criticism, her guilt over being responsible for the sexual abuse as a child and the sexual abuse to her sister, and a long-term comparison of herself with her sister's superior abilities and attractiveness. Also, she had never been emotionally close to anyone as she grew up until her first boyfriend and his family, and she lost these at the time of the breakup. Mia's anxiety traits and her tendency to catastrophize and be easily distracted are further predisposing factors.

Precipitating factors include Mia's being unwell generally and specifically receiving the systemic cortisone, a drug that suppresses adrenal production of precursor sex hormones, notably the precursors of testosterone. Therefore, for perhaps 2 years, beginning 18 months into her current relationship, Mia had abnormally low testosterone activity in her body's cells.

Perpetuating factors include the fact that Mia was unaware of normative and circular patterns of sexual response in women, and she was waiting and hoping for spontaneous desire to become sexually active again. Rather than guiding Bob as to the type of stimuli that might have given her pleasure and then arousal, Mia bypassed these and rushed to intercourse simply wanting to speed up the experience. Mia's ongoing low self-esteem and her currently unfulfilled career and study plans fueled her feeling of being substandard. She was, at times, overwhelmed by the thought of losing this relationship. Additionally, her ongoing anxiety and tendency to be distracted plus the more recent use of the SSRI further reduced her response and desire.

Protective factors include Mia's positive feelings for her partner, the fact that the disorder is acquired rather than lifelong, and her motivation to understand her situation and move on even though some effort is required. A positive prognostic sign is that Mia stated at the outset, "I know there will be no magic pill!"

Therapy

Psychoeducation was given to both partners, and they constructed Mia's own sex response cycle showing the breaks or interruptions (see Figure 5–4).

Previously unaware that women (and men) sometimes agree to or initiate sexual activity without sensing at that point any spontaneous desire, Mia was initially unable to write her own list of "incentives" for engaging in sexual activity. Understanding the normal need for sexual stimuli and a satisfactory appropriate context, the couple were more than willing to follow some modified sensate focus exercises over 4 weeks. Mindfulness techniques (to help with the difficulty of staying focused and attending to stimuli) were discussed in detail (the clinician provided literature and then contact information about local classes). The clinician explained that mindfulness-based psychoeducation has been shown to have benefit, particularly in women with past histories of sexual abuse (Brotto et al. 2008). In addition, Mia participated in brief cognitive therapy, in which her unhealthy cognitions about her own sexuality were challenged. Mia was also encouraged to visualize herself as a competent and

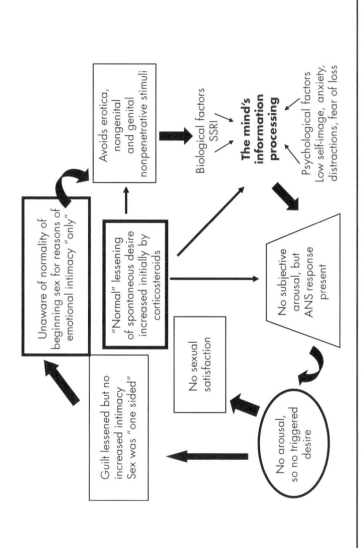

Figure 5–4.   Mia's sexual response cycle.

Note.   ANS=autonomic nervous system; SSRI=selective serotonin reuptake inhibitor.

confident sexual woman while being sexual with her partner, given recent evidence showing that adopting positive sexual schema can significantly enhance subjective sexual arousal (Middleton et al. 2008). Although individual therapy for the past sexual abuse was considered, this was decided against because Mia felt that she did not dwell on it; she did not have flashbacks, nightmares, or other symptoms of posttraumatic stress disorder; and she did not have a history of diagnosed clinical depression, self-harm, substance abuse, or promiscuity.

The clinician wished either to treat the anxiety more effectively with medication or preferably to use nonpharmacological means and discontinue the SSRI. Mia agreed with the latter option, and some brief sessions involving making thought records proved very helpful. Included were her negative and catastrophizing thoughts about her sexuality.

In Mia's case, the combination of psychoeducation, cognitive-behavioral therapy, sensate focus therapy, and mindfulness—together with removing the sexually negative medication—allowed a rewarding return of sexual pleasure that could trigger desire.

Conclusion

Women most commonly explain their sexual difficulties in terms of low desire. However, most women do not distinguish sexual desire from subjective sexual arousal/excitement. Women have multiple reasons or incentives for initiating and agreeing to sex, and desire, as in "drive," "hunger," or "lust," is an infrequent reason for many women in long-term relationships. Thus, in practical terms, the lack of sexual motivation of all types, plus or minus difficulty in becoming subjectively aroused and triggering desire once into the experience, is what typically causes women to seek help. Assessment needs to be in depth and include past and present psychosexual, medical, and mood details from both partners. Management includes explaining women's sexual response cycles and identifying points of weakness in the patient such that she can see the logic of her situation; sometimes, that explanation is all that is needed because the necessary changes become obvious to the couple. Specific therapy includes cognitive-behavioral therapy, sex therapy, mindfulness, and psychotherapy approaches. Aside from local or systemic estrogen for lost genital response and subsequent lack of sexual motivation, drug therapy is investigational. As such, medications should be considered only after psychosexual issues have been addressed with the standard and emerging psychological therapies. Given that women usually remain sexually active providing they have a functional partner, any drug requirement will be indefinite. Long-term safety data are therefore urgently needed for both hormonal and nonhormonal drugs.

Key Points

- The circular model of sexual response cycle is useful as a basis for assessment.
- The clinician works with the patient or couple to identify points of weakness or interruption of the cycle.
- The clinician shares the formulation of the problem or disorder with the couple.
- The first step of therapy is to address mental health issues, including low self-image and relationship difficulties.
- The next step is to use combinations of psychoeducation, cognitive-behavioral therapy, sex therapy, and mindfulness as first-line therapy.
- Aside from estrogen supplementation for lost genital sensitivity and reduced elasticity and vaginal lubrication, medical adjuncts remain investigational.
- Testosterone supplementation should be attempted only in research settings because of the many unknowns, including the following:
  - Which women are androgen deficient
  - Whether total androgen activity, as measured by androgen metabolites, correlates with any aspect of women's sexual dysfunction
  - Whether testosterone has any benefit for women with desire/interest disorder, which is typically associated with combined or subjective arousal disorder

- Safety of long-term treatment
- Safety of concomitant long-term estrogen treatment
- The role of production of sex steroids in the brain and adaptations with age and with menopause, as well as the consequences of exogenous sex steroids on that production
- The role of androgen receptor sensitivity and its possible change with age

References

American Psychiatric Association: Diagnostic and Statistical Manual of Mental Disorders, 4th Edition, Text Revision. Washington, DC, American Psychiatric Association, 2000

Arnow BA, Millheiser L, Garrett A, et al: Women with hypoactive sexual desire disorder compared to normal females: a functional magnetic resonance imaging study. Neuroscience 158:484–502, 2009

Bancroft J, Loftus J, Long JS: Distress about sex: a national survey of women in heterosexual relationships. Arch Sex Behav 32:193–208, 2003

Barlow DH: Causes of sexual dysfunction: the role of anxiety and cognitive interference. J Consult Clin Psychol 54:140–148, 1986

Barton DL, Wender DB, Sloan JA, et al: Randomized controlled trial to evaluate transdermal testosterone in female cancer survivors with decreased libido: North Central Cancer Treatment Group Protocol N02C3. J Natl Cancer Inst 99:672–679, 2007

Basson R: The female sexual response: a different model. J Sex Marital Ther 26:51–65, 2000

Basson R: Human sex response cycles. J Sex Marital Therapy 27:33–43, 2001

Basson R: Sexual desire and arousal disorders in women. N Engl J Med 354:1497–1506, 2006

Basson R: Women's sexual function and dysfunction: current uncertainties, future directions. Int J Impot Res 20:466–478, 2008

Basson R, Weijmar Schultz W: Sexual sequelae of general medical disorders. Lancet 369:409–424, 2007

Basson R, McInnes R, Smith MD, et al: Efficacy and safety of sildenafil citrate in women with sexual dysfunction associated with female sexual arousal. J Womens Health Gend Based Med 11:367–377, 2002

Basson R, Leiblum S, Brotto L, et al: Definitions of women's sexual dysfunctions reconsidered: advocating expansion and revision. J Psychosom Obstet Gynaecol 24:221–229, 2003

Baumeister RF, Catanese KR, Vohs KD: Is there a gender difference in strength of sex drive? Theoretical views, conceptual distinctions and a review of relevant evidence. Pers Soc Psychol Rev 5:242–273, 2001

Bhasin S, Enzlin P, Coviello A, et al: Sexual dysfunction in men and women with endocrine disorders. Lancet 369:597–611, 2007

Braunstein GD: Management of female sexual dysfunction in postmenopausal women by testosterone administration: safety issues and controversies. J Sex Med 4 (4 Pt 1):859–866, 2007

Braunstein GD, Sundwall DA, Katz M, et al: Safety and efficacy of a testosterone patch for the treatment of hypoactive sexual desire disorder in surgically menopausal women. Arch Intern Med 165:1582–1589, 2005

Brotto LA, Basson R, Luria M: A mindfulness-based group psychoeducational intervention targeting sexual arousal disorder in women. J Sex Med 5:1646–1659, 2008

Cain VS, Johannes CB, Avis NE, et al: Sexual functioning and practices in a multiethnic study of midlife women: baseline results from SWAN. J Sex Res 40:266–276, 2003

Carson JW, Carson KM, Gil KM, et al: Mindfulness-based relationship enhancement. Behav Ther 35:471–494, 2004

Clayton AH, Warnock JK, Kornstein SG, et al: A placebo-controlled trial of bupropion SR as an antidote for selective serotonin reuptake inhibitor–induced sexual dysfunction. J Clin Psychiatry 65:62–67, 2004

Clayton A, Kornstein S, Prakash A, et al: Changes in sexual functioning associated with duloxetine, escitalopram, and placebo in the treatment of patients with major depressive disorder. J Sex Med 4:917–929, 2007

Davis SR, Moreau M, Kroll R, et al: Testosterone for low libido in postmenopausal women not taking estrogen. N Engl J Med 359:2005–2017, 2008a

Davis S, Papalia MA, Norman RJ, et al: Safety and efficacy of a testosterone metereddose transdermal spray for treating decreased sexual satisfaction in premenopausal women: a randomized trial. Ann Intern Med 148:569–577, 2008b

Dennerstein L, Dudley E, Burger H: Are changes in sexual functioning during midlife due to aging or menopause? Fertil Steril 76:456–460, 2001

Dennerstein L, Koochaki P, Barton I, et al: Hypoactive sexual desire disorder in menopausal women: a survey of Western European women. J Sex Med 3:212–222, 2006

Diamond LE, Earle DC, Heiman JR, et al: An effect on the subjective sexual response in premenopausal women with sexual arousal disorder by bremelanotide (PT-141), a melanocortin receptor agonist. J Sex Med 3:628–638, 2006

Farquar CM, Harvey SA, Yu Y, et al: A prospective study of three years of outcomes after hysterectomy with and without oophorectomy. Obstet Gynecol 194:714–717, 2006

Hartmann U, Philippsohn S, Heiser K, et al: Low desire in midlife and older women: personality factors, psychosocial development, present sexuality. Menopause 11:726–740, 2004

Hawton K, Catalan J, Fagg J: Low sexual desire: sex therapy results and prognostic factors. Behav Res Ther 29:217–224, 1991

Hofling M, Lindén Hirschberg A, Skoog L, et al: Testosterone inhibits estrogen/progesterone-induced breast cell proliferation in postmenopausal women. Menopause 14:183–190, 2007

Ishunina TA, Swaab DF: Alterations in the human brain in menopause. Maturitas 57:20–22, 2007

Ito TY, Polan ML, Whipple B, et al: The enhancement of female sexual function with ArginMax, a nutritional supplement, among women differing in menopausal status. J Sex Marital Ther 32:369–378, 2006

Janssen E, Everaerd W, Spiering M, et al: Automatic processes and the appraisal of sexual stimuli: toward an information processing model of sexual arousal. J Sex Res 37:8–23, 2000

Kaplan HS: Hypoactive sexual desire. J Sex Marital Ther 3:3–9, 1979

Labrie F, Bélanger A, Bélanger P, et al: Androgen glucuronides, instead of testosterone, as the new markers of androgenic activity in women. J Steroid Biochem 99:182–188, 2006

Laumann EO, Nicolosi A, Glasser DB, et al: Sexual problems among women and men aged 40–80 y: prevalence and correlates identified in the Global Study of Sexual Attitudes and Behaviors. Int J Impot Res 17:39–57, 2005

Leiblum SR, Koochaki PE, Rodenberg CA, et al: Hypoactive sexual desire disorder in postmenopausal women: U.S. results from the Women's International Study of Health and Sexuality (WISHeS). Menopause 13:46–56, 2006

Levine SB: The nature of sexual desire: a clinician's perspective. Arch Sex Behav 32:279–285, 2003

Masters WH, Johnson V: Human Sexual Response. Boston, MA, Little, Brown, 1966

McCall K, Meston C: Differences between pre- and postmenopausal women in cues for sexual desire. J Sex Med 4:364–371, 2007

Meston CM: The effects of state and trait self-focused attention on sexual arousal in sexually functional and dysfunctional women. Behav Res Ther 44:515–532, 2006

Meston CM, Buss DM: Why humans have sex. Arch Sex Behav 36:477–507, 2007

Middleton LS, Kuffel SW, Heiman JR: Effects of experimentally adopted sexual schemas on vaginal response and subjective sexual arousal: a comparison between women with sexual arousal disorder and sexually healthy women. Arch Sex Behav 37:950–961, 2008

Nijland EA, Weijmar Schultz WCM, Nathorst-Boös J, et al: Tibolone and transdermal E_2/NETA for the treatment of female sexual dysfunction in naturally menopausal women: results of a randomized active-controlled trial. J Sex Med 5:646–656, 2008

Nurnberg HG, Hensley PL, Heiman JR, et al: Sildenafil treatment of women with antidepressant-associated sexual dysfunction. JAMA 300:395–404, 2008

Prause N, Janssen E, Hetrick WP: Attention and emotional responses to sexual stimuli and their relationship to sexual desire. Arch Sex Behav 37:934–949, 2008

Pridal CG, LoPiccolo J: Multielement treatment of desire disorders, in Principles and Practice of Sex Therapy, 3rd Edition. Edited by Leiblum SR, Rosen RC. New York, Guilford, 2000, pp 57–81

Regan P, Berscheid E: Belief about the state, goals and object of sexual desire. J Sex Marital Ther 22:110–120, 1996

Safarinejad MR: Evaluation of the safety and efficacy of bremelanotide, a melanocortin receptor agonist, in female subjects with arousal disorder: a double-blind placebo-controlled, fixed dose, randomized study. J Sex Med 5:887–897, 2008

Sanders SA, Graham CA, Milhausen RR: Predicting sexual problems in women: the relevance of sexual excitation and sexual inhibition. Arch Sex Behav 38:241–251, 2008

Sarwer DB, Durlak JA: A field trial of the effectiveness of behavioral treatment for sexual dysfunctions. J Sex Marital Ther 23:87–97, 1997

Schover LR: Androgen therapy for loss of desire in women: is the benefit worth the breast cancer risk? Fertil Steril 90:129–140, 2008

Segraves RT: Bupropion sustained release for the treatment of hypoactive sexual desire disorder in premenopausal women. J Clin Psychopharmacol 24:339–342, 2004

Segraves R, Balon R, Clayton A: Proposal for changes in diagnostic criteria for sexual dysfunctions. J Sex Med 4:567–580, 2007

Shifren JL, Davis SR, Moreau M, et al: Testosterone patch for the treatment of hypoactive sexual desire disorder in naturally menopausal women: results from the INTIMATE NM1 Study. Menopause 13:770–779, 2006

Singer B, Toates FM: Sexual motivation. J Sex Res 23:481–501, 1987

Tamimi RM, Hankinson SE, Chen WY, et al: Combined estrogen and testosterone use and risk of breast cancer in postmenopausal women. Arch Intern Med 166:1483–1489, 2006

Taylor MJ, Rudkin L, Hawton K: Strategies for managing antidepressant-induced sexual dysfunction: systematic review of randomised trials. J Affect Disord 88:241–254, 2005

Teplin V, Vittinghoff E, Lin F, et al: Oophorectomy in premenopausal women: health-related quality of life and sexual functioning. Obstet Gynecol 109:347–354, 2007

Tiefer L, Hall M, Tavris C: Beyond dysfunction: a new view of women's sexual problems. J Sex Marital Ther 28 (suppl 1):225–232, 2002

Trudel G, Marchand A, Ravart M, et al: The effect of a cognitive-behavioral group treatment program on hypoactive sexual desire in women. Sexual and Relationship Therapy 16:145–164, 2001

West SL, D'Aloisio AA, Agans RP, et al: Prevalence of low sexual desire and hypoactive sexual desire disorder in a nationally representative sample of U.S. women. Arch Intern Med 168:1441–1449, 2008

Whalen RE: Sexual motivation. Psychol Rev 73:151–163, 1966

Whipple B, Brash-McGreer K: Management of female dysfunction, in Sexual Function in People With Disability and Chronic Illness: A Health Professional's Guide. Edited by Sipski ML, Alexander CJ. Gaithersburg, MD, Aspen, 1997, pp 509–534

Wierman ME, Basson R, Davis et al: Androgen therapy in women: an Endocrine Society Clinical Practice guideline. J Clin Endocrinol Metab 91:3697–3710, 2006

Wild RA: Endogenous androgens and cardiovascular risk. Menopause 14:609–610, 2007

Witting K, Santtila P, Varjonen M, et al: Female sexual dysfunction, sexual distress, and compatibility with partner. J Sex Med 5:2587–2599, 2008

Woo JST, Brotto LA, Gorzalka BB: The role of sex guilt in the relationship between culture and women's sexual desire. Manuscript under review

6

Male Hypoactive Sexual Desire Disorder

Stephen B. Levine, M.D.

Samia Hasan, M.D.

Miriam Boraz, Ph.D.

The primary characteristic of male hypoactive sexual desire disorder (HSDD) is the disinclination to behave sexually. The diagnosis of HSDD is not often made in general psychiatric settings despite its frequent presence. Like most sexual dysfunction diagnoses in these settings, the patient's sexual disinterest typically is unrecognized. When noted, it may be ignored or viewed as irrelevant to the presenting problem, of too low a priority to merit immediate attention, or as a symptom of another psychiatric condition. The diagnosis is much more frequently considered in settings that provide therapy for couples, where it may be the chief complaint.

Although the problem of limited sexual energy and diminished sexual motivation has been known for centuries in many societies (Shah 2002), the use of the term *low libido* for this problem is only 100 years old. Physicians are now expected to respond to this complaint by ruling out hypogonadism (McVary 2007). When serum testosterone levels are normal, physicians typically assume the origin of the problem to be psychosocial. Psychiatrists and other mental health professionals, however, should be prepared to go beyond this organic versus psychological dualism to consider these five overlapping categories:

1. A pattern of no pathological significance
2. A symptom of another, more fundamental psychiatric disorder
3. A symptom of relationship alienation
4. A symptom of a physical abnormality
5. A symptom of HSDD

The treatment of patients with HSDD begins with an understanding of the complex nature of sexual desire. The appealing goal of providing an effective medication quickly comes up against the fact that sexual life and its problems comprise biological, individual psychological, interpersonal, and cultural elements (Levine 2007). A dualistic medical model of etiology and treatment often is inadequate to address HSDD.

Is the Prevalence of Male HSDD Known?

HSDD became a DSM-III psychiatric diagnosis in response to the recognition that Masters and Johnson's (1970) excitement and orgasmic phase model of sexual dysfunction failed to account for those individuals who were not motivated to have sex with their partners. The sexual response paradigm was amended by adding sexual desire as the first crucial step (Kaplan 1977; Lieff 1977). When HSDD first appeared in DSM-III (American Psychiatric Association 1980), its prevalence was unstudied.

In epidemiological studies, researchers carefully define criteria for what constitutes a so-called case and then use a specified sampling method to estimate the prevalence of the problem in some population group (Kessler et al. 2005). Definitions of a case and sampling methods vary from study to study, making generalizations from the literature difficult. None of the authors of major epidemiological studies of psychiatric disorders have sought to define any sexual disorder (Narrow et al. 2002).

The most comprehensive epidemiological study of sexuality to date is the 1992 National Health and Social Life Survey, in which 3,432 men and women were interviewed for 90 minutes and administered brief questionnaires (Laumann et al. 1994). The ages of the subjects ranged from 18 to 59 years. The survey found that 9.8% of 1,511 men who resided in households had no sex with a partner during the previous year and 17.6% had sex a few times—that is, 27.4% had sex three or fewer times. Among those who had no sex in the previous year, 39.5% rated themselves as very happy, 36.7% rated themselves as generally satisfied, and 33.8% rated themselves as unhappy. Of the total sample of 1,511 men, 139 were unhappy about their sexual frequency. When examined by age, approximately 15% of the male sample at all ages stated that they lacked interest in sex (Laumann et al. 2001); this study is the usual source of the quotation of a 15% male prevalence of HSDD (Balon 2007), but other studies converge on this number as well. For example, a survey of sexual behaviors of men ages 57–85 years demonstrated that approximately 75% of the reasonably physically healthy subjects acknowledged a continuing sexual interest (Lindau et al. 2007). In survey research, "interest in sex" sounds like desire, but ultimately it may not mean what clinicians and patients mean by "sexual desire."

Today, the prevalence of HSDD is estimated to be about 35% among women (West et al. 2008), more than twice that among men. This estimate is reflected in two facts: no placebo-controlled medication trials for HSDD have exclusively targeted men and no peer-reviewed journal articles have focused on male HSDD. In contrast, many trials and articles have focused on women's HSDD (see Chapter 5, "Disorders of Sexual Desire and Subjective Arousal in Women"). The presumed lower prevalence of HSDD among men is thought to be a consequence of men's more constant and recurring sexual interest throughout the life cycle (Beck 1995). In clinical settings, men are much more likely to complain about arousal difficulties (erectile dysfunction) than about lack of sexual desire. Women, in contrast, complain to physicians more frequently about lack of desire (Basson 2006).

The actual prevalence of HSDD in either sex remains uncertain for several reasons. The diagnostic criteria of desire and arousal diagnoses are difficult to distinguish from one another in people of either sex (Levine 2006). When desire, arousal, and orgasmic problems coexist in the same patient, the decision about the most basic dysfunction is arbitrary. The DSM-IV-TR diagnostic criterion of a deficiency in erotic fantasies (American Psychiatric Association 2000) describes more women's than men's clinical presentations of HSDD. Also, the loss of sexual desire may represent an adaptive response to long-standing personal or partner sexual disappointment rather than a disorder (Riley and May 2001).

According to DSM-IV-TR criteria, the lack of sexual interest alone is not sufficient to diagnose HSDD. The patient must be distressed or perceive the consequences of his pattern to be negative for him. The problem cannot be thought to be symptomatic of another psychiatric disorder, such as current severe depression, heroin addiction, or a past or current medication regimen.

Uncertainty exists about the prevalence of HSDD because the methods of community-based sampling provide no room for sophisticated diagnostic nuances, and the many nuances experienced in clinical settings provide little confidence about where to draw the lines between disorder, variation, and normality, and between one disorder and another.

Diagnostic Caveats

Variations in Masculinity and Religiosity

The word *male* refers to biological sex, but it also refers to gender identity—that is, how a man sees his masculinity. Biological sex closely matches gender identity in most men. However, among feminine men, solitary cross-dressers, men who want to become women, and men who periodically portray themselves as women in public, the word *male* only describes their biological sex. Another group of men, comprising priests who aspire to celibacy and the profoundly religious who believe that sexual desire is inconsistent with moral purity, has a different version of masculine identity that puts them in constant opposition to their personal manifestations of desire. Males from these groups often report having little interest in and energy for sexual expression. When they seek psychiatric attention, the clinician correctly perceives their gender identity or their religiosity to be a fundamental issue. Their low level of sexual desire is a definable pattern, but it is rarely perceived to be an indication of HSDD.

Case Example 1

Patrick left the Roman Catholic priesthood and married several years later. During courtship and in the early months of marriage, he and Colleen had satisfying sexual activity weekly. They gradually settled into a pattern of monthly and, thereafter, less frequent sex. He explained eventually that "it was one thing to abandon my commitment to celibacy and another thing to have frequent sexual behavior. I still vaguely feel it is wrong for me, even though I know it is not."

Not All Men Who Complain of Low Libido Have Low Libido

In the sexual life of any two people, a discrepancy is likely to surface between the individuals' preferred frequencies of sexual behavior together. All couples negotiate these differences in some way. One person initiates or requests sexual opportunity, and the other person responds. This intensely private, often nonverbal interpersonal process may reflect many things, including the quality of each individual's contentment with the other.

Although male patients typically refer to their own subjective experience and behavior when complaining of low libido, occasionally a man presents his partner's view. In these situations, the man fails to initiate sexual behavior and refuses his partner's sexual initiations, and the partner is the source of his help seeking. The partner's view is that any normal man in his situation ought to want to behave sexually and, therefore, his behavioral deficit is presented as low libido. He compliantly allows the partner to maintain this belief.

Case Example 2

Ben and Betty were referred for marital and sexual therapy by their respective individual therapists. Both patients were being treated for depression with medication and individual psychotherapy. Betty's frequent jealous questioning of Ben about his life outside of the marriage depressed and angered him. He explained his HSDD as being due to consistently low testosterone levels and his continued need for a selective serotonin reuptake inhibitor (SSRI). After 2 years of infrequent marital therapy sessions, Betty discovered that Ben had been having an active sexual relationship with an associate at work. His desire for the associate was intense, and his frequency was whenever they could be together. Ben lied to his wife, individual and conjoint therapists, internist, and endocrinologist before his wife's discovery of his ongoing sharing of genital photos with the other woman ended their marriage. To maintain the façade, Ben had allowed himself to undergo a liver biopsy to investigate his idiopathic hypogonadism.

All men with patterns of low sexual desire should be skillfully asked if there is a type of partner, a specific partner, a type of sexual behavior, or a social context that ignites his sexual interest. Most patients have never been asked to reveal such intimate information, and some will be hesitant to fully reveal this information. Nonetheless, through the men's responses to these questions, psychiatrists may learn about some hidden gender identity issues, homosexual desire that is unknown to the partner, paraphilia, ongoing and past affairs, marital alienation, pornography addiction, intrafamilial sexual abuse, and other manifestations of the inner life of these men. Only rarely does a man display no evidence of a conscious erotic life. From the answers to these questions, the clinician may be led away from the diagnosis of HSDD, or at least may realize that the erotic energy of male HSDD is quite different from the erotic disinterest of women's HSDD (an observation not reflected in DSM-IV-TR).

Incorrect Equations

To minimize the danger of making an egregious assessment error, clinicians should be aware of the falsity of these six statements:

1. Absent or infrequent sexual behavior with the partner = absent or infrequent sexual behavior
2. Absent or infrequent sexual behavior with a partner = absence of masturbation
3. The complaint of limited sexual energy = absence of masturbation
4. "That is the whole story, doctor" = the entire story
5. A man's declaration that he feels free to talk in front of his partner = he feels free to discuss his sexual history in front of the partner
6. A clinician's experience of the patient as masculine = the patient may not be dealing with an unconventional gender identity issue, homoeroticism, or a paraphilia

Nature of Sexual Desire

Clinical Measurement of Sexual Desire as Hypoactive

Clinically, the strength of sexual desire is often "measured" by accepting the patient's and the partner's personal accounts. Their story about low sexual desire is typically summarized with the quantitative-sounding word *hypoactive*. In research settings, low desire may be assessed in three ways: 1) by a brief history; 2) by a numerical score based on a retrospective questionnaire that employs numerous questions, each of which can be scored over a range, such as from 1 to 5; 3) by having the subject fill out a daily diary or a questionnaire. In both clinical and research endeavors, clarity is needed about what exactly is being measured.

A Definition of Sexual Desire

The diagnosis of HSDD was created before the publication of any in-depth consideration of the nature of sexual desire (Kaplan 1979, 1995; Leiblum and Rosen 1988). Sexual desire can be defined using a mathematical allusion: *"sexual desire is the sum of the forces that lean a person toward and away from sexual behavior"* (Levine 2006, p. 71). This definition asserts that three forces interact to generate the strength of a person's fluctuating levels of sexual desire at any particular time:

1. Biological sexual energy, now called *drive*
2. Degree of willingness to bring one's body to a specific partner for sexual behavior, now called *motivation*
3. One's cultural sensibilities about the normality and morality of sexual behavior, now spoken of as *sexual values*

Because drive, motivation, and values involve interacting biological, psychological, and social forces, asserting that desire is high, average, or low or rating desire as 40, 25, or 15 on a 50-point scale does not tell a clinician how much each component is contributing to an assessment. The three elements of desire may be in opposition to one another. Sexual desire is inherently conflicted for many people during some of their lives. These predictable conflicts have been referred to as the paradoxes of sexual desire (Levine 2003).

Manifestations of Sexual Desire

Sexual desire is clinically inferred by some combination of the following (Baumeister et al. 2001):

1. Masturbation
2. Attempts to initiate sexual behavior with a partner
3. Erotic fantasies—that is, thoughts about oneself in sexual interaction (These thoughts may occur during waking periods or during dreams; they may be reveries or thoughts about other people's bodies without the dreamlike intensity. Erotic fantasies can be stimulated by drive, memories, imagination, and pornography.)
4. Sexual attraction to others
5. Genital sensations of arousal, which often include some tumescence, accompanying the erotic thoughts (Men often identify these sensations as "horniness.")

Some men consider information about these manifestations to be extremely private. Others have internal prohibitions against acknowledging their manifestations of desire even to themselves. These variations are routinely seen in men who belong to the same subculture and form the basis for variations across cultures. Obtaining accurate information about sexual desire can be a considerable challenge even when the patient and the clinician belong to the same cultural group.

Case Example 3

Whitney worked in therapy individually and conjointly for over 2 years trying to understand and reverse his acquired HSDD. He consistently reported a complete absence of sexual drive manifestations and a marked aversion for sex with his wife or "anyone." One day, he casually reported that he had been masturbating once or twice a week for years while thinking about other women. Shocked, I said to Whitney, "Gee, I thought you said that you had no inclination to masturbate and felt that you could live the rest of your life without any sexual expression." "Did I say that?" Whitney asked. "Many times," his stunned wife quickly added. He replied, "Well, I am not dead. I don't have any desire to have sex with other women. That is morally wrong. I still can't bring myself to have any kind of sex with you. Maybe I just did not want to hurt you more than I have already done. I don't know."

Culture

The range of sexual drive manifestations for men at a particular age—for example, between 20 and 30 years of age—is often assumed to be the same for men of all cultures. However, men in different cultures do not have the same motivation to behave sexually. Some cultures are macho, some prohibit all sexual expression prior to marriage, and some are polygamous. Some cultures are highly educated, and others are mired in poverty. These vital variations create different values. The values component of sexual desire works by motivating or inhibiting masturbation and partner-related sexual behaviors and punishing individuals whose discovered sexual behaviors are culturally unacceptable. Culture also works, however, to limit what a man permits himself to know about himself.

Absence of Normative Data on Sexual Desire in Men as They Age

Designating the boundary between normal sexual desire and HSDD within a particular culture might be possible if trustworthy age-stratified data sets were available that quantified *all* of the manifestations of sexual desire (Balon et al. 2007). HSDD would be declared as that below 1 or 2 standard deviations from the mean. Although sexual desire apparently declines from youth through middle age to older age, no comprehensive longitudinal desire data are available to demonstrate this decline. However, cross-sectional data support this decline in desire (McKinlay and Feldman 1994). Also, much cross-sectional animal and human data support the decline in sexual frequency over time (Bancroft 2007).

Constitutional Endowment for Sexual Drive

If valid and reliable data sets were available on the longitudinal pattern of a large diverse group of men over many decades, cutoffs could be provided for low, ordinary, and high sexual constitutional endowments (Martin 1981). If people actually fall into only three categories, a clinician would then be able to state that a patient's HSDD is built on a constitutional platform of low, ordinary, or high sexual energy.

Uncertain Road From Criteria to Psychiatric Diagnosis

The numerous overlapping ways of creating criteria for psychiatric disorders makes defining any disorder a daunting task (Zachar and Kendler 2007). Although much of DSM-IV-TR is practical and has clinical utility, validity is not guaranteed (Kendell and Jablensky 2003). When patients with concerns about their low libido seek assistance, the clinician might assume that their complaint fulfills the criteria of personal distress or significant negative interpersonal consequence. Sometimes, however, the patient is motivated less by distress or relationship consequence and more by the idea that help is available. Similar to women who sought clinical help when the media led them to believe that testosterone replacement would eradicate their loss of sexual interest, men may also arrive at psychiatrist's offices looking for the wonder drug after misunderstanding media reports about some promising medication that is not yet available. Patients' distress is not to be dismissed, but some of these patients have accommodated to their diminished desire. The promise of a new medication feels to them like seeking the fountain of youth. Those who market phosphodiesterase type 5 (PDE5) inhibitors have been shocked to discover that some men with erectile dysfunction abandon the cure that they initially so eagerly sought and that only a minority of the men presumed to have erectile problems actually sought the cure. As men's sexual energies lessen in the last third of life, their high levels of distress may not be long lasting (Bancroft 2007).

Motivations for Seeking Assistance for Low Sexual Interest

The source of the seeking of clinical assistance for low libido seems to be most often the patient's female partner, next the patient himself, and rarely a professional who has dealt with the patient in some other clinical context. A married man usually seeks assistance because of fears about his partnership. He may be afraid that if he does not improve, his partner will abandon him, seek another sex partner, restart an affair, or grow more hostile. He may think that she will lose respect for him because he did not try to get better and that either of them may have an even greater sense of despair about their future as a couple.

Single men may worry that they will never be able to find or sustain a relationship with a partner. They may briefly hope that the origin is organic and curable, even though they may intuitively know better. They may finally feel ready to deal with their sexual avoidance. Identifying some of these motives during the initial encounter often generates patients' trust in the therapist's competence.

Subcategories of HSDD

The diagnostic criteria in DSM-IV-TR indicate that the clinician should specify three subtypes of HSDD: 1) lifelong or acquired, 2) situational or generalized, and 3) due to psychological or due to combined factors. Lifelong HSDD is usually about constitutional endowment of sexual drive, although the internalization of antisexual values, as can be seen in very religious individuals (see Case Example 1 earlier in this chapter), makes the issue of endowment difficult to discern. Most cases of HSDD fall into the acquired category.

Many cases of HSDD are situational, although this fact may be guarded from the partner and the clinician. Although patients may answer all of the doctor's questions, they may not provide all the relevant details. They may feel the need to mislead their partner by hiding their secret lives or they may be too embarrassed, at first, to share what they know.

Case Example 4

Amy and Adam had individual sessions and two conjoint ones before the reasons for his 3-year pattern of sexual avoidance and unreliable erections became clearer. In response to the clinician's failure to understand something that was said, the couple exchanged a long permission-giving look at each other. Amy eventually said, "The problem began when I refused to continue to indulge his wish to have us both dress up in full-length slips as a prelude to foreplay.…I want to be with a man who wants to *be* a man, not one who wants to pretend that he is a woman!"

Generalized acquired cases of low sexual desire are quite common in psychiatric practice simply because many commonly prescribed psychiatric medications (e.g., SSRIs, serotonin-norepinephrine reuptake inhibitors, prolactin-elevating antipsychotic medications, lithium) tend to inhibit sexual drive and motivation. Also, interest in sexual expression is often curtailed by the onset of new serious illness. The mechanisms for this form of generalized acquired low desire are various combinations of direct illness effects, including treatment effects from medication, radiation, or surgery; psychological reactions to being ill; and spousal reactions to the ill partner. Psychiatrists should not be surprised, for example, by the high prevalence of male HSDD among oncologists' patients. Generalized acquired diminished interest in sex among men who have become depressed is not typically diagnosed as HSDD; it is regarded as a symptom of depression. HSDD is typically diagnosed after the other symptoms of major depressive disorder improve but sexual desire remains diminished.

The third DSM-IV-TR distinction, psychological versus combined factors, requires the clinician to try to establish the origin of the problem. No guideline exists for how to make this distinction. Through the use of these three subtypes of HSDD, the writers of DSM-IV-TR prepare clinicians to expect a diversity of circumstances associated with diminished sexual interest.

Significance of Low Drive

Generalized HSDD means that the pattern of low sex drive exists in all contexts. To arrive at this diagnosis, the clinician asks the patient about the circumstances in which he has sexual energy and seeks evidence that the patient does not think about sex, does not react to others with erotic responses, does not initiate solitary or partner sex, lacks consistent interest in the sexual dimensions of life, and is unusually comfortable about not having sex for long periods of time. In terms of sexual energy, the patient is relatively asexual (Prause and Graham 2007). When the patient presents this clinical story, the clinician questions how long this pattern has been present and whether it was different earlier in life. Such a history differentiates a relative or absolute sexual drive deficiency from a disorder based on a hidden motivation to avoid sex with a partner. When a patient has a history of generalized HSDD, the clinician should consider biological rather than psychological causes. If the man has been sterile, the doctor should be suspicious that he might have a subtle genetic abnormality with early-onset sexual drive diminution.

Early Prototype for Psychogenic HSDD

The complaint of low desire often represents a lack of motivation for sexual behavior with the partner. Freud described a common form of psychic impotence characterized by the patient's erectile failures and subsequent avoidance of lovemaking with a new wife (Freud 1912/1968): "This singular disturbance affects men of strongly libidinous natures, and manifests itself in a refusal by the executive organs of sexuality to carry out the sex act, although before and after they may show themselves to be intact and capable of performing the act, and although a strong psychical inclination to carry it out is present" (p. 179). Today, these classic cases are recognized as acquired situational HSDD. Even though a couple may have had one or more children together, the men complain of the decided lack of pleasure from sex with the wife. Typically, the marriage quickly becomes asexual, and each partner is faced with the temptations of infidelity because the usual multiple benefits of sex within marriage are lacking. Freud thought that these men's lives were paralyzed by their unconscious oedipal longings. When these men become engaged or married, their maternal incest taboo is transferred to the unfortunate partner. The man is then gripped by a motivation to avoid making love to his loving, receptive, and baffled wife. This classic pattern of normal drive and an unconsciously forbidden but socially appropriate partner is still encountered.

Modern Recurring Sources of Acquired Situational HSDD

Three other variations on partner avoidance also occur:

1. *The pornography casualty.* A man has so consistently used pornography that he has inadvertently scripted his sexuality to young sex-loving women about whom he knows nothing. He has spent his young adulthood attempting to hook up with new partners without much psychological intimacy. His fiancée or wife is a *person* to him—too complex, respected, and emotionally real to arouse him. He longs for the simple imagery that excites him without the experience of nervousness.
2. *The Don Juan casualty.* A man has consistently used seduction of women to entertain himself. Quite proud of his accomplishments, he views sex as sport and may pride himself on the large number of female friends he can occasionally call to get together sexually. He marries a woman he considers terrific but has little desire for her. This is often seen in marriages between a young woman and a much older man who regards his wife as

a "prize." In some psychiatric circles, a Don Juan is referred to as a phallic narcissist or as suffering from a Madonna-whore complex (Freud 1905/ 1953). This character type has been known cross-culturally in literature and music for centuries.

3. *The practical marriage casualty.* An ambitious man marries for material, social, or family gain without any genuine attraction or other internal signs of falling in love. Although the fiancée is a loving person, the man realizes during sex that he has been false to her and to himself. This can be seen when arranged marriages do not work successfully.

Clinical Challenge of Acquired Situational HSDD Prototypes

1. *The faithful husband who seems unwilling to make love with his wife but masturbates in response to sexual drive manifestations or to prevent their appearance.* The therapist's role is to find out why he is motivated to avoid sex with his partner. Here are three possibilities:

    a. Either he has rejected her because he has lost respect for her as a person, or she has rejected him because she has lost respect for him as a person.

    b. Her physical appearance or her illness has robbed him of his sexual ardor for her.

    c. He no longer wants to submit himself to her complaints about his sexual capacities.

2. *The unfaithful husband who is currently or has been recently involved in a sexually satisfying affair and is unable to explain to his wife why he has little interest in sex with her.* The therapist's role is to learn about the affair and help the man consider his options with the therapist. The therapist should neither lie to the wife nor inform her without the patient's consent.

3. *The single man with a hidden sexual identity variation who has numerous depressive and anxiety symptoms.* Careful questioning reveals his erotic gender transformation fantasies, homoerotic desires, or paraphilic preoccupations. When his erotic unconventionality is socially abhorrent to

him, he rarely masturbates in an attempt to accommodate to a life alone without being bothered by sex. Such a man will appear to have generalized HSDD. The therapist seeks to find out if the patient is constitutionally deficient in drive or simply suppressing his sexual impulses because of his moral quandary. After growing comfortable with the therapist, many of these men eventually reveal their alternating periods of abstinence and compulsive masturbation and are then reclassified as having situational HSDD.

4. *The married man with a hidden sexual identity variation.* Some men are able to court and marry, only to fall into a similar circumstance as in the previous category.

Hypogonadism

Testosterone production by the testes is the result of physiological processes in the hypothalamus and the pituitary gland (Federman 2006). Subnormal serum testosterone levels due to testicular disease are labeled *primary hypogonadism*, whereas subnormal testosterone levels due to hypothalamic or pituitary dysfunction are known as *secondary hypogonadism*. Testosterone levels normally decline by decade in the last 50 years of the life cycle (Morelli et al. 2007) and have been found to decline at a rate of 1%–2% per year (Harman et al. 2001). Hypogonadism can be classified according to age at onset:

- *Very early onset*—occurs in fetal life and produces major sexual differentiation problems, such as occurs in androgen insensitivity syndromes.
- *Early onset*—manifests itself in delayed puberty and has less devastating central nervous system and peripheral effects than in, for example, Klinefelter's syndrome.
- *Postpubertal onset*—manifests in mild insidious onset of a lower libido, such as may occur with trauma to the testes.
- *Late onset* (also called testosterone deficiency syndrome)—manifests in older men and is thought to be the cause of sexual dysfunction (particularly erectile dysfunction), mood disturbance, weight loss, and sleep disturbance. Evidence is mounting that many of these men can be restored to sexual desire and potency with testosterone replacement (Yassin and Saad 2007).

Differential Diagnosis

The differential diagnosis of adult-onset hypogonadism typically includes drug-induced, prolactin-secreting pituitary adenoma (Schlechte 2003), liver disease, thyroid disease, hemochromatosis, panhypopituitarism, AIDS, testicular trauma, substance abuse, prostate radiation, cancer chemotherapy, and various organ system failure syndromes (Bhasin et al. 2007).

Emerging Concepts of Hypogonadism

As molecular geneticists deduce the individual protein building blocks of hormone synthesis of luteinizing hormone, follicle-stimulating hormone, gonadotropin-releasing hormone, testosterone, and cell membrane receptors (Bhasin 2007; Lofrano-Porto et al. 2007; Raivio et al. 2007), medicine can look forward to glimpsing the sources of variation in constitutional endowments of sexual drive. Similar insights are to be expected as evidence mounts about the intracellular effects on cytoplasmic and nuclear RNA/DNA synthesis mechanisms of testosterone. Currently, medicine deals primarily with serum levels of testosterone and its correlates.

Treatment of Male HSDD

Medications for Low Drive

In Search of a Medication

When a medication is found that can safely stimulate sexual desire, it is likely to provide a better understanding of the anatomy, neuroendocrinology, and biochemistry of sexual drive. It may also change how physicians discuss sexual desire and its problems. Compounds have been identified that stimulate sexual drive, but each has posed other significant clinical problems, such as nausea, hypertension, and dependence. The PDE5 inhibitors, which have been shown to increase the frequency of sexual behavior in men by improving erectile dysfunction, have been shown *not* to stimulate desire on the basis of the desire domain scores on the International Index of Erectile Function (Goldstein et al. 1998). This recurrent finding indicates that improved potency increases the motivation to have sex but, over time, does not generate new levels of sexual drive.

The search for a medication treatment for HSDD is a search for a sexual drive stimulator. A drive-enhancing drug might act without visual, auditory, olfactory, or social contextual stimuli. On the basis of our current understanding, the drug is expected to act within several specific nuclei within the hypothalamus (Pfaus et al. 2007). Such a drug might shed light on the mechanism of increased sexual drive found among many patients with mania, alcohol or substance use disorders, and Parkinson's disease (Korpelainen et al. 1998).

A drive-enhancing drug will pose certain public health issues that will further illuminate important cultural aspects of sexual desire. The drug will have a specific duration of action—minutes, hours, or a day. During this time, the increased sexual energy will shape behavior (masturbation, sex with established partner, or sex with another partner). Depending on the sexual identity of the patient, the partner may involve a woman, a man, or a minor. The sexual behavior may be conventional or paraphilic. Thus, a sexual drive–stimulating drug may create much discussion about social values concerning sexual expression and may receive intense media discussion before and after it is approved by the U.S. Food and Drug Administration.

Medication trials of sexual desire agents thus far are in Phase II or Phase III trials involving women only. Clinicians might expect that if a strong signal of efficacy and safety emerge from the studies of bremelanotide, a melanocortin peptide, and of flibanserin, a $5\text{-}HT_{1A}$ serotonin receptor agonist and $5\text{-}HT_{2A}$ serotonin receptor antagonist, then additional studies may enroll men with low sexual energy.

Testosterone as a Treatment for HSDD in the Absence of Hypogonadism

Because testosterone has been available in several forms for seven decades, physicians have provided this hormone to men complaining of low libido. Despite decades of anecdotal experience, the clinical efficacy of testosterone in this usage in uncertain, and no modern scientific evidence is available to support its lasting impact on patients. A rise in testosterone level from intramuscular injection, for instance, can be expected to lower endogenous testosterone production because of the feedback mechanisms between serum testosterone levels and hypothalamic and pituitary hormones. A concern is that providing excessive dosages of androgen might have deleterious effects on the liver, prostate, bone marrow, breast, blood pressure, or sleep mechanisms

(Wespes and Schulman 2002). A community-based study of the relationship between low libido and testosterone levels demonstrated only a modest probability that men complaining of low libido would exhibit low testosterone (Travison et al. 2006). The prudent practice would be to avoid providing androgen in any form to men with normal testosterone levels.

Studies are being done of the treatment of men with erectile dysfunction and low libido whose morning total testosterone levels are less than 300 ng/dL. In one study, sexual desire increased with placebo, but the greatest improvements in sexual desire were seen when testosterone levels exceeded 600 ng/dL (Seftel et al. 2004).

Bupropion

Used initially to counter the sexual effects of SSRIs, bupropion was studied in several pharmaceutical company trials exploring its use in treating women with HSDD who were not depressed (Segraves et al. 2001, 2004). Another study that provided a moderate signal of efficacy failed to separate the data by gender (Coleman et al. 2001). Bupropion, which causes no sexual dysfunctional side effects, can be an effective antidepressant. Whether it can assist nondepressed men with increasing and maintaining their sexual drives remains to be convincingly demonstrated.

Androgenic Compounds

After 70 years of testosterone treatment of men with sexual complaints, the current popular avenue of administration is a gel rubbed onto the skin (Nieschlag 2006). The lack of large controlled efficacy trials, however, leaves this treatment of late-onset testosterone deficiency in the controversial category.

Psychotherapy

Maurice (2005) reviewed evidence for the existing treatments of male HSDD. No specialized form of psychotherapy—cognitive-behavioral therapy, psychodynamic therapy, sex therapy, psychodrama—has claimed a strong capacity to help men and their partners with this problem. Therapy is frequently available for men alone, with their partners, or in groups of other men with limited sexual interest in their partners (as is commonly seen among the so-called sex addicts) to deal with the underlying problem, which most often is not the absence of sexual drive but rather the motivation to avoid the partner. The clinician's therapy is a process to help the patient understand what is motivating the avoidance. Although these processes do not generate case reports or controlled studies, they do help men and their partners understand the underlying issues, whether they are interpersonal (e.g., partner alienation due to disrespect) or developmental (e.g., paraphilic requirements not being fulfilled by partner). The patient may consider the work with the therapist to be valuable even though the problem is only better understood. This paradox between the helped patient and the failure of the therapy to "cure" the problem reintroduces the clinician to the fact that sexual life is affected by biological, social, cultural, and private psychological forces, which limit medication efficacy.

After Careful Scrutiny, Does Male HSDD Exist?

The answer to whether male HSDD exists is "it depends." When patients first go to a primary care physician, urologist, or endocrinologist, the physician will rule out or treat hypogonadism. Medical treatment by these physicians often precludes further consideration of the psychological, interpersonal, and cultural aspects of the problem. In our clinical experience, many successfully treated patients still have their symptom after becoming eugonadal. The mental health professionals who see a eugonadal man with low libido often have a choice of perceiving the basic problem as HSDD or as a pattern of low desire due to depression, marital alienation, or SSRI treatment. If the patient is diagnosed with HSDD, the depression, marital alienation, drug therapy, and so on, are considered to be comorbidities rather than explanations. Clinicians have to recognize the low desire pattern and evaluate the distress and the likely contributing factors because it is the distress and its attendant hope for a better sexual life that enable the patient to delve into and eventually overcome his motivations to avoid sex with his partner.

Case Example 5

Ten years after being diagnosed and treated for a prolactin-secreting pituitary tumor, Charles, now in his mid-30s, returned to talk about entering psychotherapy. Bromocriptine returned his sexual drive manifestations to him, but his sexual life was not improved. He revealed that he had been too embarrassed a decade ago to reveal that he had long struggled with masochistic erotic imagery. He routinely thinks of being humiliated through bondage and domination by a woman. "I know where this comes from: my mother was an extremely impulsive, demeaning, critical woman who abused me until I was well into high school. I need to get beyond this because I am ashamed, and my new best-of-my-life partner wants nothing to do with this behavior. I don't want to spend my life masturbating to my imagery, occasionally sneaking off to a dominatrix, and lying to my partner about my low level of sexual interest. Can you help me?"

The clinician replied, "I usually try to help this problem by arranging individual psychotherapy." After discussing the patient's ability to pay, the doctor arranged a referral for low-fee psychotherapy with an experienced therapist who had an interest in sexual abuse and its consequences. The patient never called.

Implications for Research

In recruiting for a research protocol for male HSDD, excluding those with marital problems, sexual identity variations, moral prohibitions against sexual expression, paraphilia, sexual addiction, and regular masturbation patterns will leave too few subjects for enrollment. Researchers have to look at the phenomenon of low desire as though it were simply low sexual drive. They cannot look too closely at the differences between adaptive responses to disappointments in a relationship, weakness of drive manifestations, and psychological motivations that prevent a man from bringing his body to his partner for sexual purposes. Researchers are seeking to prove that a sexual drive generator exists and that it can safely create its manifestations in diverse men. An effective drug will increase sexual drive and sexual arousability. Its efficacy could be demonstrated in gay, paraphilic, and gender-atypical men. The study endpoints might be masturbation increases and partner sex increases regardless of the gender of the partner or the nature of the sexual act engaged in. The increase in unconventional behaviors may be a political or public relations problem for drug company sponsors.

Key Points

- In diagnosing male HSDD, the clinician needs to 1) make sure the patient's complaint focuses on desire for sex rather than arousal or orgasm problems and 2) ascertain whether the problem involves drive manifestations or motivation to avoid sex.

- The clinician needs to categorize the complaint based on 1) whether the pattern has been present since adolescence; 2) whether the pattern is global or situational; 3) when and under what conditions the problem has disappeared; and 4) what social, medical, psychiatric, and developmental circumstances preceded the onset of the problem.
- If the problem is global, involving drive manifestations, whether lifelong or acquired, the patient should be carefully screened for medical conditions. Morning total testosterone level is the first step to ascertaining a hypogonadal state. Low testosterone level can be repeated, along with prolactin levels, to rule out a pituitary adenoma.
- Therapy is based on the clinician's understanding of the patient's history and social circumstances: 1) remove offending medications; 2) recommend individual, conjoint, or group psychotherapy; 3) consider psychopharmacology for comorbid psychiatric diagnoses; and 4) consider enrollment in a clinical trial of a prosexual compound.

References

American Psychiatric Association: Diagnostic and Statistical Manual of Mental Disorders, 3rd Edition. Washington, DC, American Psychiatric Association, 1980

American Psychiatric Association: Diagnostic and Statistical Manual of Mental Disorders, 4th Edition, Text Revision. Washington, DC, American Psychiatric Association, 2000

Balon R: Sexual dysfunctions, in Gabbard's Treatments of Psychiatric Disorders, 4th Edition. Edited by Gabbard GO. Washington, DC, American Psychiatric Publishing, 2007, pp 643–646

Balon R, Segraves RT, Clayton A: Issues for DSM-V: sexual dysfunction, disorder, or variation along normal distribution: toward rethinking DSM criteria of sexual dysfunction. Am J Psychiatry 164:198–200, 2007

Bancroft JH: Sex and aging. N Engl J Med 357:820–822, 2007

Basson R: Clinical practice: sexual desire and arousal disorders in women. N Engl J Med 354:1497–1506, 2006

Baumeister RF, Catanese KR, Vohs KD: Is there a gender difference in strength of sex drive? Theoretical views, conceptual distinctions, and a review of the evidence. Pers Soc Psychol Rev 5:242–273, 2001

Beck JG: Hypoactive sexual desire disorder: an overview. J Consult Clin Psychol 63:919–927, 1995

Bhasin S: Experiments of nature—a glimpse into the mysteries of the pubertal clock. N Engl J Med 357:929–932, 2007

Bhasin SP, Enzlin P, Coviello A, et al: Sexual dysfunction in men and women with endocrine disorders. Lancet 369:597–611, 2007

Coleman CC, King BR, Bolden-Watson C, et al: A placebo-controlled comparison of the effects on sexual functioning of bupropion sustained release and fluoxetine. Clin Ther 23:1040–1058, 2001

Federman DD: The biology of human sex differences. N Engl J Med 354:1507–1514, 2006

Freud S: Three essays on the theory of sexuality (1905), in The Standard Edition of the Complete Psychological Works of Sigmund Freud, Vol 7. Translated and edited by Strachey, L. London, Hogarth Press, 1953, pp 123–245

Freud S: On the universal tendency to debasement in the sphere of love (1912), in The Standard Edition of the Complete Works of Sigmund Freud, Vol 11. Translated and edited by Strachey L. London, Hogarth Press, 1968, pp 179–190

Goldstein I, Lue TF, Padma-Nathan H, et al; Sildenafil Study Group: oral sildenafil in the treatment of erectile dysfunction. N Engl J Med 338:1397–1404, 1998

Harman SM, Metter EJ, Tobin JD, et al: Longitudinal effects of aging on serum total and free testosterone levels in healthy men: Baltimore Longitudinal Study of Aging. J Clin Endocrinol Metab 86:724–731, 2001

Kaplan HS: Hypoactive sexual desire. J Sex Marital Ther 3(1):3–9, 1977

Kaplan HS: Disorders of Sexual Desire and Other New Concepts and Techniques in Sex Therapy. New York, Brunner/Mazel, 1979

Kaplan HS: The Sexual Desire Disorders: Dysfunctional Regulation of Sexual Motivation. New York, Brunner/Mazel, 1995

Kendell R, Jablensky A: Distinguishing between the validity and utility of psychiatric diagnoses. Am J Psychiatry 160:4–12, 2003

Kessler RC, Chiu WT, Dumler O, et al: Prevalence, severity and comorbidity of 12-month DSM-IV disorders in the National Comorbidity Survey Replication. Arch Gen Psychiatry 62:617–627, 2005

Korpelainen JT, Hiltunen P, Myllylä VV: Moclobemide-induced hypersexuality in patients with stroke and Parkinson's disease. Clin Neuropharmacol 21:251–254, 1998

Laumann EO, Gagnon JH, Michael RT, et al: The Social Organization of Sexuality: Sexual Practices in the United States. Chicago, IL, University of Chicago Press, 1994

Laumann EO, Paik A, Rosen RC: Sexual dysfunction in the United States: prevalence and predictors, in Sex, Love, and Health in America: Private Choices and Public Policies. Edited by Laumann EO, Michael RT. Chicago, IL, University of Chicago Press, 2001, pp 352–376

Leiblum SR, Rosen RC: Sexual Desire Disorders. New York, Guilford, 1988

Levine SB: The nature of sexual desire: a clinician's perspective. Arch Sex Behav 32:279–285, 2003

Levine SB: Demystifying Love: Plain Talk for the Mental Health Professional. New York, Routledge, 2006

Levine SB: The first principle of clinical sexuality. J Sex Med 4:853–854, 2007

Lieff HI: What is new in sex research? Inhibited sexual desire. Medical Aspects of Human Sexuality 2:94–95, 1977

Lindau ST, Schumm LP, Laumann EO, et al: A study of sexuality and health among older adults in the United States. N Engl J Med 357:762–774, 2007

Lofrano-Porto A, Barra GB, Giacomini LA, et al: Luteinizing hormone beta mutation and hypogonadism in men and women. N Engl J Med 357:897–904, 2007

Martin CE: Factors affecting sexual functioning in 60–79-year-old married males. Arch Sex Behav 10:399–420, 1981

Masters WH, Johnson V: Human Sexual Inadequacy. Boston, MA, Little, Brown, 1970

Maurice WL: Male hypoactive sexual desire disorder, in Handbook of Sexual Dysfunction. Edited by Balon R, Segraves RT. New York, Taylor & Francis, 2005

McKinlay JB, Feldman HA: Age-related variation in sexual activity and interest in normal men: results from the Massachusetts Male Aging Study, in Sexuality Across the Life Course. Edited by Rossi AS. Chicago, IL, University of Chicago Press, 1994, pp 261–285

McVary KT: Clinical practice: erectile dysfunction. N Engl J Med 357:2472–2481, 2007

Morelli A, Corona G, Filippi S, et al: Which patients with sexual dysfunction are suitable for testosterone replacement therapy? J Endocrinol Invest 30:880–888, 2007

Narrow WE, Rae DS, Robins LN, et al: Revised prevalence estimates of mental disorders in the United States: using a clinical significance criterion to reconcile 2 surveys' estimates. Arch Gen Psychiatry 59:115–123, 2002

Nieschlag E: Testosterone treatment comes of age: new options for hypogonadal men. Clin Endocrinol (Oxf) 65:275–281, 2006

Pfaus JF, Giuliano F, Gelez H: Bremelanotide: an overview of preclinical CNS effects on female sexual function. J Sex Med 4 (suppl 4):269–279, 2007

Prause N, Graham CA: Asexuality: classification and characterization. Arch Sex Behav 36:341–356, 2007

Raivio T, Falardeau J, Dwyer A, et al: Reversal of idiopathic hypogonadotropic hypogonadism. N Engl J Med 357:863–873, 2007

Riley A, May K: Sexual desire disorders, in Treatments of Psychiatric Disorders, 3rd Edition. Edited by Gabbard GO. Washington, DC, American Psychiatric Press, 2001, pp 1849–1871

Schlechte JA: Clinical practice: prolactinoma. N Engl J Med 349:2035–2041, 2003

Seftel AD, Mack RJ, Secrest AR, et al: Restorative increases in serum testosterone levels are significantly correlated to improvements in sexual functioning. J Androl 25:963–972, 2004

Segraves RT, Croft H, Kavoussi R, et al: Bupropion sustained release (SR) for the treatment of hypoactive sexual desire disorder (HSDD) in nondepressed women. J Sex Marital Ther 27:303–316, 2001

Segraves RT, Clayton A, Croft H, et al: Bupropion sustained release for the treatment of hypoactive sexual desire disorder in premenopausal women. J Clin Psychopharmacol 24:339–342, 2004

Shah J: Erectile dysfunction through the ages. Br J Urol Int 90:433–441, 2002

Travison TG, Morley JE, Araujo AB, et al: The relationship between libido and testosterone levels in aging men. J Clin Endocrinol Metab 91:2509–2513, 2006

Wespes E, Schulman CC: Male andropause: myth, reality, and treatment. Int J Impot Res 14 (suppl 1):S93–S98, 2002

West SL, D'Aloisio AA, Agans RP, et al: Prevalence of low sexual desire and hypoactive sexual desire disorder in a nationally representative sample of U.S. women. Arch Intern Med 168:1441–1449, 2008

Yassin AA, Saad F: Improvement of sexual function in men with late-onset hypogonadism treated with testosterone only. J Sex Med 4:497–501, 2007

Zachar P, Kendler KS: Psychiatric disorders: a conceptual taxonomy. Am J Psychiatry 164:557–565, 2007

7

Female Sexual Arousal Disorders

Lori A. Brotto, Ph.D.

Rosemary Basson, M.D., FRCP

Jane S. T. Woo, M.A.

Arousal was the focus of Masters and Johnson's studies of human sexual response when they invited couples into their St. Louis, Missouri, laboratory and monitored their physiological patterns of sexual arousal. This research generated their model of the human sexual response cycle (Masters and Johnson 1966). Helen Singer Kaplan's research added an initial phase of desire (Kaplan 1979). Thus, it was assumed that both women and men experience sexual desire, followed by increasing levels of genital sexual arousal, peaking in orgasm. These concepts shaped the definition and criteria for female sexual arousal disorder (FSAD) in the third edition of *Diagnostic and Statistical Manual* (DSM-III; American Psychiatric Association 1980) taxonomy.

During the past three decades, new information about the complex pathophysiology of women's impaired sexual arousal has emerged, but treatment of arousal disorder remains challenging. Given the enormous strides forward in comprehensive understanding of the etiology, treatment, and prognosis of genital sexual arousal disorder in men (erectile dysfunction) and the approval of sildenafil citrate in the United States (1998) and Canada (1999), a surge of research interest has been shown in women's arousal and its lack.

Definitions

In the current edition of DSM, DSM-IV-TR (American Psychiatric Association 2000), FSAD is defined entirely based on the woman's report of genital vasocongestion. Criterion A is "Persistent or recurrent inability to attain, or to maintain until completion of the sexual activity, an adequate lubrication-swelling response of sexual excitement"; Criterion B notes that "the disturbance causes marked distress or interpersonal difficulty"; and Criterion C adds that the dysfunction "is not better accounted for by another Axis I disorder… and is not due exclusively to the direct physiological effects of a substance… or a general medical condition" (p. 544). The "Associated Features and Disorders" section of DSM-IV-TR indicates that "the individual with female sexual arousal disorder may have little or no subjective sense of sexual arousal" (p. 543). Because this descriptor is not recognized as essential to the diagnosis of FSAD, epidemiological studies have focused almost exclusively on problematic genital arousal, in terms of vaginal dryness or dyspareunia, and not on the much more common presenting complaint of problematic subjective sexual arousal. Also, the common complaint of lost genital sexual sensitivity has not received adequate attention.

In 2002, the American Urological Association Foundation convened an international committee of experts in the field of women's sexuality to reconsider the DSM-IV-TR definitions of women's sexual dysfunction. The committee, in their report published in 2003 (Basson et al. 2003), proposed that FSAD be divided into three subtypes: 1) genital sexual arousal disorder, with a focus on inadequate or absent genital lubrication or swelling and loss of genital sexual sensitivity, despite the ability to become subjectively sexually aroused from nongenital stimuli; 2) subjective sexual arousal disorder, a new arousal disorder subtype, which was to be considered when the patient had absent or diminished feelings of sexual arousal (excitement or pleasure) from any type of sexual stimulation, even though lubrication and other genital responses were reported as present; and 3) combined sexual arousal disorder, which was described as difficulties both in genital arousal and in subjective sexual arousal. When the patient's concern was limited to dryness or discomfort on the basis of insufficient lubrication, the diagnosis recommended was dyspareunia. Although these proposed revisions represent a marked improvement from the definitions currently adopted in DSM-IV-TR, they are not yet part of the accepted nomenclature.

Persistent genital arousal disorder (PGAD) was included by the 2003 International Consensus Committee as a provisional diagnosis to be studied further, and was defined as "spontaneous, intrusive, and unwanted genital arousal (e.g., tingling, throbbing, pulsating) in the absence of sexual interest and desire. Any awareness of subjective arousal is typically but not invariably unpleasant. The arousal is unrelieved by one or more orgasms and the feelings of arousal persist for hours or days" (Basson et al. 2003). As research into PGAD is only just beginning, much less is known about its pathophysiology, treatment, and prognosis. Moreover, PGAD is not currently adopted in the DSM-IV-TR classification of sexual dysfunctions.

Given the well-documented overlap between problematic subjective sexual arousal and loss of sexual desire in women (e.g., Dennerstein et al. 2006), some have suggested that these two phenomena are indistinguishable. Therefore, we covered subjective sexual arousal disorder in Chapter 5, "Disorders of Sexual Desire and Subjective Arousal in Women." In this chapter, we focus only on genital sexual arousal—both its impairment (FSAD) and its excess (PGAD).

Practice Point

The currently recommended definitions of sexual arousal disorders focus on loss of genital sexual arousal (congestion/lubrication and sensitivity), loss of subjective sexual arousal, or a combination of both. This is in contrast to the DSM-IV-TR definition of sexual arousal disorder, which focuses only on lack of genital congestion/lubrication.

Disorders of Genital Sexual Arousal

Female Sexual Arousal Disorder

Epidemiology and Correlates

In various national probability studies, researchers have attempted to assess the prevalence of problematic genital arousal. Unfortunately, the majority of surveys have excluded women who are not in a sexually active relationship, thereby possibly missing women with sexual difficulties that preclude a relationship. The survey reports are often unclear about which aspect of arousal is being reported as difficult or absent, and the prevalence of genital sexual arousal disorder as currently defined is unclear.

When both vaginal dryness and "problems with arousal" are addressed, the former is usually more common: in England, 28% of 980 women ages 18–75 years reported recent lubrication difficulties, and 17% reported problematic arousal (Dunn et al. 1999). Among women older than 40 enrolled in a U.S. health maintenance organization, approximately 17% reported problematic arousal, not further classified (Addis et al. 2006). In a study of multiethnic perimenopausal American women, difficulties with arousal (not specified) ranged from some 20% in Caucasian and African American women to 40%–50% in Chinese, Japanese, and Hispanic women. However, pain was always or sometimes present in 20%–30% of women, and inadequate genital lubrication may have been the major etiology (Cain et al. 2003). Cross-cultural comparisons of women ages 40–80 indicated that women living in East Asia, Southeast Asia, and the Middle East had significantly higher rates of lubrication difficulties (23.0%–37.9%) than European and North American women (16.1%–27.1%) (Laumann et al. 2005). An interesting curvilinear effect of age was found such that women in their 50s were more likely to have lubrication difficulties than women in their 40s or women in their 70s (odds ratio = approximately 2.0). This contrasts with large earlier studies of Swedish women, in which the prevalence of ongoing lubrication problems progressed from 8% of women in their 40s to 26% in their late 60s (Fugl-Meyer and Fugl-Meyer 1999). A more recent study of women in this age range also found progressively worsening sexual symptoms (composite) with age (Lutfey et al., in press). Other correlates of impaired genital arousal in the Global Study of Sexual Attitudes and Behaviors were higher education and depression (Laumann et al. 2005). When distress was also assessed, the prevalence of lubrication difficulties that cause marked distress was 8%–9%, and "impaired physical response" (the latter combining genital and subjective aspects) plus marked distress was 3%–8% (Bancroft et al. 2003), emphasizing the importance of assessing associated personal and relationship distress. The prevalence of lost genital sexual sensitivity is unclear. Studies that include "inhibited enjoyment" (e.g., Dunn et al. 1999) or "sex not pleasurable" (e.g., Laumann et al. 2005) may be tapping into this. Researchers need to identify the different aspects of arousal in future epidemiological studies, just as clinicians need to do in the clinical setting for optimal assessment and management.

Biological Factors Involved in Etiology

Genital congestion is controlled by the autonomic nervous system and can be conceptualized as an immediate reflex response to erotic stimuli. However, when this genital congestion is measured by a vaginal photoplethysmograph (Sintchak and Geer 1975), the data typically demonstrate desynchrony between physiological sexual arousal and mental sexual excitement (van Lunsen and Laan 2004). Biological factors known to interfere with the genital arousal response and leading to the clinically common symptom of "genital deadness," as well as impaired lubrication, include estrogen deficiency and various medical diseases involving the pelvic autonomic nerves, such as spinal cord injury, multiple sclerosis, and diabetes mellitus. Nerve-sparing techniques during radical hysterectomy significantly lessen disruption to genital sexual arousal compared with non-nerve-sparing techniques (Pieterse et al. 2008). Androgen deprivation may also be associated with loss of genital sexual sensitivity, although the available data are primarily from research on nonhuman animals. Table 7–1 provides a more comprehensive list of biological factors involved in genital arousal.

Psychological Factors Involved in Etiology

Psychological and relational factors have been linked with genital sexual arousal in women. Measurement of genital arousal is typically reserved for the research setting, where techniques include vaginal photoplethysmography, which is used after a certain cognitive or behavioral manipulation, and vaginal pulse amplitude, which is measured by a tampon-shaped probe. Anxiety, by

Table 7–1. Biological factors involved in genital sexual arousal

Biological factor	Comments	References
Hormonal factors		
Estrogen	Peripheral estrogens are necessary for vaginal integrity and function and genital sexual sensitivity.	Bachmann et al. 1999; Traish and Kim 2006
Androgens	Endogenous testosterone levels correlate with genital arousal in cycling women. Women given sublingual testosterone have increased genital sexual arousal.	Schreiner-Engel et al. 1981
Prolactin	Hyperprolactinemia is associated with sexual desire, arousal, and orgasm dysfunction and is not explained by depression.	Kadioglu et al. 2005
Diabetes	Women with diabetes show impairments in genital arousal and lubrication.	Enzlin et al. 1998
Nitric oxide (NO)	Sildenafil improves genital arousal.	Basson and Brotto 2003; Berman et al. 2003; Caruso et al. 2001
	Reduced production of NO in diabetes is associated with reduced genital congestion.	Saenz de Tejada et al. 2005
Vasoactive intestinal polypeptide (VIP)	Neutral endopeptidase (NEP) degrades VIP, a major neurotransmitter allowing vasodilatation in the vagina. NEP inhibitors are being investigated. However, most women with arousal disorders have normal genital congestion.	Ottesen 1983; Pryde et al. 2006
Autonomic nervous system	Damage to autonomic nerves from spinal cord injury or radical hysterectomy or diabetes disrupts genital arousal.	Berard 1989; Maas et al. 2004
	Optimal level of sympathetic nervous system activity is necessary for genital sexual arousal.	Meston 2000

increasing sympathetic nervous system activity, significantly increases genital arousal (Palace and Gorzalka 1990), as shown when women are exposed to anxiety-evoking film stimuli. Cognitive distraction and self-focused, nonsexual attention also modulate genital arousal.

Based on the cognitive model of sexual response (Barlow 1986), which suggests that sexual arousal difficulties arise from distraction away from sexual cues and heightened attention to nonsexual cues, the dichotic listening paradigm (Elliott and O'Donahue 1997; Salemink and van Lankveld 2006) reveals that distraction is associated with lower levels of genital sexual arousal. Interestingly, however, there is likely an interaction of trait characteristics of the individual with state-evoked attention in that state induction of self-focused attention significantly interferes with genital arousal, but only among those women with high levels of trait self-focused attention. Among women with low trait self-focused attention, an experimental manipulation that increased self-focused attention had no effect on vaginal pulse amplitude (van Lankveld and Bergh 2008).

A more cognitively focused manipulation that encouraged sexually healthy depressed and nondepressed women to "try on" positive versus negative sexual schema prior to viewing erotic stimuli showed that genital sexual arousal was higher when subjects adopted a positive sexual schema than when they adopted a negative sexual schema (Kuffel and Heiman 2006). Among women with FSAD, positive sexual schema induction significantly improved genital sexual arousal (Middleton et al. 2008); however, false physiological feedback (i.e., telling women they had a strong genital arousal response) surprisingly decreased genital arousal in women with FSAD (McCall and Meston 2007). The authors speculated that this information generated stress for the women with FSAD, given that it conflicted with their beliefs about their genital arousal difficulties. Other researchers have shown that stress, both acute and chronic, significantly interferes with genital sexual arousal among sexually healthy women (ter Kuile et al. 2007), but this has not been empirically studied among women with FSAD.

Anticipation of pain significantly influences genital arousal in women and has implications for treating arousal difficulties among women with dyspareunia. Brauer et al. (2007) compared the vaginal pulse amplitude of women with superficial dyspareunia and sexually functional women while viewing two erotic film clips. During one of the two erotic films, women were told that they would likely receive a painful stimulus, although no pain stimulus was actually administered because the researchers were primarily interested in the threat of pain (and not of pain itself). All women participated in both conditions, the order of which was counterbalanced. Women with and without dyspareunia in the pain threat condition had lower vaginal pulse amplitude than those in the no threat condition, indicating that threat of pain had a dampening effect on genital sexual arousal, regardless of the woman's diagnosis. Thus, the anticipation of pain may be etiologically linked to reduced arousal in at least some women with sexual arousal difficulties.

Interestingly, although a strong link exists between depression and sexual arousal disorder (Avis et al. 2005; Kennedy et al. 1999; Laumann et al. 2005), the experimental induction of positive mood via the use of music did not significantly improve genital sexual arousal in sexually healthy, nondepressed women (Laan et al. 1995). Further research is needed to determine if this or other experimental paradigms that aim to heighten mood are effective for women with sexual dysfunction.

Sexual abuse is also associated with difficulties in genital arousal. Women with a history of childhood sexual abuse showed impaired genital arousal to sympathetic activation, whereas nonabused women showed the expected enhancement of vaginal pulse amplitude (Rellini and Meston 2006). One possible explanation is that abused women may have a chronically altered hypothalamic-pituitary-adrenal axis. Moreover, women with past sexual abuse reported negative affect during physiological arousal (L.A. Berman et al. 2001). Sexual genital congestion may produce sensations reminiscent of those experienced during the sexual abuse itself (Rellini 2008).

Cultural factors are also linked with genital arousal symptoms. Young women of East Asian descent have more frequent difficulties with genital arousal (Brotto et al. 2005). Among perimenopausal women, African American and Hispanic women had the lowest levels of sexual arousal (unspecified), followed by Chinese and Japanese women, followed by Caucasian women; Hispanic women also had the lowest amount of physical sexual pleasure (Avis et al. 2005).

Effects of Age Versus Effects of Menopause on Genital Arousal

Age and menopausal effects on genital arousal are difficult to tease apart, and both have been associated with changes in lubrication and genital arousal (Avis et al. 2005; Laumann et al. 1999). In the Melbourne Women's Midlife Health Project, women transitioning through menopause were compared with an age-matched premenopausal group and an age-matched postmenopausal group (Guthrie et al. 2004). Sexual responsivity was affected by aging as well as menopause, independently. However, although estradiol levels were associated with dyspareunia and arousal, estrogen's effects were less pronounced than effects of prior sexual function and partner status. The investigators suggested that psychosocial factors related to attitudes and partner status may, in fact, be more predictive of sexual response than any other biological or hormonal factor (Dennerstein and Hayes 2005).

Persistent Genital Arousal Disorder

Although PGAD is not currently adopted by the DSM-IV-TR classification system, research is currently under way to determine if PGAD might be a disorder for inclusion in DSM-V. A persistent sexual arousal syndrome was first described by Leiblum and Nathan (2001) as a condition in which unsolicited and unrelenting sexual arousal persisted for hours or days. Moreover, the symptoms did not remit spontaneously and did so only occasionally after orgasm. No obvious triggers for the arousal (e.g., viewing an erotic stimulus) were usually apparent, and the persistent genital arousal was not associated with sexual desire. Finally, the persistent arousal was viewed as unwanted, intrusive, and embarrassing. This entity is very different from hypersexuality, which features markedly heightened sexual desire. Since the first description of the syndrome in 2001, Leiblum has conducted a small number of investigations to better define the characteristics, correlates, and treatment of this persistent arousal. Leiblum renamed the condition "persistent genital arousal disorder" to reflect the finding that the genital arousal sensations were qualitatively different from those occurring during genuine sexual arousal (Leiblum 2006) and to legitimize the need for this condition to be classified as a sexual dysfunction.

No consensus exists on the etiology of PGAD. It is thought to have neurological, vascular, pharmacological, and psychological correlates. In an online Internet survey of women with PGAD, Leiblum et al. (2005) identified 6 of 364 women who linked their PGAD onset to antidepressant discontinuation. In a follow-up publication, Leiblum and Goldmeier (2008) presented the personal accounts of five women with PGAD induced by discontinuation of selective serotonin reuptake inhibitors (SSRIs). This "connection," however, might simply reflect the widespread use of SSRIs; any mechanism by which such antidepressant withdrawal could lead to the onset of PGAD is unknown. Other triggers for PGAD identified by women in the online survey were cesarean section surgery, pressure on the genitals (e.g., as in bicycle riding), increases and decreases in hormonal therapies, past sexual abuse, excessive masturbation as a child, and neurological damage. Whether these identified triggers are indeed associated with PGAD onset, as opposed to being coincidental events, is at present unknown.

Leiblum and Chivers (2007) have postulated a psychological model whereby spontaneous genital arousal is interpreted catastrophically (or at least negatively), which functions to heighten sympathetic nervous system activity and further enhance the genital arousal. In support of this theory was the finding that 88% of women who met criteria for PGAD in the online study also monitored their genital arousal (Leiblum et al. 2005). Subjective distress may well be the necessary ingredient allowing symptoms from exaggerated genital congestion to intensify such that women are diagnosed with PGAD. Nondistressed women may normalize their easy and excessive genital arousal.

Assessment of Reduced or Persistent Genital Arousal

Assessment of reduced or persistent genital arousal follows a biopsychosocial framework in which the predisposing, precipitating, and perpetuating factors implicated in etiology are explored with the woman and her partner (if possible). Assessment is intertwined with treatment such that emerging information continues to inform the progression of treatment for both FSAD and PGAD. As described in more detail in Chapter 5, "Disorders of Sexual Desire and Subjective Arousal in Women," the sexual response cycle described by Basson (see Figure 7–1) is a helpful guide for clarifying whether the difficulty relates to subjective versus genital arousal, and whether sexual desire and interest are present or absent.

The clinician can ask the patient how much genital swelling/lubrication response occurs. However, the clinician must remember that women's awareness of genital congestion is highly variable, such that a woman's perceived reduction in genital arousal is not necessarily detected if measured by conventional research tools, such as the vaginal photoplethysmograph (van Lunsen and Laan 2004). It is important for the clinician to ask the woman if she experiences subjective arousal to nongenital stimuli (physical, written, visual, fantasy, etc.). Confirmation of such subjective arousal but lack of arousing sexual sensations from genital stimulation indicates the diagnosis of genital arousal disorder. The degree of distress should be ascertained, as well as the woman's motivation for seeking treatment at the present time. Clarifying the duration (lifelong or acquired) and onset (gradual or sudden) of the complaint may suggest a particular etiology. The clinician should also clarify whether the problematic arousal is generalized (i.e., takes place in all situations) or situational (e.g., is associated with partnered sex but not with self-stimulation; takes place only with a certain partner, certain location, or during certain activities).

In addition to obtaining information from the couple, we recommend an individual assessment of each partner to explore developmental history, psychosexual history (including history of sexual or physical abuse), psychiatric history and present issues, masturbation, arousal in situations that do not involve the partner, and feelings about the partner and commitment to the relationship.

Practice Point

In assessing a woman for FSAD or PGAD, the clinician should do the following:

- Clarify subjective versus genital arousal difficulties.
- Determine the patient's degree of distress and motivation for seeking treatment at present.
- Clarify the presence or absence of sexual desire/interest.
- Use the Basson sexual response cycle (Figure 7–1) as a guide for assessment, clarifying where the woman experiences "breaks" in her response cycle.

- Determine response to various erotic and nonerotic stimuli.
- Determine whether duration is lifelong or acquired, and whether onset is generalized or situational.

The use of objective and physiological assessment tools in the evaluation of women's genital arousal may also be helpful to complement the biopsychosocial interview. Prior to assessing the woman, the clinician may ask her to complete a self-report questionnaire, such as the 19-item Female Sexual Function Index (FSFI; Rosen et al. 2000), which distinguishes subjective arousal from lubrication, or the 22-item Brief Index of Sexual Functioning for Women (BISF-W; Taylor et al. 1994), which includes an assessment of sexual pleasure. The Sexual Satisfaction Scale for Women (Meston and Trapnell 2005) is a 30-item measure of sexual satisfaction found to differentiate women with and without sexual arousal disorder. Although a self-report measure should not be used alone for making a diagnosis of any sexual dysfunction, when used as a preassessment screen, such a measure can inform the in-person interview.

Measures of genital arousal have been used almost exclusively in the research setting. Vaginal photoplethysmography (Sintchak and Geer 1975), pelvic magnetic resonance imaging (Maravilla and Yang 2008), a labial thermistor clip (Payne and Binik 2006), and thermal imaging (Kukkonen et al. 2007) are all commonly used research techniques for the assessment of genital arousal in women with sexual dysfunction. In the research setting, plethysmography (Meston and Worcel 2002) and magnetic resonance imaging (Yang et al. 2008) have been found to be sensitive to effects of pharmaceutical agents in instances where patients reported no effects on genital arousal. Color Doppler ultrasonography was found not to be a specific measure of sexual arousal because it was found to be influenced by other emotions (Kukkonen et al. 2006).

A careful genital examination is needed to assess loss of genital response. Conditions that can impair sensitivity, such as lichen sclerosis, can be excluded. Estrogen lack can be identified from pallor, loss of elasticity, and moisture. A marked loss of pubic hair and shrinkage of the clitoris suggest reduced androgen production.

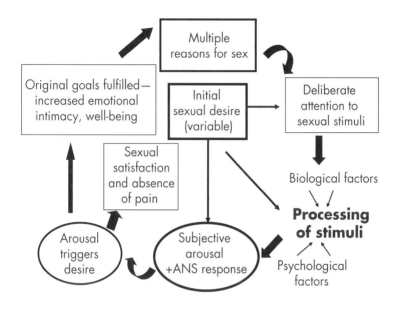

Figure 7–1.   Sexual response cycle.

Note.   ANS=autonomic nervous system.

Source.   Reprinted from Basson R: "Female Sex Response: The Role of Drugs in the Management of Sexual Dysfunction." *American College of Obstetrics and Gynecology* 98:350–352, 2001. Used with permission of Lippincott Williams & Wilkins.

Treatments for Female Sexual Arousal Disorder

Treatments for FSAD can be divided into psychological, hormonal, nonhormonal pharmaceutical, and physical aids. A first strategy in treatment is to address any current lifestyle, medical, and medication-related reasons for the lack of genital arousal. Sufficient levels of physical exercise, sleep, nutrition, and hydration, as well as the absence of smoking and excessive alcohol use, are important. The clinician should assess the patient's full array of currently used prescription and nonprescription medications that might be contributing to the impaired genital arousal, and consider dosage changes or medication substitutions. Over-the-counter lubricants, such as Astroglide, are a reasonable first-line treatment, particularly if loss of lubrication is the patient's primary complaint. Nonhormonal vaginal moisturizers, such as Replens, might also be administered.

Psychological Treatments

As described in Chapter 5, "Disorders of Sexual Desire and Subjective Arousal in Women," all female patients can benefit from psychoeducation, which combines education and didactic information with elements of psychological therapy (e.g., cognitive and/or behavioral interventions). One component of psychoeducation may be identifying specific myths that the woman has about sexual arousal (e.g., "my lubrication must be prompt and sufficient") and attempting to replace such beliefs with more accurate information. Psychoeducation also involves providing women with prevalence figures on arousal disorders and known information about their correlates.

Heiman (2002) summarized the psychological efficacy literature for female sexual dysfunction and concluded that no psychological treatment studies had been published in which FSAD was the primary complaint. Instead, treatment outcome studies have focused on women who had genital arousal complaints but who reported loss of sexual desire, anorgasmia, or dyspareunia as the presenting complaint.

Recently, a mindfulness-based cognitive-behavioral treatment was found to significantly improve several domains of sexual response and mood among women with FSAD related to gynecological cancer treatment (Brotto et al. 2008b) and among women with mixed desire and arousal complaints (Brotto et al. 2008a). Mindfulness training encourages women to practice deliberate attentiveness in nonsexual areas of their lives and is a very useful way of helping women to challenge their tendency to become distracted while attempting to be sexual. Once women have some practice being "present" in such nonsexual areas, they can be encouraged to practice awareness with their own bodies during prescribed body scan exercises, and eventually when being sexual both alone and with a partner. We have found that deliberate attention to the body can intensify the actual physiological genital arousal response, as well as the perception of genital arousal (Brotto et al. 2008a; Brotto et al. 2008b). Qualitative feedback from sex therapy participants suggested that the mindfulness components specifically were most useful to them (Brotto and

Heiman 2007). However, because these studies lacked a control group, the extent to which improvements were attributable to mindfulness, to other components of the treatment, or to nonspecific treatment effects, remains to be tested in the future.

A central goal of cognitive-behavioral therapy in treating FSAD is encouraging the woman to seek out her own "evidence for" and "evidence against" irrational thoughts about sexual arousal, and guiding her to replace these with more balanced and accurate beliefs. On the basis of the finding that genital sexual arousal is improved by cognitive schema induction, as well as situational variation in self-focused attention such that attention is redirected toward sexually exciting aspects of a situation (e.g., van Lankveld and Bergh 2008), psychological techniques targeting cognitive schema and self-focused attention might have promise for improving FSAD. The behavioral component of cognitive-behavioral therapy may involve the prescription of specific "homework" exercises, designed to heighten the patient's genital arousal. Erotica and vibrators may be combined with imagery work and fantasy training to boost both genital and subjective sexual arousal responses; this intervention has been found effective in women with FSAD secondary to gynecological cancer (Brotto et al. 2008b).

In the domain of sex therapy, sensate focus exercises are featured. Although these exercises are commonly used in the treatment of FSAD, their efficacy specifically for women with FSAD has never been explored (Heiman 2002). Sensate focus involves at least three discrete stages of touching between a couple, with progressively increasing touching directed to the genitals and breasts. For the woman with impaired genital arousal, deliberate attention to her existing arousal while minimizing anxiety and nonsexual distractions is a primary treatment goal.

Hormonal Treatments

When estrogen deficiency is implicated in etiology, the patient is given estrogen, either systemically or locally (i.e., topically), with a preference given to local treatment (Long et al. 2006). If estrogen administration alone is insufficient, investigational topical testosterone (2%; 0.5 mL two times per week around the clitoris) is sometimes added. In a small study of postmenopausal women, dehydroepiandrosterone was found to significantly improve physical sexual excitement, but only in women older than age 70 (Baulieu et al. 2000). In a randomized double-blind study of tibolone, a synthetic steroid with estrogenic, androgenic, and progestogenic effects, genital arousal of postmenopausal women significantly increased during fantasy (but not during erotic film exposure) (Laan et al. 2001). However, tibolone was determined to be not approvable by the U.S. Food and Drug Administration (FDA) in 2006.

As noted in Chapter 5, "Disorders of Sexual Desire and Subjective Arousal in Women," recent trials of systemic testosterone have not targeted women with impaired genital response. If an investigational trial of androgens is considered, the clinician must provide patient counseling about the potential benefits versus potential hazards of its use.

Nonhormonal Pharmaceutical Treatments

Various nonhormonal pharmaceutical treatments have been assessed in women with FSAD; however, none have been approved by the FDA, and all remain investigational in North America at the time of this writing (June 2008). Given the important role for nitric oxide in mediating clitoral smooth muscle relaxation, the phosphodiesterase type 5 (PDE5) inhibitors, such as sildenafil citrate, have been speculated to improve women's genital arousal. When an estrogen-replete woman has autonomic nerve damage related to, for example, radical hysterectomy or multiple sclerosis, the use of a PDE5 inhibitor might be suitable (Dasgupta et al. 2004; Rees et al. 2007). The PDE5 inhibitor sildenafil citrate (Viagra) has been found to be useful for women with FSAD due to diabetes (Caruso et al. 2006) and in women with spinal cord injury (Sipski et al. 2000). The use of a PDE5 inhibitor in women with FSAD unrelated to autonomic nerve damage remains unclear: although sildenafil has been found to be effective in studies of premenopausal (Caruso et al. 2001) and postmenopausal (Berman et al. 2003) women with FSAD who did not have hypoactive sexual desire disorder, PDE5 inhibitors may be effective only for women with a measurable reduction in genital arousal (Basson and Brotto 2003). Moreover, a case report on tadalafil (Ashton and Weinstein 2006) and a recent randomized trial of sildenafil in women with SSRI-associated anorgasmia showed reversal of sexual dysfunction with a PDE5 inhibitor (Nurnberg et al. 2008). However, Pfizer, the maker of sildenafil, has ceased funding trials of sildenafil in women due to lack of sufficient efficacy.

The dopaminergic and noradrenergic antidepressant bupropion has been found to significantly increase sexual arousability and sexual response among nondepressed premenopausal women with sexual desire disorder (Segraves et al. 2004). It has not yet been tested among women with a primary complaint of loss of genital arousal, however. Other investigational agents found to significantly improve genital arousal in women are the combination of L-arginine (nitric oxide precursor) and yohimbine (alpha-2 blocker) (Meston and Worcel 2002), oral phentolamine (Rubio-Aurioles et al. 2002), and the dopaminergic agent apomorphine (Caruso et al. 2004). The dietary supplement ArginMax, a proprietary combination of ginkgo biloba, ginseng, damiana, L-arginine, vitamins, and minerals, was found to significantly improve vaginal dryness in perimenopausal women (Ito et al. 2006). Zestra, a botanical massage oil, was found to significantly increase genital sexual arousal, pleasure from sexual arousal, and genital sensations among women with FSAD in one placebo-controlled trial (Ferguson et al. 2003). Multicenter studies on the effects of Zestra are currently under way.

Physical Aids

In addition to a possible pharmacological treatment for FSAD, therapy directed at increasing the intensity of the stimulus with the use of a physical aid can be very helpful. The EROS Clitoral Therapy Device is an FDA-approved handheld device with a suction cup that is placed over the clitoris, and then a mild vacuum increases blood flow to the clitoris. In a study that did not include a control group, use of the device for 3 months was found to significantly improve sexual arousal and other aspects of sexual response among cervical cancer patients with FSAD associated with radiotherapy and stenosis of the vagina (Schroder et al. 2005). As part of a larger treatment program, the use of vibrators, erotica, and fantasy in women with arousal disorder associated with gynecological cancer treatment was found to enhance self-reported sexual arousal and genital sensations, and showed a trend toward improving physiological sexual arousal (Brotto et al. 2008b). Although these aids are commonly prescribed in the sex therapy setting and presumed to be effective at enhancing genital arousal, no controlled trials proving their efficacy have been published.

Practice Point

For a patient with arousal disorder—that is, one who feels "genital deadness" but can be aroused by nongenital stimuli—the clinician should do the following:

- Assess estrogen status, and prescribe local (or systemic) estrogen as appropriate.
- Encourage more intense means of stimulation, both physical and mental.
- Encourage means to attend to sexual stimuli, including mindfulness techniques and sensate focus exercises.

Treatment for Persistent Genital Arousal Disorder

To date, no studies have been published on treatment efficacy for PGAD, and the available information on treatments is taken from published case reports or clinical suggestions. Leiblum has argued that a first-line treatment approach should emphasize self-management, anesthetics to numb the genital area, and pelvic floor muscle control. Following from the psychological theory of PGAD, given that these women show increased monitoring of and attention to genital and nongenital physical sensations, treatments aimed at reducing such self-focused attention, challenging interpretations of genital arousal, and reducing overall anxiety may be useful (Leiblum and Chivers 2007). Although no controlled trials have been reported, Leiblum (2007) provided case reports of women who experienced relief from PGAD with various psychotropic medications, including valproic acid, gabapentin, and escitalopram.

Case Example

Mary, a 60-year-old nurse, has been married to Thomas, a 61-year-old business entrepreneur, for the past 38 years. Her presenting complaint was loss of genital sexual sensations from sexual touching or from other sexual stimuli for the past 10 years, since her non-nerve-sparing radical hysterectomy without oophorectomy for cervical cancer. Prior to her cancer treatment, she experienced high levels of physical and subjective sexual arousal when sexually active, and she regularly reached orgasm. Since her surgery, genital arousal (swelling, sexual sensations of throbbing, tingling) and orgasm no longer occurred; however, she maintained subjective sexual arousal when she deliberately fantasized. Systemic estrogen therapy, which had been prescribed since menopause at age 41, was continued throughout her treatment for cancer, apart from a 3-month cessation when she received radiotherapy.

Mary reported some relevant issues during the developmental and psychosexual history taking. She grew up with "Victorian" parents who, by her description, did not acknowledge sexuality. Despite this, Mary was very sexually active throughout her teenage years and into her early 20s. She met Thomas when she was 21 in the Swiss Alps where he was a ski instructor. She was immediately attracted to his physical attributes and to his seeming assertiveness. They dated for a few months and married soon after. Their sexual encounters were frequent for the first 5 years of their marriage, which Mary recalls as "passionate." Being certain she did not want children, Mary persevered with birth control measures. Complications from oral contraceptives were followed by pelvic inflammatory disease from an intrauterine device, and Mary believed she was infertile. Thus, her subsequent pregnancy was truly distressing. Her now 36-year-old son inherited deafness from Thomas's side of the family. Caring for their son became the focus for both partners. Not until his later teens did the parents find out that their son was one of a group of deaf children who were repeatedly sexually abused in their school environment. When being sexual with Thomas, Mary often worried that her son, who lived with them, might walk in. With the stress of caring for their deaf child, Mary developed major depressive disorder in her 30s and was treated with amitriptyline successfully; she still takes the medication. Her depression worsened as she learned about the sexual abuse of her son and culminated in a suicide attempt at age 35.

Contrary to the experience of many women with gynecological cancer, Mary experienced a renewed wish to live after receiving her diagnosis of cervical cancer. However, due to the significant side effect of diarrhea for 4 years from her chemotherapy, her sexual self-image deteriorated and she began to avoid sexual activity, which had become unrewarding. Thomas developed prostate cancer a few years later, and his subsequent unreliable erections decreased his desirability in her eyes. Because of his erectile dysfunction, they ceased all nonintercourse sexual activities that Mary had previously found highly arousing, and attempts at intercourse became the main focus of their sexual encounters. In the background, their shared family business was failing and Mary had to step in to save it. As a result, she perceived Thomas more and more as a passive man, which further decreased her desire for him.

Mary's diagnosis was female sexual arousal disorder: using the newer terminology, her diagnosis would be genital sexual arousal disorder (note the preserved subjective arousal from fantasy).

Treatment involved identifying maladaptive beliefs, such as "A man must take charge sexually in order for me to have a sexual arousal response," and replacing them with more balanced thoughts. To challenge Mary's belief that her genital arousal response was completely absent following hysterectomy, she was encouraged to participate in mindfulness exercises during which she became aware of sensations in her body while breathing, while visually inspecting her body, and later while attempting sexual activity with Thomas. Mary was initially quite resistant to treatment suggestions, and she felt that her conservative sexual upbringing prevented her from fully participating in treatment. However, a follow-up email from the therapist 2 weeks after her first session provided the impetus (and permission) to engage in the various exercises suggested. She began to use a vibrator and erotic stimuli to boost her existing genital arousal response, and then to deliberately focus on and notice these sensations with her mind. After normalizing her lack of spontaneous desire, Mary found herself considering sexual activity despite not feeling sexually excited in the moment. On a few occasions, this led to her anticipating sexual activity with Thomas, making a deliberate effort to notice her body's sensations when they began sexual activity, and the net result was the perception of a strong genital arousal response, which culminated in an orgasm during direct clitoral manual stimulation from Thomas (Mary had not had an orgasm for several years). With mutual enthusiasm, the couple went on to learn how to use intracavernosal injection of prostaglandin E1 to manage the erectile dysfunction, and both partners experienced continued sexual improvement. Upon follow-up 6 months later, Mary reported a significant increase in her perceived genital arousal. She continued to practice mindfulness, both in general life and when being sexual. She no longer believed she was deficient in sexual arousal; instead, she learned that the capacity for this response was very much under her control.

Key Points

- Symptoms of impaired genital arousal may or may not be associated with measurable deficit.

- Therapy aims to increase the woman's awareness of and pleasure from the congestion that is occurring by 1) increasing the stimulus intensity (sex therapy, vibrators, EROS Clitoral Therapy Device) and 2) increasing her ability to attend (sensate focus therapy, mindfulness techniques).

- When estrogen deficiency is involved, local supplementation is usually effective in restoring lubrication, swelling, elasticity, and sensitivity.

- When autonomic nerve damage is present (i.e., when actual deficit in congestion is likely), vasoactive drugs including PDE5 inhibitors are sometimes used on an investigational basis.

- PGAD is poorly understood, but the associated distress can be immense. Clinician awareness of the syndrome is important to allow at least supportive therapy.

References

Addis IB, Van den Eeden SK, Wassel-Fyr CL, et al: Sexual activity and function in middle-aged and older women. Obstet Gynecol 107:755–764, 2006

American Psychiatric Association: Diagnostic and Statistical Manual of Mental Disorders, 3rd Edition. Washington, DC, American Psychiatric Association, 1980

American Psychiatric Association: Diagnostic and Statistical Manual of Mental Disorders, 4th Edition, Text Revision. Washington, DC, American Psychiatric Association, 2000

Ashton AK, Weinstein W: Tadalafil reversal of sexual dysfunction caused by serotonin enhancing medications in women. J Sex Marital Ther 32:1–3, 2006

Avis NE, Zhao X, Johannes CB, et al: Correlates of sexual function among multi-ethnic middle-aged women: results from the Study of Women's Health Across the Nation (SWAN). Menopause 12:385–398, 2005

Bachmann GA, Ebert GA, Burd ID: Vulvovaginal complaints, in Treatment of the Postmenopausal Woman: Basic and Clinical Aspects, 2nd Edition. Edited by Lobo RA. Baltimore, MD, Lippincott Williams & Wilkins, 1999, pp 195–201

Bancroft J, Loftus J, Long JS: Distress about sex: a national survey of women in heterosexual relationships. Arch Sex Behav 32:193–208, 2003

Barlow DH: Causes of sexual dysfunction: the role of anxiety and cognitive interference. J Consult Clin Psychology 54:140–148, 1986

Basson R, Brotto LA: Sexual psychophysiology and effects of sildenafil citrate in oestrogenised women with acquired genital arousal disorder and impaired orgasm: a randomized controlled trial. Br J Obstet Gynaecol 110:1014–1024, 2003

Basson R, Leiblum S, Brotto L, et al: Definitions of women's sexual dysfunction reconsidered: advocating expansion and revision. J Psychosom Obstet Gynaecol 24:221–229, 2003

Baulieu EE, Thomas G, Legrain S, et al: Dehydroepiandrosterone (DHEA), DHEA sulfate, and aging: contribution of the DHEAge Study to a sociobiomedical issue. Proc Natl Acad Sci U S A 97:4279–4284, 2000

Berard EJJ: The sexuality of spinal cord injured women: physiology and pathophysiology—a review. Paraplegia 27:99–112, 1989

Berman JR, Berman LA, Toler SM, et al: Safety and efficacy of sildenafil citrate for the treatment of female sexual arousal disorder: a double-blind, placebo controlled study. J Urol 70:2333–2338, 2003

Berman LA, Berman JR, Bruck D, et al: Pharmacotherapy or psychotherapy? Effective treatment for FSD related to unresolved childhood sexual abuse. J Sex Marital Ther 27:421–425, 2001

Brauer M, ter Kuile MM, Janssen SA, et al: The effect of pain-related fear on sexual arousal in women with superficial dyspareunia. Eur J Pain 11:788–798, 2007

Brotto LA, Heiman JR: Mindfulness in sex therapy: applications for women with sexual difficulties following gynaecologic cancer. Sexual and Relationship Therapy 22:3–11, 2007

Brotto LA, Chik HM, Ryder AG, et al: Acculturation and sexual function in Asian women. Arch Sex Behav 34:613–626, 2005

Brotto LA, Basson R, Luria M: A mindfulness-based group psychoeducational intervention targeting sexual arousal disorder in women. J Sex Med 5:1646–1659, 2008a

Brotto LA, Heiman JR, Goff B, et al: A psychoeducational intervention for sexual dysfunction in women with gynecologic cancer. Arch Sex Behav 37:317–329, 2008b

Cain VS, Johannes CB, Avis NE, et al: Sexual functioning and practices in a multiethnic study of midlife women: baseline results from SWAN. J Sex Res 40:266–276, 2003

Caruso S, Intelisano G, Lupo L, et al: Premenopausal women affected by sexual arousal disorder treated with sildenafil: a double-blind, cross-over, placebo-controlled study. Br J Obstet Gynaecol 108:623–628, 2001

Caruso S, Agnello C, Intelisano G, et al: Placebo-controlled study on efficacy and safety of daily apomorphine SL intake in premenopausal women affected by hypoactive sexual desire disorder and sexual arousal disorder. Urology 63:955–959, 2004

Caruso S, Rugolo S, Agnello C, et al: Sildenafil improves sexual functioning in premenopausal women with Type I diabetes who are affected by sexual arousal disorder: double-blind, crossover, placebo-controlled pilot study. Fertil Steril 85:1496–1501, 2006

Dasgupta R, Wiseman OJ, Kanabar G, et al: Efficacy of sildenafil in the treatment of female sexual dysfunction due to multiple sclerosis. J Urol 171:1189–1193, 2004

Dennerstein L, Hayes RD: Confronting the challenges: epidemiological study of female sexual dysfunction and the menopause. J Sex Med 2 (suppl 3):118–132, 2005

Dennerstein L, Koochaki P, Barton I, et al: Hypoactive sexual desire disorder in menopausal women: a survey of Western European women. J Sex Med 3:212–222, 2006

Dunn KM, Croft PR, Hackett GI: Association of sexual problems with social, psychological, and physical problems in men and women: a cross-sectional population survey. J Epidemiol Community Health 53:144–148, 1999

Elliott AN, O'Donahue WT: The effects of anxiety and distraction on sexual arousal in a nonclinical sample of heterosexual women. Arch Sex Behav 26:607–624, 1997

Enzlin P, Mathieu C, Vanderschueren D, et al: Diabetes mellitus and female sexuality: a review of 25 years' research. Diabet Med 15:807–808, 1998

Ferguson DM, Steidle CP, Singh GS, et al: Randomized, placebo-controlled, double blind, crossover design trial of the efficacy and safety of Zestra for Women in women with and without female sexual arousal disorder. J Sex Marital Ther 29 (suppl 1):33–44, 2003

Fugl-Meyer AR, Fugl-Meyer SS: Sexual disabilities, problems and satisfaction in 18–74 year old Swedes. Scandinavian Journal of Sexology 2:79–105, 1999

Guthrie JR, Dennerstein L, Taffe JR, et al: The menopausal transition: a 9-year prospective population-based study. The Melbourne Women's Midlife Health Project. Climacteric 7:375–389, 2004

Heiman JR: Psychologic treatments for female sexual dysfunction: are they effective and do we need them? Arch Sex Behav 31:445–450, 2002

Ito TY, Polan ML, Whipple B, et al: The enhancement of female sexual function with ArginMax, a nutritional supplement, among women differing in menopausal status. J Sex Marital Ther 32:369–378, 2006

Kadioglu P, Yalin A.S, Tiryakioglu O, et al: Sexual dysfunction in women with hyperprolactinemia: a pilot study report. J Urology 174:1921–1925, 2005

Kaplan HS: Disorders of Sexual Desire. New York, Brunner/Mazel, 1979

Kennedy SH, Dickens SE, Eisfeld BS, et al: Sexual dysfunction before antidepressant therapy in major depression. J Affect Disord 56:201–208, 1999

Kuffel SW, Heiman JR: Effects of depressive symptoms and experimentally adopted schemas on sexual arousal and affect in sexually healthy women. Arch Sex Behav 35:163–177, 2006

Kukkonen TM, Paterson L, Binik YM, et al: Convergent and discriminant validity of clitoral color Doppler ultrasonography as a measure of female sexual arousal. J Sex Marital Ther 32:281–287, 2006

Kukkonen TM, Binik YM, Amsel R, et al: Thermography as a physiological measure of sexual arousal in both men and women. J Sex Med 4:93–105, 2007

Laan E, Everaerd W, van Berlo R, et al: Mood and sexual arousal in women. Behav Res Ther 33:441–443, 1995

Laan E, van Lunsen RH, Everaerd W: The effects of tibolone on vaginal blood flow, sexual desire and arousability in postmenopausal women. Climacteric 4:28–41, 2001

Laumann EO, Paik A, Rosen RC: Sexual dysfunction in the United States: prevalence and predictors. JAMA 281:537–544, 1999

Laumann EO, Nicolosi A, Glasser DB, et al: Sexual problems among women and men aged 40–80: prevalence and correlates identified in the Global Study of Sexual Attitudes and Behaviors. Int J Impot Res 17:39–57, 2005

Leiblum SR: Persistent genital arousal disorder: what it is and what it isn't. Contemporary Sexuality 40:8–13, 2006

Leiblum SR: Persistent genital arousal disorder: perplexing, distressing, and underrecognized, in Principles and Practice of Sex Therapy, 4th Edition. Edited by Leiblum SR. New York, Guilford, 2007

Leiblum SR, Chivers M: Normal and persistent genital arousal in women: new perspectives. J Sex Marital Ther 33:357–373, 2007

Leiblum SR, Goldmeier D: Persistent genital arousal disorder in women: case reports of association with anti-depressant usage and withdrawal. J Sex Marital Ther 34:150–159, 2008

Leiblum SR, Nathan SG: Persistent sexual arousal syndrome: a newly discovered pattern of female sexuality. J Sex Marital Ther 27:365–380, 2001

Leiblum SR, Brown C, Wan J, et al: Persistent sexual arousal syndrome: a descriptive study. J Sex Med 2:331–337, 2005

Long CY, Liu CM, Hsu SC, et al: A randomized comparative study of the effects of oral and topical estrogen therapy on the vaginal vascularization and sexual function in hysterectomized postmenopausal women. Menopause 13:737–743, 2006

Lutfey KE, Link CL, Rosen RC, et al: Prevalence and correlates of sexual activity and function in women: results from the Boston Area Community Health (BACH) survey. Arch Sex Behav (in press)

Maas CP, ter Kuile MM, Laan E, et al: Objective assessment of sexual arousal in women with a history of hysterectomy. Br J Obstet Gynaecol 111:456–462, 2004

Maravilla KR, Yang CC: Magnetic resonance imaging and the female sexual response: overview of techniques, results, and future directions. J Sex Med 5:1559–1571, 2008

Masters WH, Johnson V: Human Sexual Response. Boston, MA, Little, Brown, 1966

McCall KM, Meston CM: The effects of false positive and false negative physiological feedback on sexual arousal: a comparison of women with or without sexual arousal disorder. Arch Sex Behav 36:518–530, 2007

Meston CM: Sympathetic nervous system activity and female sexual arousal. Am J Cardiol 86(2A):30F–34F, 2000

Meston CM, Trapnell P: Development and validation of a five-factor sexual satisfaction and distress scale for women: the Sexual Satisfaction Scale for Women (SSS-W). J Sex Med 2:66–81, 2005

Meston CM, Worcel M: The effects of yohimbine plus L-arginine glutamate on sexual arousal in postmenopausal women with sexual arousal disorder. Arch Sex Behav 31:323–332, 2002

Middleton LS, Kuffel SW, Heiman JR: Effects of experimentally adopted sexual schemas on vaginal response and subjective sexual arousal: a comparison between women with sexual arousal disorder and sexually healthy women. Arch Sex Behav 37:950–961, 2008

Nurnberg HG, Hensley PL, Heiman JR, et al: Sildenafil treatment of women with antidepressant-associated sexual dysfunction. JAMA 300:395–404, 2008

Ottesen B: Vasoactive intestinal polypeptide as a neurotransmitter in the female genital tract. Am J Obstet Gynecol 147:208–224, 1983

Palace EM, Gorzalka BB: The enhancing effects of anxiety on arousal in sexually dysfunctional and functional women. J Abnorm Psychol 99:403–411, 1990

Payne KA, Binik YM: Reviving the labial thermistor clip. Arch Sex Behav 35:111–113, 2006

Pieterse QD, Kenter GG, Eilers PH, et al: Vaginal blood flow after radical hysterectomy with and without nerve sparing: a preliminary report. International Journal of Gynecologic Cancer 18:576–583, 2008

Pryde DC, Maw GN, Planken S, et al: Novel selective inhibitors of neutral endopeptidase for the treatment of female sexual arousal disorder: synthesis and activity of functionalized gutaramides. J Med Chem 49:4409–4424, 2006

Rees P, Fowler CJ, Maas CP: Sexual function in men and women with neurological disorders. Lancet 369:512–525, 2007

Rellini AH: Review of the empirical evidence for a theoretical model to understand the sexual problems of women with a history of CSA. J Sex Med 5:31–46, 2008

Rellini AH, Meston CM: Psychophysiological sexual arousal in women with a history of child sexual abuse. J Sex Marital Ther 32:5–22, 2006

Rosen R, Brown C, Heiman J, et al: The Female Sexual Function Index (FSFI): a multidimensional self-report instrument for the assessment of female sexual function. J Sex Marital Ther 26:191–208, 2000

Rubio-Aurioles E, Lopez M, Lipezker M, et al: Phentolamine mesylate in postmenopausal women with female sexual arousal disorder: a psychophysiological study. J Sex Marital Ther 28 (suppl 1):205–215, 2002

Saenz de Tejada I, Angulo J, Cellek S, et al: Pathophysiology of erectile dysfunction. J Sex Med 2:26–39, 2005

Salemink E, van Lankveld JJDM: The effects of increasing neutral distraction on sexual responding of women with and without sexual problems. Arch Sex Behav 35:179–190, 2006

Schreiner-Engel P, Schiavi RC, Smith H, et al: Sexual arousability and the menstrual cycle. Psychosom Med 43:199–214, 1981

Schroder M, Mell LK, Hurteau JA, et al: Clitoral therapy device for treatment of sexual dysfunction in irradiated cervical cancer patients. Int J Radiat Oncol Biol Phys 61:1078–1086, 2005

Segraves RT, Clayton A, Croft H, et al: Bupropion sustained release for the treatment of hypoactive sexual desire disorder in premenopausal women. J Clin Psychopharmacol 24:339–342, 2004

Sintchak G, Geer JH: A vaginal plethysmograph system. Psychophysiology 12:113–115, 1975

Sipski ML, Rosen R, Alexander CJ, et al: Sildenafil effects on sexual and cardiovascular responses in women with spinal cord injury. Urology 55:812–815, 2000

Taylor JF, Rosen RC, Leiblum SR: Self-report assessment of female sexual function: psychometric evaluation of the Brief Index of Sexual Functioning for Women. Arch Sex Behav 23:627–643, 1994 ter Kuile MM, Vigeveno D, Laan E: Preliminary evidence that acute and chronic daily psychological stress affect sexual arousal in sexually functional women. Behav Res Ther 45:2078–2089, 2007

Traish AM, Kim NN: Modulation of female genital sexual arousal by sex steroid hormones, in Women's Sexual Function and Dysfunction: Study, Diagnosis and Treatment. Edited by Goldstein I, Meston CM, Davis SR, et al. New York, Taylor & Francis, 2006, pp 181–193

van Lankveld J, Bergh S: The interaction of state and trait aspects of self-focused attention affects genital, but not subjective, sexual arousal in sexually functional women. Behav Res Ther 46:514–528, 2008

van Lunsen RHW, Laan E: Genital vascular responsiveness in sexual feelings in midlife women: psychophysiologic, brain and genital imaging studies. Menopause 11:741–748, 2004

Yang CC, Cao YY, Guan QY, et al: Influence of PDE5 inhibitor on MRI measurement of clitoral volume response in women with FSAD: a feasibility study of a potential technique for evaluating drug response. Int J Impot Res 20:105–110, 2008

Recommended Readings

Hanh TN: The Miracle of Mindfulness: A Manual on Meditation. Boston, MA, Beacon Press, 1976

Heiman JR, LoPiccolo J: Becoming Orgasmic: A Sexual and Personal Growth Program for Women. New York, Simon & Schuster, 1988

Kabat-Zinn J: Full Catastrophe Living: Using the Wisdom of Your Body and Mind to Face Stress, Pain, and Illness. New York, Dell, 1990

Kabat-Zinn J: Wherever You Go, There You Are. New York, Hyperion, 1994

8

Male Erectile Disorder

Alan Riley, M.Sc., M.B., B.S., MRCS, FFPM

Elizabeth Riley, B.Sc. (Hons)

For the majority of men, their self-perception of masculinity is intimately focused on their penis and what they can do with it (Riley 2003). Loss of erectile capacity can have a profound negative effect on a man's sense of self and quality of life (Latini et al. 2002, 2007; Litwin et al. 1998). Convincing evidence indicates that restoration of erectile function by appropriate treatment results in enhanced self-esteem, reduced psychological morbidity, and increased emotional well-being, not only for the man but also for his sexual partner (Cappelleri et al. 2006; Fisher et al. 2005b; Paige et al. 2001; Willke et al. 1997). The introduction of "user-friendly," effective, and safe therapies for the restoration of erectile function means that more men can now be treated by clinicians outside of the specialty of urology. In this chapter, we review the management of male erectile disorder.

Definition of Male Erectile Disorder

The term *impotence* is no longer used to describe the inability to have an erection because the term lacked specificity, being used by some authors to include other disturbances of male sexual function. Now the favored terms are *erectile dysfunction* and *male erectile disorder*. *Erectile dysfunction*, defined as the inability to attain and maintain penile erection sufficient for satisfactory sexual performance (National Institutes of Health Consensus Development Panel on Impotence 1993), has become the favored term.

The main diagnostic criterion for male erectile disorder, provided in DSM-IV-TR (American Psychiatric Association 2000), is a "persistent or recurrent inability to attain, or to maintain until completion of the sexual activity, an adequate erection" (p. 547); this definition is not dissimilar to the erectile dysfunction definition of the National Institutes of Health Consensus Development Panel on Impotence (1993). However, additional diagnostic criteria are included in DSM-IV-TR: "The disturbance causes marked distress or interpersonal difficulty," and "the erectile dysfunction is not better accounted for by another Axis I disorder (other than a sexual dysfunction) and is not due exclusively to the direct physiological effects of a substance (e.g., a drug of abuse, a medication) or a general medical condition" (p. 547).

Although DSM-IV-TR elevates male erectile disorder to a diagnosis, in practice it is probably better considered a symptom because it always has an underlying cause or contributing factors, be they psychological, physical, pharmacological, or, more commonly, a combination of such disturbances.

DSM-IV-TR describes subtypes of sexual dysfunctions, including male erectile disorder, to indicate the onset and context of the dysfunction. Consideration of the following subtypes of erectile dysfunction is essential in arriving at the diagnosis.

Onset

Lifelong type: The erectile dysfunction has always been present (i.e., the patient has not experienced normal erectile function). This type is also known as primary erectile dysfunction.

Acquired type: The erectile dysfunction develops after a period, however short, of normal erectile function. This type is also known as secondary erectile dysfunction.

Context

Generalized type: The erectile dysfunction occurs in all types of sexual behavior.

Situational type: The patient experiences erectile dysfunction only in some types of sexual activity (e.g., with a partner but not during masturbation, or with one partner but not another).

Etiological Classification of Erectile Dysfunction

Erectile dysfunction is classified as psychogenic, organic, or mixed psychogenic and organic. At one time, the vast majority of cases of erectile dysfunction were considered to be psychogenic, and few were classified as organic. With the greater understanding of the pathophysiology of penile erection and the development of improved investigatory procedures that occurred in the late 1980s and early 1990s, the etiological classification pendulum swung in favor of underlying organic causes. Erectile dysfunction is now considered to be organic in up to 80% of cases. The major etiological and risk factors for erectile dysfunction are given in Table 8–1.

Generally, the diagnosis of psychogenic erectile dysfunction is made by exclusion, when all other causes have been excluded. The more intensively a patient is investigated, the more organic abnormalities are discovered, but the presence of an organic disease does not confirm a causal relationship with erectile dysfunction. For example, a man who presents with erectile dysfunction and is found to have diabetes mellitus would be classified as having organic erectile dysfunction, but his erectile dysfunction could equally have been caused by any of the psychological factors that operate to induce erectile dysfunction in individuals without diabetes. Hence, even if organic comorbidity is discovered, the patient should still be assessed for other causes of erectile dysfunction.

Factors in the history and description of the erectile dysfunction may help to distinguish organic from psychogenic causes. Usually, erectile dysfunction of organic origin is of gradual onset, is consistent, and is present under all circumstances, including night and awakening erections. In contrast, psychogenic erectile dysfunction may have an abrupt onset and is situational and inconsistent, with varying degrees of erection occurring under different cir-

Table 8–1. Etiological factors and risk factors for erectile dysfunction

Cardiovascular disease
Atherosclerosis
Hypertension
Peripheral vascular disease

Neurological disease
Multiple sclerosis
Post cerebral stroke

Metabolic or endocrine disease
Diabetes mellitus
Hyperlipidemia
Hypogonadism
Hyperprolactinemia
Thyroid disease
Metabolic syndrome

Trauma
Pelvic nerve and vascular injury (e.g., from pelvic fracture, bicycling)
Spinal cord injury

Intrapenile conditions
Peyronie's disease
Cavernosal fibrosis (e.g., after priapism)
Cavernous veno-occlusive dysfunction
Penile fracture

Psychiatric disease
Depression
Acute anxiety (performance anxiety, fear of failure)

Iatrogenic factors
Surgical trauma to pelvic nerves (e.g., prostatectomy)
Pelvic radiotherapy
Pharmacotherapy (see Table 8–2)

Table 8–1.   Etiological factors and risk factors for erectile dysfunction *(continued)*

Other medical conditions
Hepatic failure
Renal failure
Respiratory disorders and sleep apnea
Lower urinary tract symptoms

Lifestyle issues
Aging
Sedentary lifestyle
Poor general health
Obesity
Relationship dysfunction
Lack of privacy for attempts at sexual intercourse (e.g., living in residential home or with relatives).
Smoking, excessive alcohol, and/or illicit drug use

cumstances. The occurrence of normal, rigid nocturnal or awakening erections points to psychogenic erectile dysfunction (Segraves et al. 1987). Psychogenic erectile dysfunction is more common in younger patients (≤40 years).

Prevalence and Incidence of Erectile Dysfunction

Erectile dysfunction is a very common problem and has become a major health care issue. Many studies on the prevalence of erectile dysfunction have been done in recent decades, with widely disparate results. Among 15 large-scale prevalence studies undertaken between 1994 and 2004, the prevalence of erectile dysfunction ranged from 10% to 64% (Porst and Sharlip 2006). The disparity in prevalence rates probably reflects differences in methodology employed and populations studied in the individual studies. The prevalence of erectile dysfunction increases with age. Data from a study of over 27,000 men across eight countries reveal the prevalence of erectile dysfunction to increase with age: 8% in men ages 20–29 years; 11%, ages 30–39 years; 15%, ages 40–49 years; 22%, ages 50–59 years; 30%, ages 60–69 years; and 37%, ages 70–75 years (Rosen et al. 2004). By the year 2025, an estimated 322 million men in the world will have erectile dysfunction (Aytac et al. 1999).

The follow-up of subjects in the Massachusetts Male Aging Study provided data on the incidence of erectile dysfunction, from the time of initial sampling (1987–1989) to 1997 (Johannes et al. 2000). The crude erectile dysfunction incidence rate was 25.9 (95% confidence interval [CI], 22.5–29.9) cases per 1,000 man-years, with the annual incidence rate increasing with each decade of life, from 12.4/1,000 (95% CI, 9.0–16.9) cases in men ages 40–49 years, to 46.4/1,000 (95% CI, 36.9–58.4) cases in men ages 60–69 years.

Erectile Dysfunction and Depression

The prevalence of sexual dysfunction among male psychiatric outpatients has been reported to be 41% (Wylie et al. 2002). Depressive symptoms have been found to be significantly associated with erectile dysfunction, after controlling for age and organic disease (Araujo et al. 1998). Results from a longitudinal study conducted over 5 years in Finland suggest that moderate or severe depression may cause erectile dysfunction, and erectile dysfunction itself may cause or exacerbate depressed mood (Shiri et al. 2007); in other words, a bidirectional relationship exists between depressive symptoms and erectile dysfunction. The association between erectile dysfunction and depression or depressive symptoms is fueled further by 1) the bidirectional relationship between depression and relationship dysfunction, which itself can be associated with erectile dysfunction, and 2) the positive association between antidepressant medication and impaired erectile function (Montgomery et al. 2002; Shores et al. 2004). Treatment of erectile dysfunction is associated with improvement of depressive symptoms (Hatzichristou et al. 2005; Muller and Benkert 2001). Other relevant findings are that depressive symptoms can occur as a consequence of low testosterone levels (Shores et al. 2004), that low testosterone levels can be associated with erectile dysfunction (Hatzichristou et al. 2005; Ojumu and Dobs 2003), and that testosterone treatment in men with low testosterone improves mood and erectile function (Wang et al. 2004).

Presentation for Treatment

A large proportion of men who experience erectile dysfunction do not present for treatment. Of those who do, concern for the sexual satisfaction of their partners is a frequent motivation (Fisher et al. 2005a). Men are unlikely to seek treatment for erectile dysfunction if they and their partners are not bothered by their condition. Many elderly men consider erectile dysfunction to be a natural consequence of aging and hence do not present for treatment. For other men, embarrassment is one of the most frequent reasons for not seeking treatment. In a telephone survey conducted in Canada, only 24% of men who had not consulted a health care professional for their erectile dysfunction responded that they intended to do so in the near future (Auld and Brock 2002). However, 80% of the men who had not sought treatment responded that they would be willing to discuss their problem if a physician initiated the discussion. Therefore, health care professionals need to broach the subject.

Ideally, inquiry about sexual functioning should be a routine part of taking a medical history in all medical specialties. Two easily asked questions are, "How is your intimate life?" and "Are you having difficulty maintaining an erection during intercourse?" (American Urological Association 2005). If erectile dysfunction is discovered, additional questions should be asked to characterize it (see "Sexual History," below). However, some health care professionals have difficulty in broaching the subject, either because of embarrassment, lack of training or lack of knowledge, or a combination of these factors. In such a situation, erectile dysfunction can be identified using a validated questionnaire, such as the Sexual Health Inventory for Men (Cappelleri and Rosen 2005). Should the clinician identify erectile dysfunction (or any other sexual difficulty) and be unable to provide proper assessment and treatment, he or she should promptly refer the patient to a health care professional who is experienced in its management.

Diagnosis and Evaluation of Erectile Dysfunction

The American Urological Association's (2005) guidelines for the management of erectile dysfunction state that the initial evaluation should include medical, sexual, and psychosocial histories, as well as laboratory assays to identify possible comorbidities. The evaluative process should include assessment not only of the man, but also of his partner, their relationship, and the social situation in which their sexual activity occurs or is attempted (see Figure 8–1).

The evaluative process should address three sets of factors involved in the onset and persistence of erectile dysfunction: predisposing, triggering, and maintaining factors (see Figure 8–2). *Predisposing factors* render the patient susceptible to developing erectile dysfunction. These factors can result from disturbances in psychosexual development or the existence of certain organic diseases (see Table 8–1). *Triggering factors* are events or experiences that precipitate the onset of erectile dysfunction in a man whose vulnerability for impairment of erectile function is increased by the presence of a predisposing factor. These factors may be physical, psychological, or sociological in nature. Once erectile dysfunction has been triggered, the development of *maintaining factors* makes it persist.

An example may clarify how these factors interact. Hypertension in a man with atherosclerosis predisposes him to the development of erectile dysfunction. Beginning antihypertensive therapy may actually trigger the onset of erectile dysfunction, either by a direct pharmacological effect or by lowering blood pressure to a level that impairs adequate perfusion pressure in the atherosclerotic vessels supplying the erectile tissue. Once the man has failed to attain or maintain his erection during attempted sexual intercourse, his fear of future sexual failure maintains the erectile dysfunction, which may persist even after the triggering antihypertensive treatment is changed or withdrawn. His fear of failure may lead the man to avoid sexual interaction with his partner, who may react by thinking he is having an affair or no longer finds her sexually arousing, leading her to avoid pursuing any intimate interaction, thereby setting the scene for the development of relationship dysfunction and adding other factors that work to maintain the erectile dysfunction. If the maintaining factors are well established by the time the patient seeks treatment for his erectile dysfunction, the results of any "quick-fix" pharmacotherapeutic approach is likely to be disappointing and may confound further the psychological responses in the patient and his partner to the impaired erectile function.

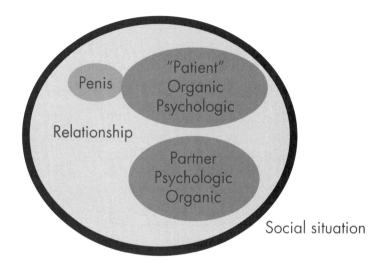

Figure 8–1. Components to be included in the assessment of a patient with male erectile disorder.

Medical History

The first step in the evaluation of erectile dysfunction is to obtain a detailed medical history. The presence of known medical and psychiatric diseases and symptoms suggestive of such diseases should be recorded, because any of these may point to an etiological factor in erectile dysfunction. In particular, cardiovascular disease (especially hypertension, ischemic heart disease, peripheral vascular disease, and cerebrovascular events), diabetes mellitus, hyperlipidemia, neurological disease, endocrine disturbances, and urogenital disorders should be asked about. The clinician should inquire about previous urogenital or spinal surgery and trauma. In addition, inquiry should be made about the presence of psychiatric illness, especially depression. The patient's use of social and illicit drugs (e.g., tobacco, alcohol, marijuana, heroin) should be recorded, because chronic use of such agents increases the risk of erectile dysfunction. The patient should also be asked about bicycle riding, including stationary bicycling, because this has been associated with perineal compression, giving rise to neurological and arterial damage that lead to erectile dysfunction (Huang et al. 2005).

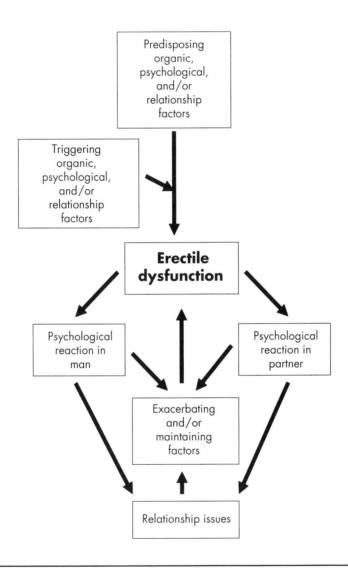

Figure 8–2.   Interaction of predisposing, triggering, and maintaining factors of male erectile disorder.

Many frequently prescribed drugs have the propensity to impair sexual function (see Table 8–2). The clinician should inquire about such drugs and assess any temporal relationship between the commencement of the medication and the onset of erectile dysfunction.

Sexual History

The clinician needs to gain experience in talking to patients about sexual functioning, because the clinician's embarrassment and use of inappropriate terminology can make the patient feel uncomfortable and inhibited, in which case the clinician will have trouble obtaining a full and reliable account of the sexual problem and its impact on his relationship with his partner. Clinicians who are not accustomed to the nonmedical words that many people use in describing sexual function and dysfunction may find Richter's (1987) book *The Language of Sexuality* helpful.

The aim of the sexual history is to establish the precise nature and characteristics of the patient's sexual difficulty, its chronology, its impact on his own and his partner's lives and their relationship, and his (and his partner's) expectations of the course of action and treatment.

The following are the most important questions to ask to detect the occurrence of erectile dysfunction:

- Are you able to attain an erection when you are stimulated sexually?
- Is your erection sufficiently hard to enable you to penetrate your partner?
- Can you maintain your erection until completion of intercourse or masturbation?
- Do you always have these problems, or do you have a normal erection in certain situations?
- Do you have nighttime erections or awake with an erection?

The clinician needs to ascertain the duration of the erectile dysfunction and ask the patient if he can date its onset to any particular event. If the patient can, the likelihood is increased that the cause is psychological. In addition, the patient should be asked about the impact of his erectile dysfunction on his sexual behavior. A common consequence of erectile dysfunction is withdrawal from intimacy and attempts at sexual activity. In one series of couples who presented for treatment of erectile dysfunction, fewer that 10% had

Table 8–2.   Drugs having the propensity to impair erectile function

Psychotropic drugs

Tricyclic antidepressants

Selective serotonin reuptake inhibitors

Major tranquilizers (especially those that increase prolactin secretion)

Antihypertensives and cardiovascular drugs

Thiazide diuretics

β-Adrenergic antagonists

Centrally acting antihypertensives

Calcium channel blockers

Digoxin

Amiodarone

Disopyramide

Spironolactone

Endocrine and metabolic drugs

Antiandrogens

Luteinizing hormone–releasing hormone analogues

Estrogens

Statins

Anabolic steroids

Alimentary system drugs

Metoclopramide

H_2 histamine antagonists, especially cimetidine

Recreational/illicit drugs

Opiates

Marijuana

Cocaine

Alcohol

Nicotine

Other drugs

Ketoconazole

experienced caressing and genital stimulation during the 4 weeks preceding clinic attendance, and the median time since these activities had taken place was nearly 3 years (Riley and Riley 2000). In a large Pan-European observational study of the management of erectile dysfunction, 13.6% of patients had not attempted sexual intercourse in the 4 weeks prior to initial clinic assessment (Riley et al. 2007). Withdrawal from intimacy and sexual activity has implications for the management of erectile dysfunction (see subsection "Sexual Counseling and Sex and Couples Therapy" later in this chapter).

Inquiring about other sexual problems is important because different sexual symptoms often coexist (Riley and Riley 2005). Two symptoms that are often confused with erectile dysfunction are loss of sexual desire and premature ejaculation, both of which can cause or result from erectile dysfunction. For example, a man with erectile dysfunction may lose his sexual desire as a defense against the repeated humiliation of failed attempts at sexual intercourse. The man who has long-standing premature ejaculation may develop erectile dysfunction because of preoccupation with trying to control his ejaculation and lack of sexual satisfaction. Conversely, the man who has difficulty maintaining his erection during intercourse may promote early ejaculation to ensure that he ejaculates before he loses his erection. Such a situation may be wrongly diagnosed as having premature ejaculation.

Another issue that should be raised with the patient concerns sexual stimulation. Some men who are seen on account of erectile dysfunction reveal the absence of effective sexual stimulation; their penises never get touched by their partners (by hand or mouth) during foreplay. Such men fail to respond to phosphodiesterase type 5 (PDE5) inhibitors that require sexual stimulation for their effect. Effective sexual stimulation can be considered as the algebraic sum of positive (sexually stimulating) and negative (sexually inhibiting) stimuli. The presence of activities and thought processes that operate to enhance or inhibit sexual response in the particular patient should be elucidated. As men age, they generally require more genitally focused and longer sexual stimulation than they did when they were younger. Furthermore, elderly men might attain full erection only at the time of ejaculation. Unless older patients recognize these normal consequences of aging, they may assume that they have erectile dysfunction or a milder form of erectile inadequacy.

Another consequence of aging is prolongation of the refractory period (the interval of time following a sexual response before another full erection is possible). For men (and their partners) who are accustomed to frequent sexual intercourse, the natural inability to attain a full erection during the long refractory period can be confused with erectile dysfunction. In this case, the man generally complains of intermittent erectile dysfunction. The clinician should ask the man to keep a diary of successful and unsuccessful sexual intercourse attempts, from which it becomes obvious that his unsuccessful attempts occur generally in the few days following a successful attempt.

History From Partner

The majority of men who seek treatment for erectile dysfunction are in heterosexual relationships. The partner often has a pivotal role in etiology, maintenance, treatment seeking, and prognosis of the erectile dysfunction. Although many female partners of men with erectile dysfunction have their own preexisting sexual difficulties, erectile dysfunction itself can have a negative effect on their sexual functioning (Çayan et al. 2004). A multinational study has shown that following the development of erectile dysfunction, female partners report significant reductions in sexual desire, arousal, orgasm attainment, and frequency of sexual activity (Fisher et al. 2005b).

In view of the high prevalence of sexual dysfunction in female partners of men who present with erectile dysfunction and the possible effect this can have on the outcome of erectile dysfunction treatment, the partner should be assessed. Ideally, the assessment, including clinical examination when appropriate, should be undertaken by face-to-face interview by a clinician with experience in the management of female sexual dysfunction.

Interviewing the partner enables the clinician to discover her thoughts on her partner's seeking and receiving treatment for his erectile dysfunction and the support and involvement in treatment she is willing to provide. Not all women are keen to reestablish sexual intercourse, seeing the occurrence of erectile dysfunction as a legitimate excuse not to do so. Also, many women consider erectile dysfunction to be a male problem and are reluctant to attend the clinic. An international advisory group identified a series of questions that can be used during consultation with the male to provide information on these issues (Dean et al. 2008); these questions are reproduced in Table 8–3.

Table 8–3.   Questions to help assess the patient's level of communication with his partner about his erectile dysfunction, and levels of partner support

Have you spoken with your partner about your erection problem?

Is your partner supportive of you getting treatment to improve your erection?

Does your partner have any concerns about the treatment?

Does your partner want to come and talk to me or to another doctor about improving your sex life together?

Do you know if your partner has any concerns about her own sexual function, or about any other health issues?

Is there anything else I should know to help me understand this problem?

Source.   Reprinted from Dean J, Rubio-Aurioles E, McCabe M, et al: "Integrating Partners Into ED Treatment: Improving the Sexual Experience for the Couple." *International Journal of Clinical Practice* 62:127–133, 2008. Used with permission.

Clinical Examination

All men who present with erectile dysfunction need to undergo a physical examination to identify underlying disease of which the sexual difficulty may be a presenting symptom or which may contribute to the maintenance of the difficulty or influence its treatment. Concomitant symptoms and features in the patient's history may highlight body systems that should be examined thoroughly. However, in the absence of such features, a focused clinical examination should include the genitourinary, endocrine, vascular, and neurological systems (Wespes et al. 2006).

Weight and height should be measured so that the patient's body mass index can be calculated, and the waist circumference should be measured. These measurements aim to identify metabolic syndrome. Blood pressure and heart rate should be recorded.

As a routine, examination of the penis is essential to exclude local abnormalities and other problems, such as Peyronie's disease, that can cause erectile dysfunction. The value of rectal examination is controversial but should be undertaken when urinary symptoms are present. Men with lower urinary tract symptoms have an increased incidence of erectile dysfunction. The testes should be palpated, and the secondary sexual characteristics, including the breasts, should be examined for evidence of hypogonadism.

Investigations

At one time, patients presenting with erectile dysfunction were subjected to extensive and often invasive investigations. Now, however, limited investigations are usually undertaken before first-line treatment is prescribed.

Blood Glucose

All patients should have their fasting blood glucose determined, if not assessed in the previous 12 months, because erectile dysfunction can be the presenting symptom of diabetes mellitus (Sairam et al. 2001). According to the World Health Organization, a fasting blood glucose of 7 mmol/L or more is highly suggestive of diabetes and requires further investigation (Alberti and Zimmet 1998).

Blood Lipids

Erectile dysfunction is a known marker for cardiovascular disease (Billups et al. 2005). For this reason, the guidelines prepared from the Second Princeton Consensus Conference on Sexual Dysfunction and Cardiac Risk emphasize the importance of evaluating and managing cardiovascular risk factors and comorbidities in patients with erectile dysfunction (Kostis et al. 2005). A fasting lipid screen (total cholesterol, low-density lipoprotein cholesterol, and high-density lipoprotein cholesterol) should therefore be undertaken for all men who present with erectile dysfunction. A suspicion of ischemic heart disease in a man presenting with erectile dysfunction should trigger further investigation (e.g., stress electrocardiogram), before commencing treatment for erectile dysfunction.

Endocrine Investigations

Most specialists consider routine screening for hypogonadism to be essential in the assessment of erectile dysfunction, even when the patient does not complain of loss of sexual desire (Buvat and Lemaire 1997). In a study of over 500 unselected men who presented with erectile dysfunction, hypogonadism and hyperprolactinemia were identified in 15.6% and 1.8%, respectively (Govier et al. 1996), but other studies have shown lower prevalence rates (Buvat and Lemaire 1997). Clinicians should always bear in mind the possible presence of hypogonadism, because testosterone deficiency is associated with increased mortality risk (Shores et al. 2006).

Although measurement of morning serum testosterone level is required for diagnosing hypogonadism, the debate is ongoing as to what actually should be measured: total testosterone, calculated free testosterone, or bioavailable testosterone. Bioavailable and free testosterone are more reliable than total testosterone for identifying hypogonadism, but these two tests are more expensive and not readily available in all laboratories. The assay should be undertaken on a morning sample of blood and repeated if out-of-range results are obtained. If the result of the repeat assay is also low, further investigation (e.g., luteinizing hormone, follicle-stimulating hormone, and prolactin) should be undertaken. Some authorities recommend including serum prolactin assay in the initial screen. This may be appropriate in psychiatric practice, because the use of neuroleptics is known to increase prolactin secretion. Further investigation and appropriate treatment are required if abnormal results are obtained.

Some clinicians include thyroid function tests in the investigation of erectile dysfunction even when symptoms of hypothyroidism or hyperthyroidism are not elucidated. Previously undiagnosed thyroid disease has been identified in men presenting with erectile dysfunction (Baskin 1989).

Specialized Procedures

A number of specialized procedures are available for investigating erectile dysfunction. These are rarely required in the initial assessment but may be useful when first-line treatment fails or for medicolegal issues.

Sometimes, establishing whether the patient has erectile potential can be helpful. The most frequently used test is observing whether the patient attains an erection following the intracavernosal injection of a vasoactive drug. This convenient, office-based procedure generally has replaced monitoring nocturnal or audiovisually stimulated penile tumescence in routine clinical practice, although the latter continues to be employed in research.

Intracavernosal injection of vasoactive drugs.   Perhaps the most widely used procedure for establishing erectile potential is the injection of a vasoactive drug, such as alprostadil (prostaglandin E_1 [PGE_1]), or a combination of drugs into the corpus cavernosum using a 27-gauge to 30-gauge needle. The standard dose of PGE_1 is 10 μg, although half this dose should be used if underlying neurological disease (e.g., multiple sclerosis, post pelvic surgery, spinal cord injury) is present, because such conditions may cause a prolonged response to PGE_1. The dose can also be increased to 20–40 μg when underlying severe organic disease (e.g., diabetes mellitus) is present. Induction of a fully rigid erection following intracavernosally injected PGE_1 confirms the integrity of the intrapenile veno-occlusive mechanism but provides no information on the other physiological processes involved in the erectile process (Elhanbly et al. 2002). Some clinicians advocate using audiovisual sexual stimulation with intracavernosal injection of vasoactive drugs as a means of overcoming psychogenic inhibition.

Invasive investigations. A series of more invasive and expensive investigations are available and are indicated when the patient fails to attain an erection in response to intracavernosal injection of a vasoactive drug, or if certain features discovered in the patient's medical history or found on examination call for further investigation. These additional investigations include color Doppler ultrasonography of the penile vasculature (allows measurement of blood flow in individually identifiable penile vessels), dynamic infusion cavernosography and pharmacocavernosometry (used to investigate veno-occlusive function), and bulbocavernous reflex latency times and somatosensory evoked potentials (used to test the integrity of the somatic-penile innervation). In addition, penile angiography is available for those men under age 50 years in whom color Doppler scanning has demonstrated an isolated arterial occlusion that may be correctable by vascular surgery.

Treatment of Erectile Dysfunction

General Considerations

Before instigating any specific treatment for erectile dysfunction, the clinician should consider the following questions. The answers should be available from the history, examination, and investigations.

- *Is the erectile dysfunction a symptom of a treatable underlying medical or psychiatric condition?* If so, this should be addressed before instigating erectile dysfunction treatment. If the erectile dysfunction is a symptom of generalized endothelial dysfunction, the patient is at increased risk of cardiovascular catastrophe.

- *Are concomitant medical conditions adequately treated or controlled?* For example, improved diabetic control may be associated with improved erectile function.
- *Is the patient taking any drug(s) that may impair sexual function?* If so, the clinician could consider changing medication(s), but a change does not always restore normal sexual function. One explanation is that the patient's drug-induced erectile dysfunction induces fear of failure, which maintains the erectile dysfunction after drug withdrawal.
- *Does the patient have any lifestyle conditions that should be addressed?* Relevant concerns include, for example, obesity, poor diet, lack of exercise, smoking, and social drug use. When a patient presents for treatment of erectile dysfunction, the clinician has an excellent opportunity to provide holistic health advice. Following such advice may have a beneficial effect on the patient's sexual functioning (Esposito et al. 2004).
- *Does the patient want treatment for erectile dysfunction?* Not all patients with erectile dysfunction want treatment. Some are satisfied merely to know the cause and the fact that they have no underlying medical diseases.
- *Is it safe for the patient to have sexual activity?* In particular, will his cardiovascular system cope with the exercise associated with sexual functioning? The Second Princeton Consensus Conference of Sexual Dysfunction and Cardiac Risk guidelines stress the importance of cardiac evaluation and provide useful advice on management of erectile dysfunction in patients with cardiac problems (Jackson et al. 2006).
- *Is it safe to prescribe treatment?* Review the patient's history and findings in light of the known contraindications and precautions of the treatment to be offered.
- *What is the partner's attitude to the problem and its treatment?* A positive and supporting attitude by the man's sexual partner is essential for the successful treatment of erectile dysfunction, but the partner's own sexual difficulties, either predating or following the onset of erectile dysfunction, may impede her ability to provide such support. In addition, the partner should be able to provide adequate penile stimulation, which is essential for the realization of the full therapeutic effect of some pharmacological

treatments. When assessment raises suspicion that the partner may not provide the support and involvement required, sexual and relationship therapy should be considered before active treatment of erectile dysfunction is instigated.

- *Does the partner have any medical problems that may impair her ability to participate in pain-free and enjoyable sexual intercourse?* Before erectile dysfunction treatment is instigated, everything must be done that will facilitate successful penile-vaginal penetration following treatment. Patients may need advice on coital positions if the partner has spinal or hip disabilities. Because most partners of men who present with erectile dysfunction are perimenopausal or postmenopausal, vaginal dryness and atrophy must be considered. Untreated urovaginal atrophy was discovered in one-third of partners of men presenting with erectile dysfunction (Riley and Riley 2000). All couples should receive advice on the use of artificial lubricants at the time of receiving erectile dysfunction treatment, and instigating such treatment may need to be delayed until the urogenital atrophy is treated with hormone replacement therapy. Particular inquiry should be made about the possibility of vaginismus, which is often overlooked in postmenopausal women (Sarrel and Whitehead 1985) and will impede successful restoration of sexual intercourse.

- *What are the patient's and partner's expectations of treating erectile dysfunction?* Many patients have unrealistic expectations of the effect that treating erectile dysfunction will have. Two common expectations are that 1) restoration of erectile function will solve long-standing relationship dysfunction and 2) treatment will enable the couple to have sexual activity similar to that which they had enjoyed in the earlier years of their relationship. These expectations are usually unmet, resulting in the patient's or couple's dissatisfaction with the treatment. The patient or couple should also be warned that successful penetration and intercourse may not occur after the first dose of erectile dysfunction treatment. Studies have shown that success rates increase as the number of treated attempts increases (McCullough et al. 2001; Schulman et al. 2004). Exactly what the treatment is likely and unlikely to do should be explained before treatment is instigated.

Treatment Options

Since time immemorial, a wide variety of forms of treatment have been used in an attempt to restore erectile function. Many patients try over-the-counter or Internet remedies before seeking professional advice. Medically approved therapeutic approaches include sex and/or couple therapy, systemic and local pharmacotherapy, mechanical devices, physiotherapy, and surgery. In the large number of clinical trials of pharmacotherapy for erectile dysfunction that have been undertaken, placebo response rates—in terms of restoration of satisfying sexual intercourse—of up to 30% (in a few instances even higher) have been reported (e.g., Olsson et al. 1996). Hence, even without treatment of proven efficacy, many men are helped by a routine consultation in which they are able to describe their problem and express their concerns and to be informed about the causes and effects of erectile dysfunction.

Sexual Counseling and Sex and Couple Therapy

In view of the disruptive influence that erectile dysfunction can have on a patient's sexual relationship, leading to withdrawal from physical intimacy and attempted sexual intercourse (Riley and Riley 2000; Riley et al. 2007), the majority of couples in which the man presents with erectile dysfunction would benefit from sexual counseling or sex and couple therapy. Because this approach requires resources that are not universally available, patients often receive other types of therapy, based on their history and wishes. However, patients with significant psychosocial problems and/or relationship difficulties should be offered sex and/or couple therapy as appropriate.

Therapists are eclectic in their therapeutic programs, drawing on sex education, communications and sexual skills training, sensate focus, systematic desensitization, and cognitive-behavioral therapy. Regardless of the program, emphasis should be given to encouraging optimal penile stimulation in nonthreatening situations. Psychotherapeutic approaches to psychogenic male erectile disorder have been well summarized by Althof (1989).

Regrettably, the outcome of sex and relationship therapy in the management of erectile dysfunction has not been evaluated in well-controlled, adequately powered, scientifically valid clinical trials. However, accounts of the therapeutic benefit have been reported based on small patient cohorts or poorly designed studies (Masters and Johnson 1970; Wylie 1997). Some studies have shown benefits from combining pharmacotherapy with sexual counseling or brief sex therapy (Banner and Anderson 2007; Gruenwald et al. 2006; Phelps et al. 2004).

Case History

George was 70 years old when he presented to his family doctor with a 4-year history of inability to attain his erection during lovemaking with his wife Carol, age 64. They had been married for 48 years. They had no relationship conflicts.

His family doctor prescribed sildenafil, with instructions to increase the dose from 50 mg to 100 mg per attempt if the lower dosage was ineffective, and to have no more than one treated attempt in 24 hours. He returned to his doctor 6 weeks later, reporting that no improvement had occurred in his erectile ability. He was referred to a urologist and underwent a thorough medical examination and extensive investigations. Although his lipid profile was atherogenic (he later started taking statins), penile arterial insufficiency was not evident. The urologist advised him to continue persevering with sildenafil "as it was sure to work now that significant organic problems had been ruled out." After a further 3 months of using sildenafil, George still saw no improvement and returned to his family doctor, who referred him to our clinic.

Both George and Carol came to our clinic. We obtained a full sexual history. The most significant fact to emerge was their lifelong lack of sexual experimentation. In their early life together, they had developed a routine sex interaction from which they had rarely deviated. Their routine was sexual intercourse on a Saturday evening, in bed in the dark. They rarely undressed together, and George had never seen his wife's vulva. They would kiss and cuddle. George would fondle Carol's breasts, and when he got his erection they would have intercourse in the missionary position. Carol's arms were always around George's neck or trunk. The whole interaction rarely lasted longer than 5 minutes. Carol never experienced orgasm during their sexual interaction and often went immediately to the bathroom and, unknown to George, masturbated to orgasm. Carol mentioned this only when George was not present.

Both George and Carol expressed embarrassment at the thought of being naked together. They said they got in the habit of not being undressed in the early days of their marriage when they lived with Carol's aging parents.

We encouraged them to gradually remove items of clothing over the course of 6 weeks. At first they were to do this in subdued light and not under the direct gaze of their partner. They were "forbidden" to touch each other, and the sessions had to be divorced from any attempted sexual interaction. We saw them at 2-week intervals during this phase of their treatment.

They progressed quickly and at the end of 4 weeks they were both comfortable being naked together. The next phase of their management plan was to encourage touching each other, excluding the genitals, when naked in the light. We suggested that they play "May I touch you?" Taking turns, one partner would touch or stroke, with varying degrees of pressure, a chosen part of the other's body, saying, for example, "May I touch your thigh?" The receiving partner would reply "yes" or "no." If yes, the touch or stroke would take place, and the receiving partner would grade the pleasure attained on a 0–10 scale. Each session would last about 30 minutes. By the end of eight sessions, George and Carol could touch each other and had learned the type and place of contact that gave pleasure. George reported that he attained erections during these sessions.

In the clinic, we talked through male and female genital anatomy using color photographs that the couple took home with them. We suggested that the couple should "examine" each other's genitals in the beam of a flashlight in subdued room light, at first just looking. When they felt comfortable doing this, they were to play "May I touch you?" focusing on the genital regions. We gave them different types of lubricants to apply to the genitals during the touching game and suggested that each guide the other in place and type of touch.

After a month, all inhibitions about being naked together had disappeared and they could touch each other's genitals without any embarrassment or anxiety. George was now experiencing good erections and, although they were told not to attempt sexual intercourse, they did so. For the first time in their life together, Carol experienced an orgasm when intercourse occurred at the end of one of these sessions.

Finally, we gave them additional advice of different types of genital stimulation, including vibration.

When seen at follow-up 3 months after conclusion of the therapeutic program, they had built on their early sexual successes and were enjoying frequent sexual caressing and intercourse. Carol continued to be orgasmic in their sexual interactions.

This case demonstrates failure of medical treatment due to lack of penile and general sexual stimulation (as described in the following section, PDE5 inhibitors work only in the presence of effective sexual stimulation) and positive results from sex therapy.

Pharmacotherapy

PDE5 inhibitors. The introduction of the PDE5 inhibitors as effective treatments has revolutionized the management of erectile dysfunction. These drugs are recommended as first-line therapy unless contraindicated by concomitant medical diseases or pharmacotherapy (American Urological Association 2005).

Mode of action of PDE5 inhibitors. The erection-facilitating property of the PDE5 inhibitors occurs within the erectile tissue of the penis. Maintaining the penis in the flaccid state is an active process dependent on contraction of the cavernosal muscle and constriction of the penile arteries and their arterioles. Sexual stimulation induces the release of nitric oxide from nonadrenergic, noncholinergic nerve terminals in the cavernous tissue, endothelial lining of the cavernous spaces, and penile arteries. The released nitric oxide stimulates the production of cyclic guanosine monophosphate (cGMP), and the increase in cGMP triggers a cascade of reactions leading to a reduction in free cytosolic Ca^{++}, which induces relaxation of the cavernosal muscle and dilatation of the penile arteries and their tributaries. Phosphodiesterase, a heterogeneous series of hydrolytic enzymes, degrades cGMP. An important member of this series is designated type 5 (PDE5). Inhibition of phosphodiesterase by a PDE5 inhibitor blocks the degradation of cGMP, leading to its accumulation in the cavernosal muscle and penile arteries and hence to magnification of the smooth muscle relaxation.

Currently licensed PDE5 inhibitors. At the time of writing, three PDE5 inhibitors—sildenafil, tadalafil, and vardenafil—are licensed, and more are being developed. Key pharmacokinetic and pharmacodynamic data relating to these drugs are given in Table 8–4. All three drugs are highly effective treatments, providing broadly similar therapeutic outcome in terms of restoration of erectile function and attainment of successful sexual intercourse. Adequately powered and methodologically valid head-to-head clinical trials have not been reported. Numerous preference studies have been undertaken, with different results, attributable in some cases to the study design. Because different patients want different features from the treatment they use (i.e., a single drug does not suit all patients), the clinician should discuss the features of each drug with the patient (and also ideally with his partner) and prescribe the product that best suits the individual's or couple's requirements or perceptions. The main difference between the treatments is duration of efficacy, which can be predicted from the different half-lives (Table 8–4). Tadalafil has the longest duration of efficacy, extending to at least 36 hours (Porst et al. 2003). A longer duration of action allows for greater dissociation between dosing and opportunity for successful intercourse and repeated attempts following a single dose. Although available data suggest that onset of therapeutic effect can occur before maximum drug plasma levels are attained, the patient needs to be informed that not all patients will respond early after dosing, to avoid disappointment and dissatisfaction with the treatment. The clinician should also advise the patient to have his first treated attempts at an interval after dosing that corresponds to time to peak concentration. An important consideration is that a heavy fatty meal impairs absorption of sildenafil and vardenafil, leading to delay in time to peak concentration by up to 1 hour. No food interaction has been reported with tadalafil.

Because PDE5 inhibitors work by magnifying the biochemical responses to sexual stimulation, patients must be advised that treated sexual attempts have to be preceded by adequate sexual stimulation.

Adverse events with the three PDE5 inhibitors are generally mild in nature and self-limited with continuous use. (Table 8–5 lists the most common adverse events.) The dropout rate due to adverse events is similar to that for placebo. Concern has been expressed about a possible causal relationship between PDE5 inhibitors and the development of nonarteritic anterior ischemic optic neuropathy (NAION). Erectile dysfunction and NAION share many common risk factors, including hypertension, diabetes mellitus, hypercholesterolemia, and cigarette smoking (Hayreh et al. 1994). The possibility of a causative association between erectile dysfunction and NAION has been critically evaluated; the conclusion is that no causal relationship exists (Hatzichristou 2005), but NAION remains a prescribing precaution for this class of drugs.

Nonresponse to PDE5 inhibitors. High discontinuation rates have been reported for erectile dysfunction treatments. In the multinational Men's Attitudes to Life Events and Sexuality epidemiological study, 58% of men with erectile dysfunction actively sought treatment, but only 16% continued to use oral therapy (Moreira et al. 2005; Rosen et al. 2004). Also, patients frequently request switching treatment (Hatzichristou et al. 2007), suggesting dissatisfaction with the treatment. Treatment dissatisfaction has many causes, including interpersonal difficulties, psychosocial issues, and lack of efficacy.

Table 8–4. Pharmacokinetics of phosphodiesterase type 5 inhibitors

	Sildenafil	Tadalafil	Vardenafil
Time to peak concentration (hours)	0.8–1	2	0.9
Peak concentration (μg/L)	560	378	18.7
Protein binding	96%	94%	94%
Half-life (hours)	2.6–3.7	17.5	3.9
Onset of action (minutes)			
Earliest	14	16	11
>50% patient response	20	30	25

Clinical trials and observational studies have confirmed that the PDE5 inhibitors are highly efficacious treatments for erectile dysfunction. However, a minority of patients, including those with severe neurological damage, severe arterial disease, extensive penile trauma with degeneration of the erectile tissue, or marked unstable diabetes may not respond to PDE5 inhibitors. In the absence of such a severe concomitant condition, nonresponse is usually due to inadequate instructions, patients' nonadherence to instructions (e.g., lack of sexual stimulation and not allowing sufficient time between dosing and attempting sex), suboptimal dosing, and lack of follow-up (Hatzimouratidis and Hatzichristou 2007). A patient should be considered a nonresponder only after he has made four sexual attempts with the highest tolerated dose used in accordance with the manufacturer's guidelines regarding timing relative to meals, alcohol ingestion, use of concomitant medications, and adequate sexual stimulation (Carson et al. 2004). By following these guidelines, 30%–50% of initial nonresponders may be converted to responders (Hatzimouratidis and Hatzichristou 2007). The conversion rate may be improved by counseling (Gruenwald et al. 2006). Allowing patients to try all three of the currently available PDE5 inhibitors improves long-term treatment compliance (Ljunggren et al. 2008).

Because the expression of PDE5 is testosterone dependent, patients with low levels of this hormone may not respond to PDE5 inhibition. Hypogonadism in men is often overlooked, even when suggestive symptoms are

Table 8–5. Most frequently reported adverse events with phosphodiesterase type 5 inhibitors

Adverse event	Sildenafil	Tadalafil	Vardenafil
Headache	12.8%	14.5%	16.0%
Dyspepsia	4.6%	12.3%	4.0%
Flushing	10.4%	4.1%	12.0%
Nasal congestion	1.1%	4.3%	10.0%
Abnormal vision	1.9%	—	<2%
Dizziness	1.2%	2.3%	2.0%
Myalgia	—	5.7%	—
Back pain	—	6.5%	—

present. The prevalence of hypogonadism (total testosterone <300 ng/dL) in men ages 45 years and older who visited primary care practices in the United States was 38.7% (Hatzichristou et al. 2007; Mulligan et al. 2006). Hypogonadal men whose erectile dysfunction is nonresponsive to PDE5 inhibitors may be converted to responders with testosterone replacement therapy (Shabsigh et al. 2004). Recent developments in transdermal formulation of testosterone have simplified testosterone replacement, but some patients still prefer to use the older injectable depot products.

Intracavernosal Injection Treatment

In intracavernosal injection treatment, the patient is taught to inject his penis with a vasoactive drug in the consulting room. When the patient is able to competently undertake the injection, he uses the treatment at home prior to sexual activity. The most frequently used drug is alprostadil; other agents include phentolamine, papaverine, and vasoactive intestinal polypeptide, or a combination of agents. Erection generally occurs within 15 minutes of injection and is not dependent on sexual stimulation. The dose needs to be titrated so the duration of the erection is no longer than 1 hour. The average response rate of alprostadil, in terms of restoration of erectile function, has been reported to be 70% or more (Flynn and Guest 1998; Porst 1996).

Intracavernosal injection of alprostadil is generally comfortable, with less than 10% of patients experiencing pain. Long-term use of this treatment can give rise to penile fibrosis. The risk of prolonged erection (erection lasting longer than 6 hours) can be reduced by dose titration; when prolonged erection occurs, it should be regarded as a medical emergency.

Transurethral Alprostadil

Transurethral administration of alprostadil to the penile erectile tissue involves inserting a small pellet of the drug into the urethral meatus by means of a disposable applicator (this product is known as MUSE, for Medicated Urethral System for Erection). A review of the literature shows this treatment to be less effective than intracorporeal injection, with an average efficacy rate of 45% (Flynn and Guest 1998).

Vacuum Constriction Devices

Vacuum constriction devices (VCDs) are often regarded as a first-line treatment for erectile dysfunction in patients who do not want to use pharmacotherapy or for whom the drugs are contraindicated. Essentially, a VCD consists of a rigid plastic cylinder that is placed over the gel-lubricated penis after a tight latex band is applied around the cylinder. The distal end of the cylinder is connected to a vacuum pump, which can be operated either manually or electrically (from batteries or mains transformer) depending on the model used. With the patient standing, the pump is activated, creating a negative pressure in the cylinder. This draws blood into the penis, which enlarges and becomes rigid as a result. When the penis is sufficiently enlarged, the latex band is slid down the cylinder and positioned around the base of the penis. A valve is then released, allowing air to enter the cylinder; the cylinder is then removed, leaving the penis enlarged and rigid. The penis is not physiologically erect, but the rigidity is usually sufficient to enable sexual intercourse. However, the penis is not rigid proximal to the constriction band, and this leads to instability at the base of the penis. This can make intromission difficult; manual assistance is usually required. Because the constriction band obstructs the inflow of blood to the penis, the penis feels cooler and looks more cyanotic than usual. The constriction band should be removed within 30 minutes to avoid penile ischemia, which may lead to irreversible damage of the erectile tissue.

The use of VCDs is contraindicated in men who have a tendency for spontaneous priapism or prolonged erections (Lewis 1997). Significant penile deformity, such as may occur with Peyronie's disease, may make application of a VCD difficult, uncomfortable, or impossible. A recent review has revealed that high levels of efficacy and satisfaction with this treatment approach have been reported in some, but not all, publications (Glina and Porst 2006), although acceptance rates tend to be low. In a study involving over 1,000 patients who were offered all erectile dysfunction treatments available at the time, 27% opted for a 2-week trial of VCD, but only 6% of the initial population finally requested this treatment modality (Graham et al. 1998).

Physiotherapy

The pelvic floor muscles have a role in the erectile process. Contraction of the ischiocavernosus muscle facilitates erection, and contraction of the bulbocavernosus muscle may be involved in maintaining erection by exerting pressure on the deep dorsal vein of the penis, thereby obstructing the outflow of blood from the erectile tissue (Rosenbaum 2007). Limited controlled studies have shown benefit in treating erectile dysfunction via pelvic floor exercises (Rosenbaum 2007).

Surgery

Arterial revascularization may be considered in those few nonsmoking patients who are under age 40 and have confirmed isolated traumatically induced arterial abnormalities (Goldstein 1996). Abnormal venous leakage from the erecting penis, a condition now called corporal veno-occlusive dysfunction, is sometimes treated surgically, but surgery is no longer recommended because of poor results at long-term follow-up (Wespes et al. 2003). Pelvic floor exercises can be used with therapeutic advantage in patients with corporal veno-occlusive dysfunction (Rosenbaum 2007).

   Surgical implantation of penile prostheses is available for patients who fail to respond to or refuse to try other therapeutic approaches. Various types of semirigid, malleable, and inflatable prostheses are available, as reviewed by Sadeghi-Nejad (2007).

Practice Points

Erectile dysfunction is not a diagnosis; it is a symptom.

An underlying cause should always be considered.

Because many sufferers of erectile dysfunction do not readily seek medical advice, health care professionals should always find the opportunity to broach the subject when patients present with other problems.

Erectile dysfunction can be an indicator of underlying epithelial dysfunction. Therefore, all men with erectile dysfunction should be screened for cardiovascular disease.

Identifying the presence of an organic abnormality does not necessarily mean that it is the cause of the erectile dysfunction. Many men have concurrent organic and psychological causes for their erectile dysfunction.

Most men who present with erectile dysfunction are in relationships. The clinician needs to take into account the partner's sexual and medical health before instigating erectile dysfunction treatment.

Most couples in which the man suffers erectile dysfunction would benefit from sexual and/or relationship counseling.

Couples in which the man has erectile dysfunction should always be advised to use an artificial lubricant when intercourse is first attempted during treatment.

When phosphodiesterase-5 inhibitors are prescribed, detailed instructions on their use should be provided, stressing the need for sexual stimulation.

Conclusion

Treating men who have male erectile disorder is a legitimate part of medical care because restoration of erectile function results in improved psychosocial functioning, enhanced quality of life, and more satisfying sexual relationships, not only for the men but also for their partners. Careful and thorough pretreatment assessment is essential and should include obtaining a detailed description of the sexual difficulty and a full medical, sexual, and psychosocial history in an attempt to identify likely etiological and risk factors for erectile dysfunction. The assessment should also include limited clinical examination and investigations, since erectile dysfunction can be the presenting symptom of underlying systemic disease.

The clinician should discuss the merits and drawbacks of all available treatments with the patient and, ideally, also the patient's sexual partner, and together they should decide on the most appropriate therapeutic approach for their particular lifestyle and sexual practices. The clinician must provide comprehensive instructions relating to the use of the treatment chosen and arrange for adequate and timely follow-up. Most patients with male erectile disorder can be managed without the need for invasive investigation, but many who opt for pharmacological or mechanical therapies would benefit from concomitant sexual and relationship counseling.

Key Points

- Erectile dysfunction is a frequently occurring problem that can cause considerable distress for the man, his sexual partner, and the relationship between them.

- Treatment of male erectile disorder is associated with enhanced self-esteem, reduced psychological morbidity, and increased emotional well-being for both sexual partners.

- Many men with male erectile disorder do not present specifically for treatment of this disorder but are likely to discuss the problem if the health care professional broaches the subject.

- Because male erectile disorder has many psychological, physical, and behavioral causes and can be the presenting symptom of serious underlying pathology, the clinician needs to obtain a full medical and sexual history, a focused clinical examination, and biochemical investigations in all men who present with this symptom. Invasive investigations are rarely required.

- Ideally, the patient's sexual partner should be involved in all stages of the management of male erectile disorder, including the initial assessment. The clinician should bear in mind that sexual or emotional problems of the partner can be factors in the cause or maintenance of male erectile disorder and can jeopardize successful therapeutic outcome.

- Before instigating specific treatment for male erectile disorder, the clinician should provide lifestyle advice and ascertain the patient's and his partner's wish for and expectations of treatment.

- Pharmacological treatments (e.g., PDE5 inhibitors, intracavernosal injection of vasoactive drugs) can provide a quick-fix therapy, but the majority of patients (and their partners) would benefit from concomitant sexual and relationship counseling.

References

Alberti K, Zimmet P: Definition, diagnosis and classification of diabetes mellitus and its complications, part 1: diagnosis and classification of diabetes mellitus provisional report of a WHO consultation. Diabet Med 15:539–553, 1998

Althof SE: Psychogenic impotence: treatment of men and couples, in Principles and Practice of Sex Therapy, Update for the 1990s. Edited by Leiblum SR, Rosen RC. New York, Guilford, 1989, pp 237–265

American Psychiatric Association: Diagnostic and Statistical Manual of Mental Disorders, 4th Edition, Text Revision. Washington, DC, American Psychiatric Association, 2000

American Urological Association: Management of erectile dysfunction. 2005. Available at: http://www.auanet.org. Accessed April 18, 2008.

Araujo AB, Durante R, Feldman HA, et al: The relationship between depressive symptoms and male erectile dysfunction: cross-sectional results from the Massachusetts Male Aging Study. Psychosom Med 60:458–465, 1998

Auld R, Brock G: Sexuality and erectile dysfunction: results of a national survey. Journal of Sexual and Reproductive Medicine 2:50–54, 2002

Aytac I, McKinlay J, Krane R: The likely worldwide increase in erectile dysfunction between 1995 and 2025 and some possible policy consequences. BJU Int 84:50–56, 1999

Banner L, Anderson R: Integrated sildenafil and cognitive-behavior sex therapy for psychogenic erectile dysfunction: a pilot study. J Sex Med 4:1117–1125, 2007

Baskin H: Endocrinologic evaluation of impotence. South Med J 82:446–449, 1989

Billups K, Bank AJ, Padmal-Nathan H, et al: Erectile dysfunction is a marker for cardiovascular disease: results of the Minority Health Institute expert advisory panel. J Sex Med 2:40–52, 2005

Buvat J, Lemaire A: Endocrine screening in 1,022 men with erectile dysfunction: clinical significance and cost-effective strategy. J Urol 158:1764–1767, 1997

Cappelleri J, Rosen R: The Sexual Health Inventory for Men (SHIM): a 5-year review of research and clinical experience. Int J Impot Res 17:307–319, 2005

Cappelleri J, Bell S, Althof S, et al: Comparison between sildenafil-treated subjects with erectile dysfunction and control subjects on the Self-Esteem and Relationship Questionnaire. J Sex Med 3:274–282, 2006

Carson C, Giuliano F, Goldstein I, et al: The "effectiveness" scale—therapeutic outcome of pharmacologic therapies for ED: an international consensus panel report. Int J Impot Res 16:207–213, 2004

Çayan S, Bozlu M, Canpolat B, et al: The assessment of sexual functions in women with male partners complaining of erectile dysfunction: does treatment of male sexual dysfunction improve female partner's sexual functions? J Sex Marital Ther 30:333–341, 2004

Dean J, Rubio-Aurioles E, McCabe M, et al: Integrating partners into ED treatment: improving the sexual experience for the couple. Int J Clin Pract 62:127–133, 2008

Elhanbly S, Schoor R, Elmogy M, et al: What nonresponse to intracavernous injection really indicates: a determination by quantitative analysis. J Urol 167:192–196, 2002

Esposito K, Giuliano F, Di Palo C, et al: Effect of lifestyle changes on erectile dysfunction in obese men: a randomized controlled trial. JAMA 291:2978–2984, 2004

Fisher W, Meryn S, Sand M, et al: Communication about erectile dysfunction among men with ED, partners of men with ED, and physicians: the Strike Up a Conversation study, part 1. J Mens Health Gend 2:64–78, 2005a

Fisher W, Rosen R, Eardley I, et al: Sexual experience of female partners of men with erectile dysfunction: the Female Experience of Men's Attitudes to Life Events and Sexuality (FEMALES) study. J Sex Med 2:675–684, 2005b

Flynn TN, Guest JF: Intracorporeal and transurethral application of alprostadil: a review of the literature. Int J Impot Res 10 (suppl 3):S47, 1998

Glina S, Porst H: Vacuum constriction devices, in Standard Practice in Sexual Medicine. Edited by Porst H, Buvat J. Boston, MA, Blackwell, 2006, pp 121–125

Goldstein I: Arterial revascularization procedures. Semin Urol 4:252–258, 1996

Govier F, McClure D, Kramer-Levien D: Endocrine screening of sexual dysfunction using free testosterone determination. J Urol 156:405–408, 1996

Graham P, Collins J, Thijssen A: Popularity of the vacuum erection device in male sexual dysfunction. Int J Impot Res 10 (suppl 3):S6, 1998

Gruenwald I, Shenfeld O, Chen J, et al: Positive effect of counselling and dose adjustment in patients with erectile dysfunction who failed treatment with sildenafil. Eur Urol 50:134–140, 2006

Hatzichristou D: Phosphodiesterase-5 inhibitors and nonarteritic ischemic optic neuropathy (NAION): coincidence or causality? J Sex Med 2:751–758, 2005

Hatzichristou D, Cuzin B, Martin-Morales A, et al: Vardenafil improves satisfaction rates, depressive symptomatology and self-confidence in a broad population of men with erectile dysfunction. J Sex Med 2:109–116, 2005

Hatzichristou D, Haro J, Martin-Morales A, et al: Patterns of switching phosphodiesterase type 5 inhibitors in the treatment of erectile dysfunction: results from the Erectile Dysfunction Observational Study. Int J Clin Pract 61:1850–1862, 2007

Hatzimouratidis K, Hatzichristou D: Phosphodiesterase type 5 inhibitors: the day after. Eur Urol 51:75–89, 2007

Hayreh S, Joos K, Podhajsky P, et al: Systemic diseases associated with nonarteritic anterior ischemic optic neuropathy. Am J Ophthalmol 118:766–780, 1994

Huang V, Munarriz R, Goldstein I: Bicycle riding and erectile dysfunction: an increase in interest (and concern). J Sex Med 2:596–604, 2005

Jackson G, Rosen R, Kloner R, et al: The second Princeton consensus on sexual dysfunction and cardiac risk: new guidelines for sexual medicine. J Sex Med 3:28–36, 2006

Johannes C, Araujo A, Feldman H, et al: Incidence of erectile dysfunction in men 40 to 69 years of age: longitudinal results from the Massachusetts Male Aging Study. J Urol 163:460–463, 2000

Kostis J, Jackson G, Rosen R, et al: Sexual dysfunction and cardiac risk (the second Princeton Consensus Conference). Am J Cardiol 96:313–321, 2005

Latini D, Penson D, Colwell H, et al: Psychological impact of erectile dysfunction: validation of a new health related quality of life measure for patients with erectile dysfunction. J Urol 168:2086–2091, 2002

Latini D, Penson D, Wallace K, et al: Clinical and psychosocial characteristics of men with erectile dysfunction: baseline data from ExCEED. J Sex Med 3:1059–1067, 2007

Lewis R: External vacuum therapy for erectile dysfunction: use and results. World J Urol 15:78–82, 1997

Litwin M, Nied R, Dhanani N: Health related quality of life in men with erectile dysfunction. J Gen Intern Med 13:159–166, 1998

Ljunggren C, Hedelin H, Salomonsson K, et al: Giving patients with erectile dysfunction the opportunity to try all three available phosphodiesterase type 5 inhibitors contributes to better long term treatment compliance. J Sex Med 5:469–475, 2008

Masters WH, Johnson V: Human Sexual Inadequacy. Boston, MA, Little, Brown, 1970

McCullough A, Siegel R, Shpilsky A: Intercourse success rates with sildenafil citrate. J Urol 165:A170, 2001

Montgomery S, Baldwin D, Riley A: Antidepressant medications: a review of the evidence for drug-induced sexual dysfunction. J Affect Disord 69:119–140, 2002

Moreira EJ, Brock G, Glasser D, et al: Help-seeking behaviour for sexual problems: the Global Study of Sexual Attitudes and Behaviours. Int J Clin Pract 59:6–16, 2005

Muller M, Benkert O: Lower self-reported depression in patients with erectile dysfunction after treatment with sildenafil. J Affect Disord 66:255–261, 2001

Mulligan T, Frick M, Zuraw Q, et al: Prevalence of hypogonadism in males aged at least 45 years: the HIM study. Int J Clin Pract 60:762–769, 2006

National Institutes of Health Consensus Development Panel on Impotence. Impotence. JAMA 270:83–90, 1993

Ojumu A, Dobs AS: Is hypogonadism a risk factor for sexual dysfunction? J Androl 24 (suppl 6):S46–S51, 2003

Olsson AM, Abramsson L, Grenabol L, et al: Peroral treatment of erectile dysfunction with sildenafil (Viagra) (UK-92-480): a double-blind, placebo-controlled, international multicenter study. Scand J Urol Nephrol 30:181–186, 1996

Paige N, Hays R, Litwin M, et al: Improvement in emotional well-being and relationships of users of sildenafil. J Urol 166:1774–1778, 2001

Phelps J, Jain A, Monga M: The PsychoedPlusMed approach to erectile dysfunction treatment: the impact of combining a psychoeducational intervention with sildenafil. J Sex Marital Ther 30:305–314, 2004

Porst H: The rationale for prostaglandin E1 in erectile failure: a survey of worldwide experience. J Urol 155:802–815, 1996

Porst H, Sharlip I: History and epidemiology of male sexual dysfunction, in Standard Practice in Sexual Medicine. Edited by Porst H, Buvat J. Oxford, UK, Blackwell, 2006, pp 43–48

Porst H, Padmal-Nathan H, Giuliano F, et al: Efficacy of tadalafil for the treatment of erectile dysfunction at 24 and 36 hours after dosing: a randomized controlled trial. Urology 62:121–125, 2003

Richter A: The Language of Sexuality. Jefferson, NC, McFarland, 1987

Riley A: The impact of erectile disorder on the man. Int J Clin Pract 57:358–359, 2003

Riley A, Riley E: Behavioural and clinical findings in couples where the man presents with erectile disorder: a retrospective study. Int J Clin Pract 54:220–224, 2000

Riley A, Riley E: Premature ejaculation: presentation and associations—an audit of patients attending a sexual problems clinic. Int J Clin Pract 59:1482–1487, 2005

Riley A, Beardsworth A, Kontomidas S, et al: Sexual intercourse frequency in men presenting for treatment of erectile dysfunction: results from the Pan-European Erectile Dysfunction Observational Study. J Sex Marital Ther 33:3–18, 2007

Rosen R, Fisher W, Eardley I, et al: The multinational Men's Attitudes to Life Events and Sexuality (MALES) study, 1: prevalence of erectile dysfunction and related health concerns in the general population. Curr Med Res Opin 20:607–617, 2004

Rosenbaum T: Pelvic floor involvement in male and female sexual dysfunction and the role of pelvic floor rehabilitation in treatment: a literature review. J Sex Med 4:4–13, 2007

Sadeghi-Nejad H: Penile prosthesis surgery: a review of prosthetic devices and associated complications. J Sex Med 4:296–309, 2007

Sairam K, Kulinskaya E, Boustead G, et al: Prevalence of undiagnosed diabetes mellitus in male erectile dysfunction. BJU Int 88:68–71, 2001

Sarrel P, Whitehead M: Sex and menopause: defining the issues. Maturitas 7:217–224, 1985

Schulman CC, Shen W, Stothard DR, et al: Integrated analysis examining first-dose success, success by dose, and maintenance of success among men taking tadalafil for erectile dysfunction. Urology 64:783–788, 2004

Segraves K, Segraves R, Schoenberg H: Use of the sexual history to differentiate organic from psychogenic impotence. Arch Sex Behav 16:125–137, 1987

Shabsigh R, Kaufman J, Steidle C, et al: Randomized study of testosterone gel as adjunctive therapy to sildenafil in hypogonadal men with erectile dysfunction who do not respond to sildenafil alone. J Urol 172:658–663, 2004

Shiri R, Koskimaki J, Tammela T, et al: Bidirectional relationship between depression and erectile dysfunction. J Urol 177:669–673, 2007

Shores M, Sloan K, Matsumoto A, et al: Increased incidence of diagnosed depressive illness in hypogonadal older men. Arch Gen Psychiatry 61:162–167, 2004

Shores M, Matsumoto A, Sloan K, et al: Low serum testosterone and mortality in male veterans. Arch Intern Med 166:1660–1665, 2006

Wang C, Cunningham G, Dobs A, et al: Long-term testosterone gel (AndroGel) treatment maintains beneficial effects on sexual function and mood, lean and fat mass and bone mineral density in hypogonadal men. J Clin Endocrinol Metab 89:2085–2098, 2004

Wespes E, Wildschutz T, Roumeguere T, et al: The place of surgery for vascular impotence in the third millennium. J Urol 170:1284–1286, 2003

Wespes E, Amar E, Hatzichristou D, et al: EAU guidelines on erectile dysfunction: an update. Eur Urol 49:806–815, 2006

Willke R, Glick H, McCarron J, et al: Quality of life effects of alprostadil therapy for erectile dysfunction. J Urol 157:2124–2128, 1997

Wylie K: Treatment outcome of brief couple therapy in psychogenic male erectile disorder. Arch Sex Behav 26:527–545, 1997

Wylie K, Steward D, Seivewright N, et al: Prevalence of sexual dysfunction in three psychiatric outpatient settings: a drug misuse service, an alcohol misuse service and a general adult psychiatric clinic. Sexual and Relationship Therapy 17:149–160, 2002

9

Female Orgasmic Disorder

Anita H. Clayton, M.D.

David V. Hamilton, M.D., M.A.

Humans, chimpanzees, bonobos, and dolphins are the only animals that have heterosexual activity when the female is not in estrus. In all of these species, sexual activity does more than ensure reproduction. It forms an important basis of social bonding, the glue that helps provide social cohesion.

These facts help to explain the distress that a woman might feel if she has female orgasmic disorder (FOD). In a sample of 1,749 U.S. women, 24% complained of problems with orgasm; their level of distress was not assessed (Laumann et al. 1994). No significant differences in the prevalence of orgasmic complaints in this population were found based on race, ethnicity, or level of education (a proxy measure of income and socioeconomic status). A more recent study found that 35% of urban Chinese women reported some kind of sexual dysfunction (Parish et al. 2007). Seventy-five percent of these women reported being unable to achieve orgasm at some point in the past year, and 11% reported an inability to achieve orgasm that persisted longer than 2 months.

A study from Morocco found that sexual dysfunction rates among Moroccan women are similar to those found in North America, Europe, and Australia (Kadri et al. 2002). Of the 728 women sampled, 29% had no education, 78% pursued no professional activity, and 58% were married. These sociodemographic factors indicate a population very different from the North American, European, Australian, and urban Chinese samples. However, 26.6% of the Moroccan participants reported having sexual dysfunction always or often during the 6 months prior to the survey. Although these studies do not allow us to compare rates of female anorgasmia, using the broader category of sexual complaints, women seem to suffer from sexual dysfunctions at about the same prevalence across different cultures.

A recent meta-analysis of epidemiological studies of the prevalence of female sexual dysfunction in cultures worldwide suggests that sexual dysfunctions are highly prevalent across cultures and that the occurrence of sexual dysfunction increases directly with age for both men and women (Derogatis and Burnett 2008). Many studies also found that although the frequency of symptoms increases with age, personal distress about those symptoms appears to diminish as individuals become older. Finally, respondents' medical problems appear to outweigh the role of culture in determining effects on sexual function.

Recent data support genetic and environmental contributions to orgasmic function. Twin studies of 4,037 women from the United Kingdom (Dunn et al. 2005) and 3,080 Australian women (Dawood et al. 2006) support a significant genetic influence on orgasmic capacity. One-third of the women reported never or infrequently achieving orgasm with intercourse, and 21% reported achieving orgasm during masturbation (Dunn et al. 2005). Genetic influences accounted for 34% and 32%, for the two studies respectively, of the variance in achieving orgasm with intercourse, with an estimated heritability of 45% and 51%, respectively, for orgasm during masturbation. These results suggest that the wide variation in orgasmic dysfunction in women has a strong genetic basis and cannot be attributed solely to sociocultural influences. However, high variability in traits is supportive evidence of a lack of selection for functionality. Whereas clitoral length is highly variable, vaginal length is not. Given the association of clitoral structures and orgasms, the marked variability in clitoral size suggests little or no evolutionary selection pressure on clitoral structure and, by inference, on female orgasm (Wallen and Lloyd 2008).

Orgasmic function is also mediated, at least in part, by personality factors. In a recent large population study (N=2,632), variations in normal personality factors were correlated with an increased prevalence of orgasmic response. Highly introverted women were found to have a 150% increase in risk of having problems with orgasm; emotionally unstable women had a 100% increase in risk. Not being open to new experiences conferred a 140% increase in the odds of disordered orgasm. Conversely, agreeableness and conscientiousness were not found to be statistically correlated with orgasmic dysfunction (Harris et al. 2008). In addition, partner or relational problems may also play a role, as demonstrated by a study of communication patterns in heterosexual couples in which the woman was experiencing FOD were poorer than in control couples, primarily, but not exclusively, when discussing sexual matters (Kelly et al. 2006).

Our objectives in this chapter are to discuss what it means to have FOD and to describe the therapies that are currently available to help overcome this problem. The discussion of the diagnosis of and treatments for FOD will be aided by putting the current approaches to this problem in historical context. We will also briefly discuss healthy sexual physiology, which will illustrate the foundations of how FOD is diagnosed and treated.

A Brief History of the Orgasm

Prior to the advent of psychoanalytic thought at the turn of the twentieth century, sexuality was considered a moral and spiritual matter. It was not specifically thought of as a medical concern. Female sexuality began to be considered as a subject of inquiry by the medical mainstream only with the advent of Sigmund Freud's psychoanalytic theory in 1897. Psychoanalytic theory conceived of the psychological development of both men and women as being primarily a constituent of early psychosexual stages. The psychological problems of adulthood were thought to be manifestations of early trauma, at a time when sexual drives had not yet been repressed, allowing for symbolization of conflicts and, ultimately, for reason itself (Freud 1924/1961).

Freud believed that a seminal event in the development of any child was the realization that men and women have different genitalia. Following the phallocentrism of his time, Freud believed that a boy's realization that women do not have penises led to *castration anxiety*. Likewise, in little girls, the lack of a penis led to *penis envy*, which Freud believed was the central fact in the development of women's personalities. In Freud's conception of the female, the clitoris was a "little penis," which inevitably led to feelings of inferiority. According to Freud, this inferiority ultimately led to a less fully developed sense of morality (Freud 1924/1961).

Freud believed that the way to psychological maturity for women was for them to "transfer" the experience of the orgasm away from the clitoris to the vagina. A clitoral orgasm was evidence that a woman had not yet overcome her penis envy and was still attempting to experience sex as a man would. The vaginal transference theory seems plainly misogynistic by contemporary standards, and even Freud envisioned a day when future biological revelations could disprove his theory of female sexuality (Freud 1920/1955). Freud's prediction did not take long to reach fruition.

In 1953, endocrinologist Alfred Jost discovered that a functional ovary was not necessary for the development of a female, whereas a functional testes, producing testosterone and antimullerian hormone, was necessary for a male to develop (Jost 1953). In the same year, Alfred Kinsey published his landmark *Sexual Behavior in the Human Female*, in which he argued that a vaginal orgasm was not possible for a normally developed human female (Kinsey 1953). These data destroyed the underpinnings of Freud's theory, as Freud himself had predicted. Following Kinsey's initial epidemiological treatises on reports of sexual behavior, the cultural climate changed enough by the 1960s to allow scientific study of sexual behaviors.

Human Sexual Response: Four-Phase Model

In their seminal treatise on human sexuality, *Human Sexual Response*, Masters and Johnson (1966) proposed a four-phase model to describe the sexual response of both men and women (see Figure 9–1); this model continues to serve as the basis for the diagnostic taxonomy of sexual disorders. To clarify the physical changes that are necessary to achieve orgasm, we should first examine more fully the sexual stages that precede it. Because the goal of this chapter is to understand orgasmic dysfunction in women, we can limit our discussion to Masters and Johnson's model of the female sexual response. As the psychological and neurophysiological basis of libido has become better understood, contemporary researchers have included desire as the first phase of the response cycle.

Desire

Sexual desire in humans is a complex neurobiological and psychological phenomenon. Beginning in the 1980s, researchers attempted to arrive at a definition of sexual desire that would allow for its study as a psychological state, conceptualizing it as an appetitive drive necessary to provoke the subsequent physical changes of the sexual excitement phase. Following this understanding, *sexual desire* is defined as the conditions of the central nervous system that are necessary to mediate the beginning of the sexual excitement phase. Few studies have been done of how people in general use the term *sexual desire* or of what the term is used to signify. Regan and Berscheid (1996) found that the general population tends to agree with the research definition; in their study, 98.5% of both men and women described *desire* as a subjective, psychological experience rather than as a physiological or behavioral sexual event. The authors found that women experience desire as a more romantic, interpersonal experience than do men. Significantly more women endorsed that love and intimacy are goals of desire, whereas significantly more men viewed sexual activity as a goal of sexual desire.

Excitement

During the excitement stage, a number of physiological changes begin in both men and women. Both experience an increase in heart rate, respiratory rate, and blood pressure, necessary for increased perfusion pressure (i.e., blood flow) in the genitals. In women, vasocongestion in the genitals results in clitoral engorgement. The labia increase in size and may change in shape. Although an overall increase in skeletal muscle tension occurs, the distal vaginal muscles relax, allowing for the expansion of the vaginal canal. Vasocongestion also leads to the production of lubrication in the estrogen-rich tissues of the vaginal canal, which also darken in color and become smoother. Finally, the breasts may increase in size, and the nipples harden and/or become erect. The clitoris withdraws under the clitoral hood, decreasing the size of the external

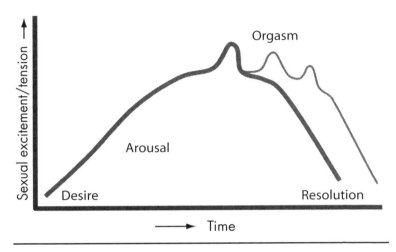

Figure 9–1.   Classical model of sexual response.

Source.   Adapted from Masters and Johnson (1966).

clitoris. Contraction of the pubococcygeus muscle reduces the size of the outer third of the vaginal canal, creating the *orgasmic platform*. Unlike Kinsey (1953), Masters and Johnson (1966) believed that the contraction of these tissues was necessary for a woman to achieve orgasm. Although the goal of identifying extraclitoral tissues able to produce orgasm may be seen as a vestige of the psychoanalytic understanding of female sexuality and sexual disorders, in their research, Masters and Johnson did not identify vaginal orgasms in any of their volunteers.

Orgasm

Orgasm is a sensation of intense pleasure accompanied by an alteration in consciousness, contraction of the genitourinary musculature, and, in some cases, involuntary vocalization (Meston et al. 2004). Masters and Johnson (1966) identified a plethora of physiological changes that occur during orgasm. Respiratory rate typically exceeds 40 respirations/minute. Blood pressure peaks with the initiation of orgasm (+30–80 mm Hg systolic, +20–40 mm Hg diastolic) and then decreases. Likewise, heart rate peaks at initiation of orgasm at 110–180 beats/minute.

Claims have been made that a woman's orgasm helps to facilitate conception. The contraction of the pubococcygeus muscle causes the uterus to descend. Beginning with orgasm, the cervical os dilates, perhaps allowing for easier flow of sexual fluids into the uterus and fallopian tubes beyond. A more controversial claim has been that the rhythmic contractions of the orgasmic platform are intended to aid in propelling seminal fluid and sperm through the cervix. As with all teleological hypotheses, this assertion has been difficult to prove.

Neuroimaging has been used to demonstrate areas of the brain that are involved in orgasm. Positron emission tomography (PET) suggests that activation of the left lateral orbitofrontal cortex is related to the level of behavioral inhibition during sexual behavior, with deactivation of the temporal lobe directly reflecting the level of sexual arousal. Regional cerebral blood flow is decreased in the prefrontal cortex and the left temporal lobe during orgasm in women. The deep cerebellar nuclei are associated with orgasm-specific muscle contractions, with the ventral midbrain and right caudate, both dopamine-containing areas, also involved (Georgiadis et al. 2006). Other PET scans, coupled with magnetic resonance imaging (MRI), have shown increased activation at orgasm, compared with preorgasm sexual arousal, in the paraventricular nucleus of the hypothalamus, periaqueductal gray area of the midbrain, hippocampus, and cerebellum (Komisaruk et al. 2002). Hormonally, spikes in prolactin and oxytocin lead to an overall sense of well-being and may act to facilitate bonding with a sexual partner. Finally, studies from the 1980s show that consciousness is not necessary for orgasm. Like men, women sometimes orgasm while they are sleeping (Fisher et al. 1983).

Many women describe orgasms as originating from the vagina, not the clitoris. In the 1940s, Ernst Gräfenberg, a German gynecologist later known for developing the intrauterine device (IUD), hypothesized the existence of tissue within the vagina that was associated with vaginal orgasm in some women. He located the area on the anterior vaginal wall, in the outer one-third or about 2 inches behind the clitoris. His assertion was roundly ridiculed and dismissed by the medical community of his time, following the psychoanalytic belief that the transference of orgasm from clitoris to vagina was due to emotional maturity, not anatomy.

In the late 1970s, a few researchers began to listen to women who continued to report having vaginal orgasms. By this time, the work of Kinsey and of

Masters and Johnson had led the medical community to believe that vaginal orgasm was not possible. Case reports began to appear in the medical literature in the early 1980s that described women not only achieving vaginal orgasms but also ejaculating from this area, which they referred to as the "G-spot," in honor of Gräfenberg. Tissue studies have identified the paraurethral glands, or Skene glands, which help lubricate the vagina, as possible sources for ejaculated fluid during orgasm in some women (Addiego et al. 1981). Perry and Whipple reported that orgasms produced through stimulation of the anterior vaginal wall generate uterine contractions, whereas those originating in the clitoris cause contractions of the pelvic muscles (Whipple and Perry 2002).

However, the existence of the G-spot remains controversial, because the anatomy and physiology have not been elucidated. Recent researchers have denied the existence of the G-spot because very few tactile (i.e., touch-receptive) nerve endings exist anywhere in the vagina (Hines 2001). They argue that the presence of such nerve bundles would make vaginal delivery of a pregnancy overwhelmingly painful. Both the glans, or head, of the penis and the clitoris contain huge numbers of these tactile nerve endings, and therefore these types of nerves have been thought necessary for orgasm. Proponents of the G-spot have countered that vaginal orgasms are mediated through pressure-sensitive nerves, not tactile nerves (Hilliges et al. 1995). This controversy has continued into the twenty-first century, with proponents alleging that to deny the existence of the G-spot is tantamount to refusing to accept the reports of those women who have vaginal orgasms (Whipple and Perry 2002).

Not only are the anatomy and physiology of vaginal orgasm and the G-spot not fully understood, but neither are those of any kind of orgasm, in either men or women. Orgasms are difficult to study, largely because of their intensely personal and subjective nature. However, it is irrefutable at this point that some women report having orgasms that originate in the vagina. The G-spot remains the current best explanation for how this happens.

Resolution

After completion of orgasm, which typically lasts several seconds, the resolution of the sexual cycle begins. Vascular engorgement begins to drain through the venous blood vessels of the pelvis, causing the clitoris and labia to return to their pre-aroused size and position. The cervix remains open for approximately 30 minutes following orgasm, and its position lowers in the vaginal canal, approximating the position of pooling semen following unprotected penile-vaginal intercourse. Heart rate, blood pressure, and respiratory rate all return to normal within minutes following orgasm.

For many women, orgasm does not necessarily mean the resolution of the sexual cycle. Women capable of multiple orgasms remain aroused following orgasm. The factors that contribute to the ability to have multiple orgasms are unknown. Women who have singular orgasms and those who have multiple orgasms are both thought to have healthy, normal sexual functioning.

Diagnosis of Female Orgasmic Disorder

DSM-IV-TR enumerates criteria for the diagnosis of all recognized psychiatric disorders, including FOD (American Psychiatric Association 2000, p. 549). The DSM-IV-TR criteria for FOD are as follows:

A. Persistent or recurrent delay in, or absence of, orgasm following a normal sexual excitement phase. Women exhibit wide variability in the type or intensity of stimulation that triggers orgasm. The diagnosis of female orgasmic disorder should be based on the clinician's judgment that the woman's orgasmic capacity is less than would be reasonable for her age, sexual experience, and the adequacy of sexual stimulation she receives.
B. The disturbance causes marked distress or interpersonal difficulty.
C. The orgasmic dysfunction is not better accounted for by another Axis I disorder (except another sexual dysfunction) and is not due exclusively to the direct physiological effects of a substance (e.g., a drug of abuse, a medication) or a general medical condition.

Furthermore, FOD is designated as lifelong or acquired, as generalized or situational, and as being due to psychological factors (e.g., depression, anxiety) or a combination of psychological and physical factors (e.g., depression or anxiety in addition to a medical illness or drug use).

The critical factor in making the diagnosis of FOD is stated in the beginning of Criterion A: the woman must experience a delay or absence of orgasm *following a normal excitement phase.* Although a lack of sexual excitement may, in turn, lead to the inability to achieve orgasm, this would not correctly be diagnosed as FOD. Libido is not necessarily a problem for a woman with

FOD alone; however, a woman might have concurrent diagnoses of FOD and hypoactive sexual desire disorder.

Another important part of Criterion A is the clinician's judgment that "the woman's orgasmic capacity is less than would be reasonable for her age, sexual experience…" Data indicate that, unlike men, women typically find it easier to have an orgasm as they age and gain sexual experience (Levin 2001). Finally, a woman must have adequate stimulation to achieve orgasm. The diagnosis of FOD would not be indicated in a woman whose sexual partner suffers from premature ejaculation, thus depriving her of sufficient stimulation to reach orgasm.

Criterion B is relatively simple. For a lack of orgasm to be a problem, it must be associated with marked distress or interpersonal difficulty. Common complaints of distress include a sense of loss, guilt, frustration, anxiety, or inadequacy. The Female Sexual Distress Scale, a validated measure of sexually related personal distress, has been used to quantify distress in research trials (Derogatis et al. 2002). A woman who is unconcerned about her lack of orgasm is not suffering from FOD. Although this lack of interest may be evidence of another psychiatric problem, such as depression, this is not necessarily the case. Multiple factors appear to play a role in a woman's choice to participate in sexual activity, among them a desire for intimacy, partner consideration, and a desire for sexual pleasure (Basson 2001). Although 48% of men reported that sex which does not result in orgasm was unsatisfying, 43% of women felt the same (Levin 2001); the difference was not statistically significant, indicating that approximately the same proportion of men and women find orgasm essential to a fulfilling sexual experience.

Criterion C is meant to provide the exclusion criteria. FOD should not be diagnosed in women with sexual difficulties due to other psychiatric conditions such as depression, anxiety, or psychosis. However, if an anorgasmic woman has a history of a depressive disorder that does not include sexual dysfunction as one of its symptoms, or if anorgasmia preceded onset of the depressive illness, then the diagnoses of FOD and a depressive disorder could both be made.

Multiple neurotransmitters must act in concert for orgasm to occur. Drugs that affect sex steroids (e.g., estrogen, prolactin; Kruger et al. 2005) or neurotransmitter function (e.g., norepinephrine, serotonin, nitric oxide; Stahl 2001) run the risk of impairing the ability to orgasm. Although all antidepressants run the risk of impairing orgasm, not all antidepressants confer the same degree of dysfunction. Studies have found that the selective seroto-nin reuptake inhibitor (SSRI) antidepressants (i.e., citalopram, escitalopram, fluvoxamine, fluoxetine, paroxetine, sertraline), along with the serotonin-norepinephrine reuptake inhibitor (SNRI) antidepressant venlafaxine, confer the greatest degree of risk, whereas antidepressants that do not exploit seroto-nin reuptake as their primary therapeutic action, including bupropion and mirtazapine (Clayton et al. 2002; Montejo et al. 2001) and transdermal sele-giline (Clayton et al. 2007a), do not significantly inhibit orgasm. The SNRI duloxetine appears to have effects intermediate to SSRIs and antidepressants with a unique mechanism of action (Clayton et al. 2007b). Sexual dysfunc-tion related to serotonin reuptake inhibitor (SRI) effects is increased in indi-viduals with the GG genotype of the serotonin 2A receptor ($5\text{-HT}_{2A}\text{-}1438$) single nucleotide polymorphism (Bishop et al. 2006). Opiate pain medica-tions among many other drugs have been associated with orgasmic dysfunc-tion, as have other sedating antianxiety and sleep medications. According to Duncan et al. (2000), some medications that make orgasm more difficult for men, including a variety of antihypertensive medications, have been found not to have an effect on women's ability to orgasm. Duncan et al. (2000) also found that smokers are less likely to report healthy sexual function, including or-gasm, than nonsmoking controls. These findings demonstrate the complexity of the necessary physiological conditions for orgasm.

A variety of medical conditions, including diabetes, cardiovascular disease, and neurological disease, also can affect a woman's ability to orgasm. The med-ical condition most often associated with orgasmic dysfunction is spinal cord injury. Prior to the mid-1990s, spinal cord injury affecting the nerves originat-ing from the lumbar area was thought to mean that orgasm was not possible. When women with spinal cord injuries affecting the lumbar area reported hav-ing normal orgasms, these were dismissed as "phantom orgasms," considered similar to the phantom pain experienced by amputees. More recent studies have found that although many women with spinal cord injuries affecting the lumbar area do experience orgasmic dysfunction, some woman with these in-juries can experience orgasms. Sipski (1995) reported that 44% of subjects with spinal cord injuries were orgasmic, whereas Jackson and Wadley (1999) found that 54% of women with spinal cord injuries reported having orgasm. In the latter study, 32% of orgasmic women with spinal cord injury had cervi-cal spine injuries, 41% had thoracic injuries, and 52% had lumbosacral injuries. These data demonstrate that the specific function of the nervous system in orgasm is not currently fully understood, and that having a spinal cord injury does not necessarily mean the end of a woman's orgasmic life.

No specific laboratory or imaging studies are recommended at this time for the clinical evaluation of orgasmic dysfunction. However, if a medical illness–related or substance-induced orgasmic dysfunction is suspected, maximizing effective treatment of the medical condition or eliminating the potential contributing substance may aid in identification of the cause of the orgasmic dysfunction.

Lastly, the specifiers used when making the diagnosis of FOD help to paint a more detailed, realistic picture of the woman suffering from FOD. Moreover, they help to differentiate potential causes of FOD, which make possible specific research into potential treatments. Although the causes of FOD are not understood, a reasonable assumption is that FOD in a woman with lifelong orgasmic dysfunction has a different cause from acquired FOD in a woman with previously healthy orgasms. The different causes may be of central importance, because they may lead to differences in treatment. Likewise, FOD that occurs in a healthy, drug- or medication-free woman is likely different from FOD occurring due to a mixture of psychological factors and spinal cord injury, for example.

Thus, FOD may be diagnosed due to psychological factors, as well as a combination of psychological and physical factors, which include drugs of abuse, medications, and medical or psychiatric illnesses or injuries. However, FOD cannot be diagnosed due to physical factors alone. DSM-IV-TR Criterion B, marked distress or interpersonal difficulty, requires that a woman have a psychological component to orgasmic dysfunction for that dysfunction to be diagnosed as FOD.

Treatment of Female Orgasmic Disorder

Psychological Approaches

Prior to the 1960s, the treatment for orgasmic dysfunction was psychoanalysis or psychoanalytically oriented psychotherapy. These techniques focused primarily on the intrapsychic and interpersonal conflicts that were thought to inhibit healthy sexual function. Case studies often depicted the anorgasmic woman as a masochist, unconsciously choosing a sexual relationship that was unsatisfying as a way of externalizing her own sense of inferiority (Lief and Friedman 2006). However, the efficacy of psychoanalytic therapy for orgasmic dysfunction is unknown. In addition, contemporary psychoanalytic and psychodynamic techniques do not continue to reflect this approach. In cases in which orgasmic dysfunction is caused by chronic relationship problems due to maladaptive personality styles, psychodynamic therapy or psychoanalysis can make an important contribution to the resolution of those personality traits and concomitant improvement in interpersonal and sexual function.

A drawback of psychodynamic and psychoanalytic therapies is that they often take quite a while to produce results. Although these therapies may produce widespread meaningful changes, including improvement in sexual experiences, the length of treatment may be daunting. For a woman with psychological difficulties limited to FOD, more specific, targeted therapies have been found to produce quicker results.

Masters and Johnson were the first researchers to observe couples having sex. They worked only with heterosexual couples in committed, reportedly monogamous relationships. They focused on the various means of stimulation, and they recognized that nonsexual problems in a couple's relationship often led to sexual dysfunction. They found that in nearly half of the couples they worked with, one or both partners experienced some form of sexual dysfunction at some time in the relationship (Masters and Johnson 1970). Happily, they found that nearly all of these difficulties were transitory and remitted with couples therapy, directed sexual therapy, or both.

For women with FOD, the most important first step is education. Many women believe that orgasm ought to be achieved by vaginal penetration with their partner's penis and that if they are unable to achieve orgasm in this fashion, then they are simply anorgasmic. Several studies have shown that the majority of orgasmic women are not able to achieve orgasm through intercourse alone, but are able to achieve orgasm through manual or oral stimulation of the clitoris and surrounding areas, including the labia minora and periurethral area. A smaller percentage of women are able to achieve orgasm through stimulation of the cervix, possibly through penetration (Heiman 2000). Duration of sexual activity is another important factor in determining if a woman is receiving adequate stimulation. Many men are able to progress through the sexual stages and achieve orgasm within just a few minutes. Although some women are able to achieve orgasm with little stimulation, far more require a significant period of directed foreplay to achieve orgasm. Open communication between sexual partners, including discussion of the possibly sensitive subject of premature ejaculation, is an important preliminary step in addressing orgasmic dysfunction.

For women who have never or rarely been able to experience orgasm, either alone or with a partner, directed masturbation has been shown to be highly effective. Written or video-based materials provide a woman with step-by-step instructions in how to stimulate herself. In some studies of directed masturbation, erotic materials have also been provided to heighten sexual excitement.

Directed masturbation was first evaluated in the 1970s, and a number of studies and case reports have shown that in women with primary anorgasmia (i.e., women who have never had an orgasm), directed masturbation almost always allowed those women to experience orgasm (Heiman 2000). Other studies have produced a more conservative efficacy rate of 65% (McMullen and Rosen 1979). These studies indicate that more than half of these women were subsequently able to have orgasm with a sexual partner as well, although this number may be low because of the short follow-up period of these studies; that is, more of these women may have been found to have orgasms with their partners if given a bit more time.

Some women are able to orgasm alone but find the pressure of a sexual encounter with a partner too anxiety provoking. Masters and Johnson (1970) addressed this problem with a technique they termed *sensate focus*, in which the goal of a sexual encounter is initially shifted away from the achievement of orgasm. Sensate focus involves dictated programmatic, progressive levels of touching, starting with nonsexual touching and progressing to more sexual touching and eventual intercourse or other genital stimulation. Studies of sensate focus have shown little evidence that the technique dramatically improves orgasmic function. In a study of 18 women unable to orgasm with their partner, sensate focus helped 2 of them to reach orgasm (Matthews et al. 1976). However, nearly all of the couples that participated in the sensate focus study found that the technique led to a greater sense of well-being, intimacy, and closeness in their relationship.

Various techniques to reduce anxiety surrounding sexual encounters fall into the category of *systematic desensitization*. These techniques include exposing women to sexually explicit material, including erotic writing, pictures, and video. The effectiveness of these techniques is difficult to determine because they have usually been studied in conjunction with some other kind of therapy.

Finally, some women experience pervasive anxiety or other mood symptoms that are also manifest during sexual activity. In cognitive-behavioral therapy, pioneered by Aaron Beck and his colleagues at the University of Pennsylvania in the 1970s and 1980s, carefully recorded thought records are used to capture the cognitions that accompany these emotions. Maladaptive thought patterns, which Beck termed "cognitive distortions," are identified and challenged. McCabe (2001) found that the use of cognitive-behavioral therapy, in conjunction with sensate focus, systematic desensitization, and directed masturbation, reduced anorgasmia from 66% to 11% in a sample of sexually dysfunctional women.

Unfortunately, the study of FOD has been limited by the lack of distinction of causality, such as separating women suffering from the disorder into groups based on diagnostic specifiers. As previously discussed, the cause of FOD in a woman who has had it her entire life is likely different from that of a woman with a change from previously healthy sexual function. Likewise, a woman whose FOD is due to psychological factors would likely require different treatment from a woman whose FOD is due to a combination of psychological factors and medical illness. Although some of the interventions discussed in this section may be used in general clinical practice, referral to a specialist in sexual therapy may be important for some women.

Pharmacotherapy

At the time of this writing (2009), the U.S. Food and Drug Administration has not approved any medications for the treatment of FOD. Various agents have been tested, and some have shown a degree of preliminary success. Small, proof-of-concept studies showed that the vasoactive agent sildenafil was somewhat effective for the treatment of FOD, although larger subsequent studies failed to demonstrate separation from placebo (Shields and Hrometz 2006). Recently, sildenafil (50–100 mg/day) was found superior to placebo in effects on arousal and orgasmic dysfunction in premenopausal women with SRI-induced arousal or orgasmic problems. Better results were seen in women with higher plasma levels of thyroxine and testosterone, which enhance nitric oxide function. Over 80% of the women complained at study baseline of concomitant decreased desire, which was unaffected by sildenafil treatment, despite the improvements in orgasmic function (Nurnberg et al. 2008).

Bupropion has been studied in women with FOD, also with mixed results (Modell et al. 2000; Segraves et al. 2006). Studies of women with SSRI-induced sexual dysfunction have demonstrated statistical improvements in desire and clinical improvements in arousal and orgasm with sustained-release bupropion (300–400 mg/day) (Clayton et al. 2004). Some of the difficulty in demonstrating superiority of new treatments over placebo may be related to difficulties defining the study population, lack of validation of outcome measures, low sensitivity of hormonal assays in women, and problems obtaining long-term safety data. Unfortunately, a safe, effective treatment for FOD remains an unaccomplished goal of medical science.

Other strategies in the management of antidepressant-associated orgasmic dysfunction include decreasing the dose of the antidepressant; changing to one less likely to cause sexual dysfunction; or adding an antidote demonstrated superior to placebo, such as bupropion (Clayton et al. 2004), buspirone (Landen et al. 1999), or sildenafil (Nurnberg et al. 2008). Maximizing treatment of conditions that cause sexual dysfunction may also lead to improvements in orgasmic capacity. Treatments under development primarily involve hormonal interventions, such as androgens (e.g., testosterone, dehydroepiandrosterone; Kingsberg and Janata 2007), melanocortins (e.g., bremelanotide; Safarinejad 2008), oxytocin (Caldwell et al. 1986), and dopaminergic agents (e.g., apomorphine; Bechara et al. 2004).

Conclusion

Orgasm remains mysterious because it is an entirely private experience. A clinician likely takes on faith that when a patient reports having an orgasm, the patient is having the same experience that the clinician knows as orgasm, in the same way that the clinician accepts the report of any emotion, whether it be love or despair. The clinician can observe changes in vital signs, neurotransmitters, and other physical factors during orgasm, but the central fact of orgasm—that is, pleasure—remains very difficult to objectify and quantify and, therefore, extremely perplexing to research and treat. Despite or perhaps because of these inherent difficulties, the clinician must listen to his or her female patients. When they complain that a lack of orgasm is causing them distress, the clinician must hear them and do whatever is possible to help. In the end, this is true of any kind of pain.

Orgasm is not "an extra" in health and overall well-being; it is part of a pleasurable, happy, healthy life. Although the understanding of orgasm dysfunction and its treatment remains relatively primitive, the approach to the problem must not be.

Key Points

- Orgasm is a subjective experience, accompanied by a number of objective, physiological changes.

- Distress is a necessary criterion for the diagnosis of FOD.

- When diagnosing FOD, the clinician must be aware of the specific patterns of presentation, such as whether the lack of orgasm is lifelong or acquired, and the context of the difficulties, including psychological, medical, and pharmacological factors that may be contributing to orgasmic dysfunction.

- A wide array of psychological and psychoeducational therapies are available for both the woman who has never experienced orgasm (primary anorgasmia) and the woman who has achieved orgasm in the past but is not able to at some later time (secondary anorgasmia).

- Currently, no reliable pharmacological therapies are available for the treatment of FOD.

References

Addiego J, Belzer EG, Comolli J, et al: Female ejaculation: a case study. J Sex Res 17:13–21, 1981

American Psychiatric Association: Diagnostic and Statistical Manual of Mental Disorders, 4th Edition, Text Revision. Washington, DC, American Psychiatric Association, 2000

Basson R: Using a different model for female sexual response to address women's problematic low sexual desire. J Sex Marital Ther 27:395–403, 2001

Bechara A, Bertolino MV, Casabé A, et al: A double-blind randomized placebo control study comparing the objective and subjective changes in female sexual response using sublingual apomorphine. J Sex Med 1:209–214, 2004

Beck AT: Cognitive Therapy and Emotional Disorders. New York, International Universities Press, 1975

Bishop JR, Moline J, Ellingrod VL, et al: Serotonin 2A-1438 G/A and G-protein Beta3 subunit C825T polymorphisms in patients with depression and SSRI-associated sexual side-effects. Neuropsychopharmacology 31:2281–2288, 2006

Caldwell JD, Prange AJ Jr, Pedersen CA: Oxytocin facilitates the sexual receptivity of estrogen-treated female rats. Neuropeptides 7:175–189, 1986

Clayton AH, Pradko JF, Croft HA, et al: Prevalence of sexual dysfunction among newer antidepressants. J Clin Psychiatry 63:357–366, 2002

Clayton AH, Warnock JK, Kornstein SG, et al: A placebo-controlled trial of bupropion SR as an antidote for selective serotonin reuptake inhibitor–induced sexual dysfunction. J Clin Psychiatry 65:62–67, 2004

Clayton AH, Campbell BJ, Favit A, et al: Symptoms of sexual dysfunction in patients treated for major depressive disorder: a meta-analysis comparing selegiline transdermal system and placebo using a patient-rated scale. J Clin Psychiatry 68:1860–1866, 2007a

Clayton A, Kornstein S, Prakash A, et al: Changes in sexual functioning associated with duloxetine, escitalopram, and placebo in the treatment of patients with major depressive disorder. J Sex Med 4:917–929, 2007b

Dawood K, Kirk KM, Bailey JM, et al: Genetic and environmental influences on the frequency of orgasm in women. Twin Res Hum Genet 9:603–608, 2006

Derogatis LR, Burnett AL: The epidemiology of sexual dysfunctions. J Sex Med 5:289–300, 2008

Derogatis LR, Rosen R, Leiblum S, et al: The Female Sexual Distress Scale (FSDS): initial validation of a standardized scale for assessment of sexually related personal distress in women. J Sex Marital Ther 28:317–330, 2002

Duncan LE, Lewis C, Jenkins P, et al: Does hypertension and its pharmacotherapy affect the quality of sexual function in women? Am J Hypertens 13:640–647, 2000

Dunn KM, Cherkas LF, Spector TD: Genetic influences on variation in female orgasmic function: a twin study. Biol Lett 1:260–263, 2005

Fisher C, Cohen HD, Schiavi RC, et al: Patterns of female sexual arousal during sleep and waking: vaginal thermo-conductance studies. Arch Sex Behav 12:97–122, 1983

Freud S: Beyond the pleasure principle (1920), in The Standard Edition of the Complete Psychological Works of Sigmund Freud, Vol 18. Translated and Edited by Strachey J. London, Hogarth Press, 1955, pp 3–72

Freud S: The dissolution of the Oedipus complex (1924), in The Standard Edition of the Complete Psychological Works of Sigmund Freud, Vol 19. Translated and Edited by Strachey J. London, Hogarth Press, 1961, pp 172–179

Georgiadis JR, Kortekaas R, Kuipers R, et al: Regional cerebral blood flow changes associated with clitorally induced orgasm in healthy women. Eur J Neurosci 24:3305–3316, 2006

Goldberg DC, Whipple B, Fishkin RE, et al: The Grafenberg spot and female ejaculation: a review of initial hypotheses. J Sex Marital Ther 9:27–37, 1983

Harris JM, Cherkas LF, Kato BS, et al: Normal variations in personality are associated with coital orgasmic infrequency in heterosexual women: a population-based study. J Sex Med 5:1177–1183, 2008

Heiman JR: Orgasmic disorders in women, in Principles and Practice of Sex Therapy, 3rd Edition. Edited by Leiblum SR, Rosen RC. New York, Guilford, 2000, pp 118–153

Hilliges M, Falconer C, Ekman-Ordeberg G, et al: Innervation of the human vaginal mucosa as revealed by PGP 9.5 immunohistochemistry. Acta Anat (Basel) 153:119–126, 1995

Hines TM: The G-spot: a modern gynecologic myth. Am J Obstet Gynecol 185:359–362, 2001

Jackson AB, Wadley V: A multicenter study of women's self-reported reproductive health after spinal cord injury. Arch Phys Med Rehabil 80:1420–1428, 1999

Jost A: Problems of fetal endocrinology: the gonadal and hypophyseal hormones. Recent Prog Horm Res 8:379–418, 1953

Kadri N, McHichi Alami KH, McHakra Tahiri S: Sexual dysfunction in women: population-based epidemiological study. Arch Womens Ment Health 5:59–63, 2002

Kelly MP, Strassberg DS, Turner CM: Behavioral assessment of couples' communication in female orgasmic disorder. J Sex Marital Ther 32:81–95, 2006

Kingsberg SA, Janata JW: Female sexual disorders: assessment, diagnosis, and treatment. Urol Clin North Am 34:497–506, 2007

Kinsey A: Sexual Behavior in the Human Female. Philadelphia, PA, WB Saunders, 1953

Komisaruk BR, Whipple B, Crawford A, et al: Brain activity (fMRI and PET) during orgasm in women, in response to vaginocervical self-stimulation. Abstr Soc Neurosci 841:17, 2002

Kruger TH, Hartmann U, Schedlowski M: Prolactinergic and dopaminergic mechanisms underlying sexual arousal and orgasm in humans. World J Urol 23:130–138, 2005

Landen M, Eriksson E, Agren E, et al: Effect of buspirone on sexual dysfunction in depressed patients treated with selective serotonin reuptake inhibitors. J Clin Psychopharmacol 19:268–271, 1999

Laumann EO, Gagnon JH, Michael RT, et al: The Social Organization of Sexuality: Sexual Practices in the United States. Chicago, IL, University of Chicago Press, 1994

Levin RJ: Sexual desire and the deconstruction and reconstruction of the human female sexual response model of Masters and Johnson, in Sexual Appetite, Desire and Motivation: Energetics of the Sexual System. Edited by Everaerd W, Laan E, Both S. Amsterdam: Royal Netherlands Academy of Arts and Sciences, 2001, pp 63–93

Lief HI, Friedman RC: History of psychologic treatments, in Women's Sexual Function and Dysfunction: Study, Diagnosis, and Treatment. Edited by Goldstein I, Meston CM, Davis SR, et al. New York, Taylor & Francis, 2006, pp 427–434

Masters WH, Johnson VE: Human Sexual Response. Boston, MA, Little, Brown, 1966

Masters WH, Johnson VE: Human Sexual Inadequacy. Boston, MA, Little, Brown, 1970

Matthews A, Bancroft J, Whitehead A, et al: The behavioral treatment of sexual inadequacy: a comparative study. Behav Res Ther 14:427–436, 1976

McCabe MP: Evaluation of a cognitive behavioral therapy program for people with sexual dysfunction. J Sex Marital Ther 27:259–271, 2001

McMullen S, Rosen RC: Self-administered masturbation training in the treatment of primary orgasmic dysfunction. J Consult Clin Psychol 47:912–918, 1979

Meston CM, Hull E, Levin RJ, et al: Disorders of orgasm in women. J Sex Med 1:66–68, 2004

Modell JG, May RS, Katholi CR: Effect of bupropion-SR on orgasmic dysfunction in nondepressed subjects: a pilot study. J Sex Marital Ther 26:231–240, 2000

Montejo AL, Llorca G, Izquierdo JA, et al: Incidence of sexual dysfunction associated with antidepressant agents: a prospective multicenter study of 1022 outpatients. J Clin Psychiatry 62 (suppl 3):10–21, 2001

Nurnberg HG, Hensley PL, Heiman JR, et al: Sildenafil treatment of women with antidepressant-associated sexual dysfunction: a randomized controlled trial. JAMA 300:395–404, 2008

Parish WL, Laumann EO, Pan S: Sexual dysfunction in urban China: a population-based survey of men and women. J Sex Med 4:1559–1574, 2007

Regan PC, Berscheid E: Beliefs about the state, goals, and objects of sexual desire. J Sex Marital Ther 22:110–120, 1996

Safarinejad MR: Evaluation of the safety and efficacy of bremelanotide, a melanocortin receptor agonist, in female subjects with arousal disorder: a double-blind placebo-controlled, fixed dose, randomized study. J Sex Med 5:887–897, 2008

Segraves RT, Clayton AH, Croft H, et al: A multicenter, double-blind, placebo-controlled study of bupropion XL in females with orgasm disorder. Paper presented at the annual U.S. Psychiatric and Mental Health Congress, New Orleans, LA, November 2006

Shields KM, Hrometz SL: Use of sildenafil for female sexual dysfunction. Ann Pharmacother 40:931–934, 2006

Sipski ML, Alexander CJ, Rosen RC: Orgasm in women with spinal cord injuries: a laboratory-based assessment. Arch Phys Med Rehabil 76:1097–1102, 1995

Stahl SM: The psychopharmacology of sex, part 2: effects of drugs and disease on the 3 phases of human sexual response. J Clin Psychiatry 62:147–148, 2001

Wallen K, Lloyd EA: Clitoral variability compared with penile variability supports nonadaptation of female orgasm. Evol Dev 10:1–2, 2008

Whipple B, Perry JD: The G-spot: a modern gynecologic myth (letter). Am J Obstet Gynecol 187:519; author reply 187:520, 2002

Recommended Readings

Clayton A: Satisfaction: Women, Sex and the Quest for Intimacy. New York, Ballantine Books, 2006

Heiman JR: Orgasmic disorders in women, in Principles and Practice of Sex Therapy, 3rd Edition. Edited by Leiblum SR, Rosen RC. New York, Guilford, 2000

Lief HI, Friedman RC: History of psychologic treatments, in Women's Sexual Function and Dysfunction: Study, Diagnosis, and Treatment. Edited by Goldstein I, Meston CM, Davis SR, et al. New York, Taylor & Francis, 2006

Meston CM, Hull E, Levin RJ, et al: Disorders of orgasm in women. J Sex Med 1:66–68, 2004

10

Delayed and Premature Ejaculation

Marcel D. Waldinger, M.D., Ph.D.

Most men feel good when they ejaculate after a prolonged time of sexual intercourse or after their female partner has had an orgasm or after she has whispered to him that it is time for him to come. If "normal" ejaculation time—that is, the time that a man can postpone his ejaculation after vaginal intromission—were defined in terms of what the average woman prefers, the definition would be vulnerable to various psychological, cultural, and sociological factors. Because defining normal ejaculation time is very difficult, defining a delayed or a premature ejaculation is also challenging. In the last two decades, and despite the difficulties, enormous progress has been made toward defining normal, delayed, and premature ejaculations.

Ejaculation Disorders in DSM-IV-TR

Ejaculation and orgasm usually occur simultaneously in men even though ejaculation and orgasm are two separate phenomena. Ejaculation occurs in the genital organs, whereas orgasmic sensation—although related to the genitals—is mainly a cerebral event and involves the whole body. The clinical syndrome of anesthetic ejaculation is a good example of how orgasm and ejaculation may exist independently of each other. Men with anesthetic ejaculation experience a normal ejaculation but have no sensation of orgasm (Williams 1985). Besides these somatic and neurobiological underpinnings, both ejaculation and orgasm are influenced by inner psychological processes.

A clear distinction between orgasm and ejaculation is not made in DSM-IV-TR (American Psychiatric Association 2000). In DSM-IV-TR, ejaculation disorders are categorized under the heading of *orgasmic disorders.* Strangely, in DSM-IV-TR, delayed ejaculation has been called "male orgasmic disorder," analogous to "female orgasmic disorder," whereas premature ejaculation has not been called "premature orgasm" (Waldinger and Schweitzer 2005). Moreover, two rather rare syndromes, anesthetic ejaculation (Williams 1985) and partial ejaculatory incompetence (Riley and Riley 1982), are not mentioned at all in DSM-IV-TR. The synonymous terminology of ejaculation and orgasm in DSM-IV-TR is not in line with current neurobiological views, which are that different neurobiological pathways and neurotransmitters are involved in ejaculation and orgasm (Waldinger and Schweitzer 2005). Therefore, based on the aforementioned arguments, the heading "Orgasmic Disorders" should be changed to "Ejaculation Disorders" in the pending DSM-V. Moreover, the term *delayed ejaculation* would be more appropriate than *male orgasmic disorder* in the pending DSM-V. In this chapter, I use the term *delayed ejaculation.*

Delayed Ejaculation

Not every complaint of having had a delayed ejaculation is the result of an ejaculatory "disorder." For example, a woman may believe her partner to have a delayed ejaculation, even though from an objective point of view he is ejaculating within a "normal" ejaculation time. On the other hand, some men complain of a delayed ejaculation because they never have an ejaculation, whether by masturbation or intercourse. These two situations are demonstrated by the following patients.

Case Example 1

Arthur is a 31-year-old plumber who has been married for 4 years to Angela, who accompanied him to his appointment. Arthur is a mentally and physically healthy man who enjoys life and has many friends. However, Arthur is convinced that he has delayed ejaculation and feels unhappy about it. Angela confirmed her husband's story, adding that she is not satisfied with their sex life because intercourse takes too much time. Angela reported that she has always had difficulty achieving orgasm by self-stimulation of the clitoris and has rarely reached orgasm by coitus. She does not like self-stimulation. After being asked for more details about the way the couple is making love, Arthur reported that he usually has an ejaculation after about 15 minutes. In his previous relationship, a delay was never a problem, but Angela has repeatedly told him that she does not like his penile thrusting for such a long time.

Case Example 2

Bob, a 41-year-old clergyman, has been married for about 12 years. Bob reported his complaint in a very clear and technical way. Whatever he does while making love, he rarely ejaculates. Sometimes, with great effort, he has been able to ejaculate after a long period of masturbation, but he has never been able to ejaculate during coitus, even after 1 hour of frequent and vigorous thrusting. His wife, who accompanied Bob to his appointment, confirmed his story and added that she is very sorry for Bob that he cannot experience the pleasurable feelings of an ejaculation and associated orgasm. She has told Bob that she suffers from 2–3 days of vaginal pain after they have sex, and she asked him to seek medical treatment to be able to ejaculate sooner.

These cases illustrate typical problems encountered in daily clinical practice. Arthur is not suffering from an objective delayed ejaculation time; coitus duration of about 15 minutes is rather normal. However, Angela did not like that duration, and she appeared to have her own sex-related difficulties. She erroneously told her husband that he was suffering from delayed ejaculation. In contrast, the complaints of Bob and his wife represent a real and severe ejaculatory disorder. Whatever Bob did, and no matter how much his wife sympathized with him, he was unable to ejaculate.

Lifelong Versus Acquired Delayed Ejaculation

Delayed ejaculation can be either lifelong (primary) or acquired (secondary). If delayed ejaculation has been present from early adulthood, the disorder is considered lifelong. In the acquired form, delayed ejaculation becomes apparent after the man has previously experienced normal ejaculatory functioning during his life. The paucity of well-designed studies on lifelong delayed ejaculation may be due in part to the rather low prevalence of the disorder but also to a frequently made misjudgment by clinicians about the negative impact on the quality of life of couples (Waldinger and Schweitzer 2005).

Delayed ejaculation is sometimes considered to be "beneficial" because a man gains sufficient time to satisfy his sexual partner to have one or multiple orgasms. However, lifelong delayed ejaculation is involuntary and may induce many emotional and practical problems for both sexual partners.

In addition to having reproduction difficulties, many men become frustrated by the lack of ejaculation and orgasm. Female sexual partners can also become victim, because they imagine that they are unattractive to their partner in facilitating ejaculation or they might think that another partner is needed. Obviously, intense thrusting for a long time may also become painful, which may result in a cumbersome sexual relationship and even in failure to conceive, which is often the main reason for couples to seek help.

Definition of Delayed Ejaculation

Delayed ejaculation means that a man finds it difficult or impossible to ejaculate, despite the presence of adequate sexual stimulation, erection, and conscious desire to achieve orgasm. In an effort to ejaculate, some men may struggle even to the complete physical exhaustion of both sexual partners. Delayed ejaculation may occur in coitus, masturbation (either by the patient or by the partner), or oral sex.

Throughout the years, a variety of terms have been used to refer to this ejaculatory disorder: retarded ejaculation, inhibited ejaculation, difficult ejaculation, late ejaculation, and ejaculatio retarda or retardata. Other terms for ejaculation failure include inability to ejaculate, no ejaculation, anejaculation, ejaculatory incompetence, impotentia ejaculandi or ejaculationis, ejaculatio deficiens or nulla, and lack (loss, failure, inability) of ejaculation (Dekker 1993).

Symptoms of Delayed Ejaculation

If ejaculation is delayed in all situations, in all sexual activities, and with all partners, the disorder is *generalized*. In contrast, the delayed ejaculation is *sit-*

uational if it is limited to certain situations or certain partners. Situational delayed ejaculation may have varied clinical presentations in that different men with the disorder are able to ejaculate by masturbation but not intravaginally, to ejaculate during sex with a man but not with a woman, to ejaculate with one particular woman but not with another, to ejaculate with the same woman on one occasion but not on the next, or to ejaculate only when the sexual act is accompanied by specific stimulation.

Prevalence of Delayed Ejaculation

Lifelong delayed ejaculation is a relatively uncommon condition in clinical practice. In many studies analyzing the distribution of sexual dysfunctions in men, delayed ejaculation is always the least expressed sexual complaint. The prevalence of delayed ejaculation differs across studies. For example, in a general U.S. male population, the prevalence was 8% (Laumann et al. 1999); in a study in Iceland, the prevalence was less than 1% in men ages 55–57 years (Líndal and Stefánsson 1993); in France, the prevalence was 4% (Spira et al. 1998); and in a Swedish study among men ages 18–74 years, the prevalence was 2% (Fugl-Meyer and Fugl-Meyer 1999). In the Swedish study, the prevalence was higher at older age. One should always realize that prevalence data may be biased by lack of accurate measurement tools.

Assessment

A complete medical and sexual history is crucial in each patient with delayed ejaculation. The clinician should clarify whether delayed ejaculation is generalized or situational (based on location, sexual activity, specific partner), whether the complaint existed from the first sexual encounters (lifelong) or occurred later in life (acquired), whether ejaculation or orgasm or both are lacking. The clinician should inquire about the frequency of delayed ejaculations and the duration of the ejaculation time.

Lifelong Delayed Ejaculation

Psychological Theories

According to the classical psychological view, lifelong delayed ejaculation is attributed to fear, anxiety, hostility, and relationship difficulties (Kaplan

1974; Munjack and Kanno 1979; Shull and Sprenkle 1980). Many different manifestations of anxiety and fear have been hypothesized, including fears of death and castration, fear of loss of self resulting from loss of semen, fear of castration by the female genitals, fear that ejaculation would hurt the female, fear of being hurt by the female, performance anxiety, unwillingness to give of oneself as an expression of love, fear of impregnating the female, and guilt secondary to a strict religious upbringing. The psychological ideas and explanations may have face validity in some individual cases, but no well-controlled studies support a generalization of any of the various psychological hypotheses. Still, despite the absence of a coherent psychological theory, anecdotal data of successful behavioral treatments illustrate that psychological and environmental factors contribute to lifelong delayed ejaculation.

Neurobiological Research

Animal experiments in the 1940s demonstrated that rats reared in isolation either are not capable of achieving ejaculation or remain sexually inactive even after repeated exposure to a receptive female (Beach 1942). In contrast, rats raised in groups with either same-sex or opposite-sex cage mates did not show these clear deficits in copulatory behavior. Importantly, in most but not all of the isolation-reared males, sexual performance gradually improved with experience. These interesting early findings suggest that early traumatic experiences may induce delayed ejaculation but also that experience and learning play a role in rat copulatory performance.

In the last few decades, animal studies have shown that central serotonergic neurotransmission, including the amount of serotonin (5-hydroxytryptamine [5-HT]) turnover and involvement of serotonergic receptors, is involved in the ejaculatory functioning in animals and men (Olivier et al. 1998; Waldinger et al. 1998a). In laboratory rats, researchers attempted to create hyposexual behavior, mimicking delayed ejaculation, by manipulating the level of sexual experience (Mos et al. 1990). For example, of sexually "naive" male rats (i.e., rats with no previous encounter with a female rat) that were exposed to female receptive rats (in estrus) for the first time during tests of 15 minutes each, 8.3% of the study sample showed no sexual activity at all. Although 82% displayed sexual activity, they failed to ejaculate during the test. The sexual performance of these sexually naive male rats improved after treatment with 5-HT_{1A} receptor agonists. In particular, two selective 5-HT$_{1A}$ receptor agonists (i.e., 8-OH-DPAT and flesinoxan) enhanced sexual behavior almost to the level of sexually experienced rats. Sexual performance was also facilitated after treatment with partial 5-HT$_{1A}$ receptor agonists (i.e., buspirone and ipsapirone), although sedation became enhanced after buspirone in higher doses. Furthermore, α_2-adrenoceptor antagonists such as yohimbine and idazoxan appear effective in shortening ejaculation time of sexually naive rats (Mos et al. 1990, 1991). These findings indicate that naive male rats are able to perform sexual activities reminiscent of sexually experienced rats in a very short time. Mos et al. (1990) also showed that males treated with 5-HT$_{1A}$ receptor agonists (i.e., flesinoxan and gepirone) were more attractive to receptive females than were placebo-treated males. Gessa et al. (1979) found that hyposexual behavior in sexually inactive rats can be reversed by the opioid receptor antagonist naloxone.

Following these findings, several studies showed that other pharmacological compounds and certain neuropeptides can act beneficially toward copulatory behavior in sexually inactive rats. For example, the 5-HT$_{1A}$ receptor agonist 8-OH-DPAT clearly increased sexual activity in rats that were sexually inactive (Haensel et al. 1991). Similarly, the erectogenic drug sildenafil (Ottani et al. 2002) and low doses of the hormone melatonin (Drago and Busa 2000) also showed reversibility of hyposexual behavior of sexually inactive rats. These pharmacological studies strongly suggest that specific neurobiological mechanisms should be held responsible for hyposexual behavior in the sexually inactive rat. Indeed, in recent years, neurobiological differences have been found between rats that are sexually inactive and rats that display normal sexual behavior. Despite the fact that more animal studies are needed, it is suggested that researchers should also study these substrates in men with delayed ejaculation and anejaculation.

Brain Imaging

Nothing is known about the brain regions involved in delayed ejaculation and anejaculation. However, a very interesting study on anejaculation was performed by Georgiadis and Holstege (2004). Eleven healthy male volunteers tried to achieve ejaculation during the positron emission tomography scan; only half of the attempts were successful. Successful ejaculation resulted in very marked increases of regional cerebral blood flow in the mesodiencephalic transition zone and the cerebellum (Holstege et al. 2003). The scans of the unsuccessful attempts showed activations in the right orbitofrontal cortex, in the left dorsal prefrontal cortex, and bilaterally in the anterior insula. Comparison with the scans of successful attempts of ejaculation showed that non-ejaculatory performance involves more cortical activity than ejaculation, especially in the left temporal pole and most anterior amygdala, structures that are important for vigilance and fear behavior. Georgiadis and Holstege (2004) concluded that higher levels of activity in the anterior temporal lobe may lead to anejaculation. Although the volunteers were not patients with persistent anejaculation, this study provides very interesting information, because the unsuccessful attempts may mimic the real-life situation of anejaculation in men who have no urogenital abnormalities.

Acquired Delayed Ejaculation

Psychological Causes

Men with psychologically induced acquired delayed ejaculation have no specific identifiable characteristics. Obviously, the ejaculation disturbance has not existed previously. In addition, the onset may occur suddenly with a situational or intermittent delay. The clinician should always look for provocative psychological trauma (e.g., the discovery of the partner's infidelity) or lack of sexual and psychological stimulation (inadequate technique or lack of attention to sexual stimuli).

Somatic Causes

A moderate but acceptable delay of ejaculation occurs during aging. Delay or failure of ejaculation may result from androgen deficiency, traumatic or surgical spinal injuries with damage of lumbar sympathetic ganglia and the connecting nerves, abdominoperineal surgery, lumbar sympathectomy, and neurodegenerative disorders, such as multiple sclerosis or diabetic neuropathy. A wide range of drugs (selective serotonin reuptake inhibitors [SSRIs], tricyclic antidepressants, antipsychotics, alpha-sympatholytics) and alcohol (either directly during acute consumption or chronically) can impair ejaculation through central and peripheral mechanisms.

Treatment

Various treatments have been used to treat men with delayed ejaculation. Vibratory and electrical stimulation, a variety of sexual exercises, and a range of psychotherapeutic techniques have been used separately or in combination (Apfelbaum 1989; Delmonte 1984; Delmonte and Braidwood 1980; Gagliardi 1976). Some men with delayed ejaculation have successfully ejaculated from vibration of the penis, but data on long-term improvements are lacking (Beckerman et al. 1993). Transrectal electrical stimulation of the internal genitals (electroejaculation) is used mainly to obtain semen from men with paraplegia. This intervention, however, is extremely painful if used in neurologically healthy men and is not an option to treat lifelong delayed ejaculation. Masturbation exercises have been extensively described as a way to treat delayed ejaculation (Kaplan 1974). Other published techniques include individual psychodynamic psychotherapy, marital therapy, rational emotive therapy, and social skills training. The overall impression is that variable results can be achieved with each technique, but controlled clinical trials are lacking. To date, most studies have had various methodological shortcomings. For example, researchers have assessed outcomes by means of one-word ratings (*improved*, *cured*, or *unchanged*), have provided no specific information on ejaculation, and have not used standardized treatments. Therefore, and due to scientific uncertainties, no firm conclusions or recommendations about treatment approaches can be given (Dekker 1993).

Physicians need to be alert with patients who are taking ejaculation-delaying drugs. With regard to antidepressant-induced ejaculation delay, five treatment strategies may be attempted: 1) waiting until the side effects spontaneously disappear, 2) reducing dosage, 3) stopping the drug a few days before intercourse (drug holidays), 4) switching to another antidepressant, and 5) using an antidote (Waldinger 1996). However, few placebo-controlled studies have investigated these strategies, and even fewer well-controlled studies have compared these strategies. In general, the best strategy is to switch to another antidepressant that is known to have less of an ejaculation-delaying effect. Although fluvoxamine has ejaculation-delaying effects, both human and animal studies have shown that of all SSRIs, fluvoxamine has the least ejaculation-delaying effects (Waldinger et al. 1998b). Other antidepressants that have no ejaculation-delaying effects are mirtazapine (Coleman et al.

2001) and bupropion (Waldinger 2007a). Vascular or neuropathic damage is usually irreversible, and the patient should be counseled to look for alternative methods to satisfy the sexual wishes of both sexual partners. Androgen deficiency requires appropriate testosterone replacement therapy. General instructions may include enjoying more time together, minimizing alcohol consumption, making love when people are not tired, and practicing pelvic floor training.

Currently, the best way to treat patients with lifelong delayed ejaculation is to inform them about existing factors that can delay their ejaculation and to instruct them through counseling. Beneficial effects through psychotherapy depend on the severity of delayed ejaculation and the individual's receptiveness to counseling. A combination of masturbation exercises and general therapeutic interventions appears to be most successful. Well-controlled clinical research of ejaculation delay requires the clinically objective investigation of intravaginal ejaculation latency time, masturbation ejaculation latency time, and oral ejaculation latency time by use of a stopwatch (Waldinger et al. 2007a).

Effective drug treatment is not yet available. Unraveling the neurobiology of ejaculation and its interaction with psychological factors is of utmost importance in furthering research aimed at finding drugs to facilitate ejaculation. In addition, for the development of drugs that facilitate ejaculation, psychopharmacological animal research remains pivotal. However, because the prevalence of lifelong delayed ejaculation is presumably rather low, and because the development of drugs in general is extremely expensive, pharmaceutical companies are unlikely to work on developing a specific drug for this indication in the near future. Therefore, at this point in time, the better option for finding drugs that help treat lifelong or acquired retarded ejaculation is to seek secondary medical uses of existing drugs on the basis of animal research information.

Premature Ejaculation

Not every early ejaculation is the result of an ejaculatory disorder. For example, a man may believe that he is ejaculating very early, even though from an objective point of view he is doing so within a normal ejaculation time. On the other hand, some men complain that early ejaculation occurs very soon after penetration at every intercourse.

Case Example 3

Colin is a 29-year-old successful businessman, married for 3 years to Cheryl, who accompanied him on his visit. Based on Colin's medical history, he appears to be both mentally and physically a healthy man, who is doing sports twice a week and who reports to have a happy marriage. This is confirmed by his wife. However, Colin complains of having premature ejaculation and feels very unhappy about it. In contrast, Cheryl says that she does not understand his complaint. She is quite satisfied with her sexual life; she regularly, but not always, experiences a coitally induced orgasm, and she has not been aware that her husband has premature ejaculation. After being asked for more details about the way the couple has intercourse, Colin reports that he usually has an ejaculation after about 10 minutes of intercourse with regular penile thrusts. He considers this time period too short, particularly when his wife does not get a coitally induced orgasm. According to his opinion, a man should be able to bring his wife to an orgasm by active thrusting.

Case Example 4

Donald is a 34-year-old teacher at a high school. His girlfriend of about 28 years of age, a teacher at the same high school, could not accompany him because she had to work. Donald is rather hesitant to talk about his sexual life, but after some reassurance, he reports to have had early ejaculations since his first sexual contacts at age 18. He had two relationships before he met his current girlfriend. With all three of them, he experienced early ejaculations at nearly every intercourse. According to Donald, he usually ejaculates within 15 seconds. He feels embarrassed and has been avoiding sexual contact for approximately 6 months. His girlfriend is rather annoyed about the low frequency of intercourse and does not understand that his early ejaculations are such a problem for him. She does not mind at all.

These two case examples represent a debate on the definition of premature ejaculation that has been ongoing since the 1970s. The best way to understand this debate is to have a look at the history of premature ejaculation.

History of Premature Ejaculation

Since the beginning of the twentieth century, premature ejaculation has been regarded by many as the expression of an unconscious psychological conflict.

However, at the same time, it has been attributed to urological disturbances, such as a too short frenulum, and many different treatments have been recommended (Waldinger 2004). A clearer understanding of the differences in etiology and treatment has resulted from the classification, introduced in 1943 by the German endocrinologist Bernhard Schapiro, of two types of premature ejaculation (Schapiro 1943), which were later termed *primary* (lifelong) premature ejaculation and *secondary* (acquired) premature ejaculation (Godpodinoff 1989).

Definition of Premature Ejaculation

Until 1980, the year in which DSM-III was published (American Psychiatric Association 1980), no official definition existed for premature ejaculation. In the first part of the twentieth century, psychoanalysts considered a man to have premature ejaculation when ejaculation occurred so quickly after vaginal penetration that a woman hardly had any chance of becoming sexually aroused. In the absence of any official definition, the generally accepted idea was that a man had premature ejaculation when he consistently ejaculated within 1 minute after penetration.

In 1970, Masters and Johnson strongly refuted a short ejaculation time as the criterion for the definition of premature ejaculation and stated that a man has premature ejaculation when he is not able to control his ejaculation to satisfy his female partner in more than 50% of intercourses. Their view influenced the first official definition for premature ejaculation, in DSM-III, in which premature ejaculation was defined solely in terms of an absence of voluntary "control," with no attention to the time that passes before a man ejaculates (the ejaculation time). However, in the following DSM-III-R (American Psychiatric Association 1987), DSM-IV (American Psychiatric Association 1994), and DSM-IV-TR editions, "control" is no longer mentioned in the definition. In these editions, premature ejaculation is defined as "persistent or recurrent ejaculation with minimal sexual stimulation before, on, or shortly after penetration and before the person wishes it" (DSM-IV-TR, p. 554). However, because little evidence-based research into ejaculation time had been conducted by the 1980s, a quantification of "short" ejaculation time was not included in the DSM definition. In contrast, the definition of premature ejaculation in ICD-10, the classification system of the World Health

Organization (1993), does mention a cutoff point for ejaculation time. According to ICD-10, a man has premature ejaculation when he ejaculates very soon (e.g., within 15 seconds) after penetration. However, the ICD-10 makes no reference to any study in which this figure had been reported as outcome data (Waldinger and Schweitzer 2006a, 2006b).

A long-unanswered question regarding the definition of premature ejaculation is what is actually meant by the criteria "shortly after penetration" (DSM-IV-TR) and "very soon after penetration" (ICD-10). To investigate the criterion of a short ejaculation time, Waldinger et al. (1994) introduced the intravaginal ejaculation latency time (IELT), which is defined as the time between vaginal penetration and intravaginal ejaculation. Moreover, Waldinger et al. (1998a) postulated that there is a continuum of the IELT in the general male population and that the IELT is neurobiologically and genetically determined. However, not until 2005 was such a variability of the IELT demonstrated in men (Waldinger et al. 2005a). In a stopwatch study, financed by Pfizer International, the IELT was measured in an unselected cohort of men in the general population of five countries (The Netherlands, United Kingdom, Spain, Turkey, and United States) during a 1-month period (Waldinger et al. 2005a). The study demonstrated for the first time that in the general male population, the IELT has a skewed distribution, with a median IELT of 5.4 minutes (confidence interval 0.55–44.1 minutes). Such a continuum of ejaculation time had previously been observed using various cohorts of laboratory male Wistar rats (Pattij et al. 2005a, 2005b). Based on this continuum, Pattij et al. (2005a, 2005b) presented a new animal model for premature ejaculation. In addition, they proposed three endophenotypes of male rats: 1) rats that always ejaculate after a very short time of copulatory behavior (i.e., rapid ejaculating rats); 2) rats that ejaculate after a normal ejaculation latency time (i.e., normal ejaculating rats); and 3) rats that ejaculate after a long ejaculation latency time (i.e., sluggish ejaculating rats). Waldinger (2002) postulated that lifelong premature ejaculation in men represents a specific phenotype and is characterized by specific symptomatology.

Patients with lifelong premature ejaculation frequently ask their treating physicians, "What exactly is a normal ejaculation time?" On the basis of the stopwatch study conducted in four European countries and the United States (Waldinger et al. 2005a), any figure under the 2.5 percentile, or the 0.5 percentile in a skewed distribution, may be regarded as abnormal or dysfunctional. In the study conducted in the four European countries and the United States, men under the 2.5 percentile had an IELT of less than 1 minute (Waldinger et al. 2005b). In other words, men with an ejaculation time of less than 1 minute have, according to the statistics, an abnormal IELT compared with the IELT of the rest of men in the general population (Waldinger et al. 2005b). This IELT of 1 minute or less was already known from a study in which a clinical cohort of Dutch men with lifelong premature ejaculation had measured their IELTs with a stopwatch over a 1-month period at every intercourse; 80% of these men ejaculated within 40 seconds and 90% ejaculated within 1 minute after vaginal penetration (Waldinger et al. 1998c). On the basis of the aforementioned findings in both human and animal research, Waldinger and colleagues postulated that lifelong premature ejaculation is mainly a neurobiological ejaculation disorder, and probably also a genetically determined one that is related to disturbances of serotonergic (5-HT) neurotransmission in the central nervous system (Waldinger 2002). In 1998, the authors defined lifelong premature ejaculation in terms of an ejaculation that occurs within 1 minute after vaginal penetration (Waldinger 2002; Waldinger et al. 1998c).

Classification of Premature Ejaculation

Since Schapiro's (1943) review, the importance of distinguishing lifelong premature ejaculation from acquired premature ejaculation has been known. Such a distinction is important because it has consequences for the appropriate treatment.

Lifelong Premature Ejaculation

Men with lifelong premature ejaculation have experienced early ejaculations in almost every contact with every sexual partner from their first sexual relations. The aforementioned stopwatch studies, as well as studies in which premature ejaculation was self-reported, have demonstrated that 90% of men with lifelong premature ejaculation ejaculate within 1 minute and that another 10% ejaculate within 1–2 minutes (Waldinger et al. 1998c, 2007). Interestingly, many years after men with premature ejaculation were treated mainly by psychoanalysts, current evidence-based research has demonstrated that the psychoanalysts' definition of premature ejaculation as occurring within 1 minute after penetration was actually correct. In 2007, the International

Society for Sexual Medicine (ISSM), in a meeting in Amsterdam, reached consensus on a new definition of lifelong premature ejaculation by accepting the 1-minute criterion. According to the ISSM, premature ejaculation is a male sexual dysfunction characterized by 1) ejaculation that always or nearly always occurs prior to or within about 1 minute of vaginal penetration; 2) the inability to delay ejaculation during all or nearly all vaginal penetrations; and 3) negative personal consequences, such as distress, bother, frustration, and/ or the avoidance of sexual intimacy (McMahon et al. 2008). Throughout their life, men with lifelong premature ejaculation usually ejaculate within the same short ejaculation time. However, about 20%–30% of these men, at some point in life after age 30 or so, begin to have an even shorter ejaculation time (Waldinger et al. 1998c, 2007). Based on this knowledge of lifelong premature ejaculation, Donald in Case Example 4 would be diagnosed with lifelong premature ejaculation.

Acquired Premature Ejaculation

Men who begin having early ejaculations at a certain age, never having had this complaint previously and having been able to delay ejaculation in the past, may be diagnosed as having acquired premature ejaculation. Men with acquired premature ejaculation are more heterogeneous as a group than are those with lifelong premature ejaculation, probably due to the different factors and dysfunctions that may lead to acquired premature ejaculation. In addition to psychological and relationship factors, hyperthyroidism, erectile difficulties, and urological problems such as prostatitis may cause acquired premature ejaculation (Althof 2006; Carani et al. 2005; Shamloul and El-Nashaar 2006; Trinchieri et al. 2007).

The characteristics of acquired premature ejaculation have not been as thoroughly investigated and described as have those of lifelong premature ejaculation. Little has been published regarding IELT quantification and patient-reported outcome (e.g., subjective experiences, such as feelings of satisfaction, that are relevant for quality of sexual life) in cohorts of men with acquired premature ejaculation. Most studies on acquired premature ejaculation used inclusion and exclusion criteria, and therefore the characteristics of a whole cohort of these men were not completely investigated. This lack of knowledge currently impairs the formulation of an evidence-based definition for this premature ejaculation subtype. Nevertheless, an expert panel on acquired premature ejaculation, meeting under the auspices of the ISSM in Hamburg in 2008, agreed on the following interim position statement:

> Acquired premature ejaculation is a subtype of premature ejaculation characterized by 1) a substantial decrease in time to ejaculation compared to a man's previous sexual experience; 2) the inability to delay ejaculation on all or nearly all vaginal penetrations; and 3) negative personal consequences, such as distress, worry, frustration, and/or the avoidance of sexual intimacy.

This expert panel agreed that further clinical research is required to obtain IELT data, as well as patient-reported outcome data, for men with acquired premature ejaculation.

Other Subtypes of Premature Ejaculation

Based on data obtained from large-scale surveys on the prevalence of premature ejaculation in the general population (Patrick et al. 2005), Waldinger and Schweitzer (2006b) postulated that in addition to lifelong premature ejaculation and acquired premature ejaculation, two other premature ejaculation subtypes can be diagnosed: natural variable premature ejaculation and premature-like ejaculatory dysfunction (Waldinger and Schweitzer 2006b, 2008; Waldinger 2006, 2007c). In *natural variable premature ejaculation*, a man only occasionally and incidentally experiences early ejaculation. This incidentally occurring early ejaculation should not be regarded as a symptom of underlying psychopathology, but instead as a manifestation of normal variation of ejaculation time. Treatment consists of psychoeducation and reassurance that no pathology is involved.

Men with *premature-like ejaculatory dysfunction* complain about premature ejaculation, although from an objective point of view, their ejaculation time is normal or even prolonged (e.g., 3–20 minutes). Treatment should consist of counseling, psychoeducation, and sometimes psychotherapy. Currently, however, no evidence-based outcome data are available regarding these treatments in this premature ejaculation subgroup. Colin from Case Example 3 probably has premature-like ejaculatory dysfunction.

Men with natural variable premature ejaculation and premature-like ejaculatory dysfunction are rarely seen at outpatient urological or sex therapy clinics. The existence of these groups of men has been derived mainly from epidemiological surveys. Because the prevalences of lifelong premature ejaculation and acquired premature ejaculation are probably rather low (about 5%–10%), the very high prevalence rates of 20%–30% of premature ejaculation in the general male population is likely determined by the large number of males who are dissatisfied with their sexual ejaculatory performance despite actually having normal ejaculation times (Waldinger and Schweitzer 2008). This becomes evident in, for example, a blinded timer device study among 474 men from five countries (Waldinger et al., in press). In this survey of the general male population from the Netherlands, United Kingdom, Spain, Turkey, and the United States, the median IELT was 6 minutes (range = 0.1–52.1 minutes). Males were asked whether they were discontented with their IELT and whether they were interested in taking active drugs to delay their ejaculation. More than a third (38%) reported that their IELT was shorter than they would have liked. Of these men, 64% (23% of the total sample) showed willingness to take medication to increase their latency time. This subpopulation of men was found to have a median IELT of 4.9 minutes, which is slightly lower than the median of 6.0 minutes of the overall population. In other words, despite their complaints of premature ejaculation, these men had just normal ejaculation time.

Drug Treatment of Premature Ejaculation

The treatment of premature ejaculation with drugs depends on the premature ejaculation subtype and the underlying etiology and pathogenesis (Waldinger 2008a). Drug treatment consists of daily and on-demand drug treatment.

Daily Drug Treatment

Evidence-based psychopharmacological research has demonstrated that use of some SSRIs, such as paroxetine 20 mg/day, sertraline 50–100 mg/day, and citalopram 20–40 mg/day, as well as clomipramine 10–20 mg/day, which is the most serotonergic of the tricyclic antidepressants, may clinically and statistically significantly delay ejaculation compared with placebo (Waldinger et al. 2004). Of all SSRIs and clomipramine, use of paroxetine 20 mg/day exerts the strongest ejaculation delay (Waldinger et al. 2004). However, the use of SSRIs and clomipramine in the treatment of premature ejaculation is off-label. The daily intake of these serotonergic antidepressants has a number of advantages over the intake of drugs a few hours before intercourse (on-demand intake). Using a daily drug strategy, sexual contact may take place at any moment of the day with about an 80% chance of a moderate to very strong ejaculation delay (Waldinger 2007b). Moreover, the daily use of drugs does not interfere with the desirable spontaneity of having sexual contact on the spur of the moment, because ejaculation will be delayed for nearly all intercourses. In addition, the risk of nausea or other gastrointestinal side effects during sexual contact is diminished after 1–3 weeks due to habituation of the gastrointestinal tract to the serotonergic component of this group of drugs (Waldinger 2007b).

The side effects of the SSRIs and clomipramine vary based on short- and long-term use (Waldinger 2007b). In the short term, SSRIs may give rise particularly to fatigue and yawning, but also to a vague feeling of nausea, flatulence, loose stools, and increased perspiration. Usually, these side effects diminish and then disappear after 2–3 weeks of daily treatment. However, over the long term, SSRIs may cause weight gain and sometimes erectile difficulties and decreased sexual desire. In addition to these serotonergic side effects, clomipramine may give rise to anticholinergic side effects, such as dry mouth, blurred vision, and constipation. The clinician needs to inform patients about these aforementioned side effects when prescribing the drugs. If the side effects are too disturbing or continue for a long time, the patient should be advised to stop taking the drugs, gradually reducing the daily dosage to prevent the occurrence of SSRI discontinuation syndrome. The clinician can then prescribe another SSRI that may cause fewer side effects.

On-Demand Drug Treatment

Compared with daily treatment with SSRIs, the on-demand use of serotonergic antidepressants a few hours before intercourse in general leads to less ejaculation delay in men with lifelong premature ejaculation. The on-demand use of these drugs, however, has an increased risk of gastrointestinal side effects (particularly nausea) a few hours after drug intake, which could potentially co-occur with the moment of intercourse. Another disadvantage of on-demand drug use is that it may have a negative effect on the spontaneity of sex. For many men and their partners, it is rather inconvenient to be thinking most of the time whether or not they dare have sex (Waldinger et al. 2007). However, despite these drawbacks, the on-demand use of clomipramine 20–40 mg, about 4–6 hours prior to coitus, may lead to a clinically relevant and satisfactory ejaculation delay, due to the drug's serotonergic and sympatholytic properties. The on-demand use of serotonergic antidepressants may also have advantages over daily treatment. On-demand use of a drug reduces the chance of interactions with other drugs, as well as interactions with alcohol. For men who have no steady partner or are content in a relationship with a rather low coitus frequency, on-demand drugs are likely preferable. Advising daily intake of SSRIs to men who have sexual contact perhaps only once or twice per month is dubious practice. For on-demand treatment, tramadol, phosphodiesterase type 5 (PDE5) inhibitors, and EMLA cream are available, but their use to treat premature ejaculation is off-label.

Tramadol. Two studies have been published on the ejaculation-delaying effect of tramadol 50–100 mg (Safarinejad and Hosseini 2006; Salem et al. 2008). The on-demand use of the drug 1–3 hours prior to coitus may lead to a delayed ejaculation. The precise cause of the induced ejaculation delay is unclear; the delay may be related to the serotonin reuptake inhibitory property of the drug, as it is rather unlikely to be caused by its antagonistic effect on the μ-receptor. Due to the drug's opioid affinity, the patient should be informed about the risk of drug dependency when taking tramadol on a more regular basis.

PDE5 inhibitors. PDE5 inhibitors, such as sildenafil, tadalafil, and vardenafil, may effectively treat the cause of premature ejaculation, particularly in the case of acquired premature ejaculation that is the result of erectile difficulties. These drugs facilitate erectile function and therefore diminish the chance that a man decides to (prematurely) ejaculate as a way to mask his difficulty to maintain his erection. Because the PDE5 inhibitors have no effect on actual ejaculation time, these drugs are not useful for men with lifelong premature ejaculation and no erectile difficulties. Although some publications have recommended PDE5 inhibitors for men with lifelong premature ejaculation, the methodology of these studies is rather weak (McMahon et al. 2006a, 2006b). Moreover, the use of PDE5 inhibitors to treat premature ejaculation has not been approved by the U.S. Food and Drug Administration (FDA).

EMLA cream.   The use of anesthetizing creams and sprays to delay ejaculation is the oldest known pharmacological method of treating premature ejaculation (Schapiro 1943). A few studies have demonstrated that creams containing lidocaine and prilocaine, such as EMLA cream, may delay ejaculation. However, few men with lifelong premature ejaculation report much success using EMLA cream, and few studies have been published on these negative treatment results. EMLA cream has not been approved by the FDA for treating premature ejaculation.

New drugs for premature ejaculation.   Since the 1990s, the SSRIs and clomipramine have become the most popular drugs used to treat premature ejaculation. However, they have not been officially registered with the FDA or the European Medicines Agency (EMEA) for the treatment of premature ejaculation; the pharmaceutical companies that have produced these drugs have never been interested in drug treatment of premature ejaculation, for marketing reasons. Likewise, the companies producing tramadol and PDE5 inhibitors have not been interested in the treatment of premature ejaculation. Currently, however, two pharmaceutical companies are interested in the registration of their drugs, dapoxetine and TEMPE, for treating premature ejaculation.

Dapoxetine.   In 2009, the EMEA registered dapoxetine for on-demand treatment of premature ejaculation in Europe. Dapoxetine, an SSRI, was originally developed by Eli Lilly as an antidepressant with a short half-life ("Dapoxetine" 2005). Because of its pharmacokinetic properties, such as its short half-life, the drug is suitable for on-demand use to treat premature ejaculation. Two placebo-controlled trials have shown that when taken 1–3 hours before intercourse, dapoxetine leads to statistically significant delay in ejaculation compared with placebo (Pryor et al. 2006). However, the extent of ejaculation delay seems to be rather weak, based on the reported drug-induced normal IELT distribution (Waldinger et al. 2008). Dapoxetine has not been approved by the FDA as a drug to treat premature ejaculation.

TEMPE.   TEMPE, an anesthesizing topical spray containing lidocaine and prilocaine, has been developed by the British company Plethora Solutions specifically to treat premature ejaculation (Dinsmore et al. 2007). The spray penetrates the skin of the glans penis immediately, whereas creams and sprays containing lidocaine and prilocaine penetrate the skin at a much slower rate. Dinsmore et al. (2007) found that the spray delays ejaculation without clinically relevant side effects. The finding that the induced geometric mean IELT is somewhat shorter than the induced mean IELT indicates that the drug has potential to delay ejaculation (Waldinger et al. 2008). TEMPE has not yet been approved by the FDA or EMEA for the treatment of premature ejaculation.

Psychological Treatment of Premature Ejaculation

Premature ejaculation was long regarded as a psychological disorder that had to be treated by psychotherapy. Various psychological treatments, including psychoanalytic (Waldinger 2006), psychosomatic (Schapiro 1943), and behavioral (Masters and Johnson 1970; Semans 1956) approaches, have been suggested, but only a few more or less well-controlled studies have investigated their results (O'Donohue et al. 1993). For many years, the outcome objective of psychological intervention has been the prolongation of the IELT. However, the majority of studies investigating psychological interventions for delaying ejaculation lack the robust methodology that has been used in drug treatment studies of lifelong premature ejaculation. A better objective for psychological intervention is likely the improvement of a mutually satisfying sexual relationship between the patient and his partner. Because premature ejaculation may lead to sexual problems for the patient's partner or to relationship problems, the clinician should assess the relationship and the partner's well-being.

A variety of psychotherapeutic approaches to premature ejaculation have been described, but their efficacy has not been evaluated in properly controlled and adequately powered trials, and the different therapeutic modalities have not been compared in formal studies. Only some men who seek treatment for premature ejaculation are likely to require in-depth psychotherapy (McMahon et al. 2006a, 2006b). Despite hard evidence on the efficacy of psychotherapy, behavioral retraining is still often practiced by sexologists. The most common behavioral treatments are the stop-start method (Semans 1956) and the squeeze technique (Masters and Johnson 1970). The basis of behavioral retraining is the hypothesis that premature ejaculation occurs because the man fails to appreciate the sensations of heightened arousal and recognize the feelings of ejaculatory inevitability.

Stop-Start Method

In 1956, Semans described a direct behavioral treatment for premature ejaculation. He developed what is now known as the stop-start method. This method was embedded within a framework of therapy that involved both the individual with premature ejaculation and his partner. The first step in the treatment is to interview each partner separately, with the aim of modifying any misconceptions the partners may have about the therapy. Also, the partners are instructed to rest, if either is fatigued, before beginning the therapy. Once "love play" is begun, the partners are instructed to touch each other and to progress toward genital stimulation. When the man begins to experience sensations indicative of an approaching ejaculation, he tells his partner, who immediately stops stimulating him. Once the subjective sensation of high arousal disappears, genital stimulation is reintroduced and again interrupted when similar sensations reappear. This cycle is repeated until the male is able to postpone ejaculation indefinitely. Upon successful postponement of ejaculation following these initial instructions, the partners are again interviewed, separately and then together, with the aim of introducing the next step, which is stimulation of the penis with the aid of lubrication. The reasoning behind this step is that the initial "dry" stimulation of the penis does not adequately match the sensations that will be felt once vaginal penetration is reintroduced. Once indefinite postponement of ejaculation is reached using the lubricant, intercourse without premature ejaculation should be possible, according to Semans. He presented the results of this treatment for 8 of an initial 14 couples. The remaining 6 were dropped from treatment or could not be followed up.

O'Donohue et al. (1993) pointed out several methodological weaknesses in Semans's study. For example, no control group was used, and assessment of change relied solely upon the self-report by the husband and wife, with more truth being attributed to what the wife reported. Although Semans did not address this issue specifically, he did demonstrate awareness of the role of social pressures (e.g., to report sexual satisfaction rather than dissatisfaction) by recommending the separate assessment of both partners (O'Donohue et al. 1993).

Squeeze Technique and Sensate Focus

The sexologist couple Masters and Johnson (1970) described a very high success rate for couples using their squeeze method. Their technique appears

similar to Semans's start-stop method in that it involves inclusion of the partner, manual stimulation of the penis prior to vaginal stimulation, and use of
a modified stop-start technique. In this technique, in addition to cessation of
movement, the partner squeezes the glans penis firmly between the thumb
and the first two fingers to reduce tumescence. During the final step of this
method, when the penis is stimulated within the vagina, the woman lifts herself off the penis and applies the squeeze until the man's arousal subsides. Masters and Johnson, like Semans, emphasized the benefits of first explaining to
the couple that their problem is readily amenable to treatment. However, they
emphasized intense daily therapy sessions and, when possible, the social seclu-
sion of the treatment couple. Their therapy was a long and involved process. Although Masters and Johnson claimed a 97% success rate with their so-called
squeeze technique for delaying ejaculation, no other investigators have been
able to replicate this very high percentage of success.

Concurrent with practicing the squeeze technique, the couple is encouraged to spend time in mutual pleasuring involving nongenital massage and
caressing, following the program known as sensate focus. This is suggested to
reduce the genital-focused interaction of the ejaculatory control process. Sensate focus requires a cooperative partner and sufficient time to follow the program properly. Moreover, manual penile stimulation must be culturally
acceptable.

Research on Behavioral Techniques

Even with the extensions of Semans's technique provided by Masters and
Johnson (1970), the few controlled studies that have been conducted have
been unable to demonstrate that these behavioral techniques can definitely
cure premature ejaculation (De Amicis et al. 1985; Hawton et al. 1986). Despite many anecdotal reports of the efficacy of this technique, as well as reports of short-term success rates ranging from 60% to almost 100% (Clarke
and Parry 1973; Masters and Johnson 1970), the methodology and design of
these studies have been weak and fail to meet the criteria of evidence-based
research. In addition, long-term maintenance of ejaculatory control induced
by these treatments has been shown to be very low (De Amicis et al. 1985).

Must one conclude that the overall efficacy of these techniques is insufficient to treat premature ejaculation? The answer is no. In my opinion, these

techniques have not been adequately studied according to the current standards of evidence-based research specifically designed to investigate premature ejaculation. The rather high dropout rate (43%) in Semans's (1956) sample and the contrasting very high success rate (97%) reported by Masters and Johnson (1970) may have been influenced by the type of premature ejaculation their patients had (Waldinger 2008b; Waldinger and Schweitzer 2008). The authors did not specify what percentage of their population had lifelong or acquired premature ejaculation, how frequently these men suffered from premature ejaculation, and how short their ejaculation time was in the majority of their intercourses (i.e., whether these men had natural variable premature ejaculation or premature-like ejaculatory dysfunction). Behavioral treatment might be much more successful in men with premature-like ejaculatory dysfunction than in men with lifelong or acquired premature ejaculation (Waldinger 2008b; Waldinger and Schweitzer 2008).

Clinical Interview of Men With Complaints of Premature Ejaculation

During the clinical interview of a man with complaints of premature ejaculation, the clinician should ask the following questions:

- *What exactly is "premature"?* Is it premature for you, for your sexual partner, or for both of you? Can you estimate the time that usually passes after you have penetrated the vagina before you get an ejaculation? Does ejaculation occur so quickly that you can count the number of penile thrusts? If so, after how many thrusts do you get an ejaculation?
- *How often do you have a premature ejaculation?* Does premature ejaculation occur always, nearly always, or only sometimes? In what percentage of attempts at having sex do you have premature ejaculation?
- *For how long have you experienced premature ejaculation?* Have you experienced early ejaculations from your first sexual encounters, or did problems with ejaculation begin only at a certain age? At what age did early ejaculations begin?
- *Do you also ejaculate outside the vagina when this has not been the purpose?* How often do you ejaculate outside the vagina? Do you ejaculate at the

moment of penetration or after only two or three strokes following penetration?

- *Whose plan was it to seek treatment?* Did you decide to seek treatment, or are you seeking treatment at your partner's request? What exactly do you expect from treatment for premature ejaculation?
- *Do you talk about premature ejaculation with your sexual partner?* What did your partner tell you? Does your partner agree that you have premature ejaculation?
- *How is your relationship with your partner in general?* Are you happy with each other? Are there any problems in the relationship? If so, do you think that your relationship in general may interfere with your sexual relationship?
- *How is your general health?* Do you have any problems getting or maintaining an erection? Have you ever had some problems with your thyroid gland or with voiding? Did you ever have complaints of prostatitis?

Because different treatments for premature ejaculation are available, the clinician should try to get an idea of the patient's willingness to accept a certain treatment. Moreover, the clinician should carefully consider whether a certain treatment is also suitable for the patient. For example, before prescribing serotonergic antidepressants, the clinician needs to ask questions about the use of other drugs that may interfere with the use of SSRIs, about previous treatments, and about contraindications for SSRI treatment. The patient should also be consulted regarding his preference for a specific treatment. To get more information about this preference, the clinician can ask the following questions:

- *What do you have in mind about treatment?* What do you know about treatment? Have you read on the Internet or in books about available treatment options? What do you expect from treatment? What are your partner's expectations?
- *Would you prefer to take a drug on a daily basis or only a few hours before intercourse?* How often do you have sexual contact? With a frequency of two or three times a week, I recommend daily treatment with a serotonergic antidepressant. What would you think of taking daily medication? With a frequency of two or three times a month, I suggest taking a drug only a few hours before intercourse. What would you think of that type of treatment?

Conclusion

Since the mid-1990s, men have shown an increasing interest in drug treatment for premature ejaculation, as well as for delayed ejaculation. Currently, however, no drugs are available to treat delayed ejaculation, and research into drug treatment for premature ejaculation has been conducted by clinicians and neuroscientists with hardly any financial support from pharmaceutical companies. A considerable number of studies have shown that daily use of some SSRIs and clomipramine delays ejaculation effectively and that the initial side effects diminish and even disappear after about 3 weeks. The on-demand use of PDE5 inhibitors is particularly useful in men who have premature ejaculation on the basis of erectile difficulties. The recent interest of the pharmaceutical industry is welcomed, but the registration of a new drug, whether it effectively or inadequately delays ejaculation, may lead to new hype that accompanies marketing strategies of the producing pharmaceutical companies. A well-known marketing strategy is to criticize effective and safe treatment strategies that have previously been accepted by the medical community (Waldinger 2008a). Therefore, prescribing physicians need to remain informed through independent studies—that is, studies conducted and written by authors other than those of the pharmaceutical company and their advisers or medical writers (Waldinger 2008a).

Apart from the developments in drug treatment for premature ejaculation, important progress has been made in the research of a better and more appropriate classification of premature ejaculation. Research into the recently proposed classification of four premature ejaculation subtypes, genetic research (Janssen et al. 2009), as well as pharmacogenetic and animal research, may contribute to a better understanding of their etiology, pathogenesis, and treatments in the next decade.

Key Points

- Various behavioral treatments are indicated for delayed ejaculation, but no hard evidence exists to support their efficacy.
- Drug treatment for delayed ejaculation is currently not available.

- Men with lifelong premature ejaculation always or nearly always ejaculate within about 1 minute after vaginal penetration.

- A physical examination is usually not required after the diagnosis of lifelong premature ejaculation has been made.

- In men with acquired premature ejaculation, a physical examination and various laboratory tests are required for confirming the diagnosis.

- In premature-like ejaculatory dysfunction, men complain of premature ejaculation, but the IELT is in the normal range or even has a long duration.

- Daily treatment with paroxetine 20 mg exerts the strongest ejaculation delay in men with lifelong premature ejaculation, but its use is off-label.

- After on-demand treatment with clomipramine, a man should wait 4–6 hours before starting intercourse.

- Psychological counseling may improve a mutually satisfying sexual relationship between the patient and his partner.

References

Althof S: The psychology of premature ejaculation: therapies and consequences. J Sex Med 3 (suppl 4):324–331, 2006

American Psychiatric Association: Diagnostic and Statistical Manual of Mental Disorders, 3rd Edition. Washington, DC, American Psychiatric Association, 1980

American Psychiatric Association: Diagnostic and Statistical Manual of Mental Disorders, 3rd Edition, Revised. Washington, DC, American Psychiatric Association, 1987

American Psychiatric Association: Diagnostic and Statistical Manual of Mental Disorders, 4th Edition. Washington, DC, American Psychiatric Association, 1994

American Psychiatric Association: Diagnostic and Statistical Manual of Mental Disorders, 4th Edition, Text Revision. Washington, DC, American Psychiatric Association, 2000

Apfelbaum B: Retarded ejaculation: a much-misunderstood syndrome, in Principles and Practice of Sex Therapy: Update for the 1990s, 2nd Edition. Edited by Leiblum SR, Rosen RC. New York, Guilford, 1989, pp 168–206

Beach FA: Comparison of copulatory behavior of male rats raised in isolation, cohabitation, and segregation. J Genet Psychol 60:3–13, 1942

Beckerman H, Becher J, Lankhorst GJ: The effectiveness of vibratory stimulation in an ejaculatory man with spinal cord injury. Paraplegia 31:689–699, 1993

Carani C, Isidori AM, Granata A, et al: Multicenter study on the prevalence of sexual symptoms in male hypo- and hyperthyroid patients. J Clin Endocrinol Metab 90:6472–6479, 2005

Clarke M, Parry L: Premature ejaculation treated by the dual sex team method of Masters and Johnson. Aust N Z J Psychiatry 7:200–205, 1973

Coleman CC, King BR, Bolden-Watson C, et al: A placebo-controlled comparison of the effects on sexual functioning of bupropion sustained release and fluoxetine. Clin Ther 23:1040–1058, 2001

Dapoxetine: LY210448. Drugs R D 6:307–311, 2005

De Amicis LA, Goldberg DC, LoPiccolo J, et al: Clinical follow-up of couples treated for sexual dysfunction. Arch Sex Behav 14:467–490, 1985

Dekker J: Inhibited male orgasm, in Handbook of Sexual Dysfunctions. Edited by O'Donohue W, Geer JH. Boston, MA, Allyn & Bacon, 1993, pp 279–301

Delmonte MM: Case reports on the use of meditative relaxation as an intervention strategy with retarded ejaculation. Biofeedback Self Regul 9:209–214, 1984

Delmonte M, Braidwood M: Treatment of retarded ejaculation with psychotherapy and meditative relaxation: a case report. Psychol Rep 47:8–10, 1980

Dinsmore WW, Hackett G, Goldmeier D, et al: Topical eutectic mixture for premature ejaculation (TEMPE): a novel aerosol-delivery form of lidocaine-prilocaine for treating premature ejaculation. BJU Int 99:369–375, 2007

Drago F, Busa L: Acute low doses of melatonin restore full sexual activity in impotent male rats. Brain Res 878:98–104, 2000

Fugl-Meyer AR, Fugl-Meyer KS: Sexual disabilities, problems and satisfaction in 18–74 year old Swedes. Scandinavian Journal of Sexology 2:79–105, 1999

Gagliardi FA: *Ejaculatio retardata*: conventional psychotherapy and sex therapy in a severe obsessive-compulsive disorder. Am J Psychother 30:85–94, 1976

Georgiadis JR, Holstege G: Ejaculation or no ejaculation: the left anterior temporal lobe decides? Program No. 214.18.2004 Abstract. Washington, DC, Society for Neuroscience, 2004

Gessa GL, Paglietti E, Quarantotti BP: Induction of copulatory behavior in sexually inactive rats by naloxone. Science 204:203–205, 1979

Godpodinoff ML: Premature ejaculation: clinical subgroups and etiology. J Sex Marital Ther 15:130–134, 1989

Haensel SM, Mos J, Olivier B, et al: Sex behavior of male and female Wistar rats affected by the serotonin agonist 8-OH-DPAT. Pharmacol Biochem Behav 40:221–228, 1991

Hawton K, Catalan J, Martin P, et al: Prognostic factors in sex therapy. Behav Res Ther 24:377–385, 1986

Holstege G, Georgiadis JR, Paans AM, et al: Brain activation during human male ejaculation. J Neurosci 23:9185–9193, 2003

Janssen PKC, Bakker SC, Réthelyi J, et al: Serotonin transporter promoter region (5-HTTLPR) polymorphism is associated with the intravaginal ejaculation latency time in Dutch men with lifelong premature ejaculation. J Sex Med 6:276–284, 2009

Kaplan HS: Retarded ejaculation, in The New Sex Therapy. Edited by Kaplan HS. New York, Brunner/Mazel, 1974, pp 316–338

Laumann EO, Paik A, Rosen RC: Sexual dysfunction in the United States: prevalence and predictors. JAMA 281:537–544, 1999

Líndal E, Stefànsson JG: The lifetime prevalence of psychosexual dysfunction among 55- to 57-year-olds in Iceland. Soc Psychiatry Psychiatr Epidemiol 28:91–95, 1993

Masters WH, Johnson VE: Human Sexual Inadequacy. Boston, MA: Little, Brown, 1970

McMahon CG, McMahon CN, Leow LJ, et al: Efficacy of type-5 phosphodiesterase inhibitors in the drug treatment of premature ejaculation: a systematic review. BJU Int 98:259–272, 2006a

McMahon CG, Waldinger MD, Rowland D, et al: Ejaculatory disorders, in Standard Practice in Sexual Medicine. Edited by Porst H, Buvat J, Standards Committee of the ISSM. Oxford, UK, Blackwell, 2006b, pp 188–209

McMahon CG, Althof S, Waldinger MD, et al: An evidence-based definition of lifelong premature ejaculation: report of the International Society for Sexual Medicine Ad Hoc Committee for the Definition of Premature Ejaculation. BJU Int 102:338–350, 2008

Mos J, Olivier B, Bloetjes K, et al: Drug-induced facilitation of sexual behaviour in the male rat: behavioural and pharmacological aspects, in Psychoneuroendocrinology of Growth and Development. Edited by Slob AK, Baum MJ. Rotterdam, The Netherlands, Medicom, 1990, pp 221–232

Mos J, Van Logten J, Bloetjes K, et al: The effects of idazoxan and 8-OH-DPAT on sexual behaviour and associated ultrasonic vocalizations in the rat. Neurosci Biobehav Rev 15:505–515, 1991

Munjack DJ, Kanno PH: Retarded ejaculation: a review. Arch Sex Behav 8:139–150, 1979

O'Donohue W, Letourneau E, Geer JH: Premature ejaculation, in Handbook of Sexual Dysfunctions. Edited by O'Donohue W, Geer JH. Boston, MA, Allyn & Bacon, 1993, pp 303–333

Olivier B, van Oorschot R, Waldinger MD: Serotonin, serotonergic receptors, selective serotonin reuptake inhibitors and sexual behaviour. Int Clin Psychopharmacol 13 (suppl 6): S9–S14, 1998

Ottani A, Giuliani D, Ferrari F: Modulatory activity of sildenafil on copulatory behaviour of both intact and castrated male rats. Pharmacol Biochem Behav 72:717–722, 2002

Patrick DL, Althof SE, Pryor JL, et al: Premature ejaculation: an observational study of men and their partners. J Sex Med 2:358–367, 2005

Pattij T, de Jong T, Uitterdijk A, et al: Individual differences in male rat ejaculatory behavior: searching for models to study ejaculation disorders. Eur J Neurosci 22:724–734, 2005a

Pattij T, Olivier B, Waldinger MD: Animal models of ejaculatory behaviour. Curr Pharm Des 11:4069–4077, 2005b

Pryor JL, Althof SE, Steidle C, et al; Dapoxetine Study Group: Efficacy and tolerability of dapoxetine in the treatment of premature ejaculation: integrated analysis of two randomized, double-blind, placebo-controlled trials. Lancet 368:929–937, 2006

Riley AJ, Riley EJ: Partial ejaculatory incompetence: the therapeutic effect of midodrine, an orally active selective alpha-adrenoceptor agonist. Eur Urol 8:155–160, 1982

Safarinejad MR, Hosseini SY: Safety and efficacy of tramadol in the treatment of premature ejaculation: a double-blind, placebo-controlled, fixed-dose, randomized study. J Clin Psychopharmacol 26:27–31, 2006

Salem EA, Wilson SK, Bissada NK, et al: Tramadol HCL has promise in on-demand use to treat premature ejaculation. J Sex Med 5:188–193, 2008

Schapiro B: Premature ejaculation: a review of 1130 cases. J Urol 50:374–379, 1943

Semans JH: Premature ejaculation: a new approach. South Med J 49:353–357, 1956

Shamloul R, El-Nashaar A: Chronic prostatitis in premature ejaculation: a cohort study in 153 men. J Sex Med 3:150–154, 2006

Shull GR, Sprenkle DH: Retarded ejaculation reconceptualization and implications for treatment. J Sex Marital Ther 60:234–246, 1980

Spira A, Bajos N, Giami A, et al: Cross-national comparisons of sexual behaviour surveys: methodological difficulties and lessons for prevention. Am J Public Health 88:730–731, 1998

Trinchieri A, Magri V, Cariani L, et al: Prevalence of sexual dysfunction in men with chronic prostatitis/chronic pelvic pain syndrome. Arch Ital Urol Androl 79:67–70, 2007

Waldinger MD: Use of psychoactive agents in the treatment of sexual dysfunction. CNS Drugs 6:204–216, 1996

Waldinger MD: The neurobiological approach to premature ejaculation (review). J Urol 168:2359–2367, 2002

Waldinger MD: Lifelong premature ejaculation: from authority-based to evidence-based medicine. BJU Int 93:201–207, 2004

Waldinger MD: The need for a revival of psychoanalytic investigations into premature ejaculation. J Mens Health Gend 3:390–396, 2006

Waldinger MD: Four measures of investigating ejaculatory performance. J Sex Med 4:520, 2007a

Waldinger MD: Premature ejaculation: definition and drug treatment. Drugs 67:547–568, 2007b

Waldinger MD: Premature ejaculation: state of the art. Urol Clin North Am 34:591–599, 2007c

Waldinger MD: New challenges: the need for independency (editorial). Sexologies 17:3–4, 2008a

Waldinger MD: Premature ejaculation: different pathophysiologies and etiologies determine its treatment. J Sex Marital Ther 34:1–13, 2008b

Waldinger MD, Schweitzer DH: Retarded ejaculation in men: an overview of psychological and neurobiological insights. World J Urol 23:76–81, 2005

Waldinger MD, Schweitzer DH: Changing paradigms from a historical DSM-III and DSM-IV view toward an evidence-based definition of premature ejaculation, part I: validity of DSM-IV-TR. J Sex Med 3:682–692, 2006a

Waldinger MD, Schweitzer DH: Changing paradigms from a historical DSM-III and DSM-IV view toward an evidence-based definition of premature ejaculation, part II: proposals for DSM-V and ICD-11. J Sex Med 3:693–705, 2006b

Waldinger MD, Schweitzer DH: The use of old and recent DSM definitions of premature ejaculation in observational studies: a contribution to the present debate for a new classification of PE in the DSM-V. J Sex Med 5:1079–1087, 2008

Waldinger MD, Hengeveld MW, Zwinderman AH: Paroxetine treatment of premature ejaculation: a double-blind, randomized, placebo-controlled study. Am J Psychiatry 151:1377–1379, 1994

Waldinger MD, Berendsen HHG, Blok BFM, et al: Premature ejaculation and serotonergic antidepressants-induced delayed ejaculation: the involvement of the serotonergic system. Behav Brain Res 92:111–118, 1998a

Waldinger MD, Hengeveld MW, Zwinderman AH, et al: A double-blind, randomized, placebo-controlled study with fluoxetine, fluvoxamine, paroxetine and sertraline. J Clin Psychopharmacol 18:274–281, 1998b

Waldinger MD, Hengeveld MW, Zwinderman AH, et al: An empirical operationalization study of DSM-IV diagnostic criteria for premature ejaculation. International Journal of Psychiatry in Clinical Practice 2:287–293, 1998c

Waldinger MD, Zwinderman AH, Schweitzer DH, et al: Relevance of methodological design for the interpretation of efficacy of drug treatment of premature ejaculation: a systematic review and meta-analysis. Int J Impot Res 16:369–381, 2004

Waldinger MD, Quinn P, Dilleen M, et al: A multinational population survey of intravaginal ejaculation latency time. J Sex Med 2:492–497, 2005a

Waldinger MD, Zwinderman AH, Olivier B, et al: Proposal for a definition of lifelong premature ejaculation based on epidemiological stopwatch data. J Sex Med 2:498–507, 2005b

Waldinger MD, Zwinderman AH, Olivier B, et al: The majority of men with lifelong premature ejaculation prefer daily drug treatment: an observational study in a consecutive group of Dutch men. J Sex Med 4:1028–1037, 2007

Waldinger MD, Zwinderman AH, Olivier B, et al: Geometric mean IELT and premature ejaculation: appropriate statistics to avoid overestimation of treatment efficacy. J Sex Med 5:492–499, 2008

Waldinger MD, McIntosh J, Schweitzer DH: A five-nation survey to assess the distribution of the Intravaginal Ejaculatory Latency Time among the general male population. J Sex Med (in press)

Williams W: Anaesthetic ejaculation. J Sex Marital Ther 11:19–29, 1985

World Health Organization: The ICD-10 Classification of Mental and Behavioural Disorders: Diagnostic Criteria for Research. Geneva, World Health Organization, 1993

11

Dyspareunia and Vaginismus

Melissa A. Farmer, B.A.

Alina Kao, B.A.

Yitzchak M. Binik, Ph.D.

Given the high reported prevalence rates of approximately 15% for sexual pain (Harlow and Stewart 2003; Laumann et al. 1999), every psychiatrist has likely treated a woman with sexual pain, whether or not the clinician has asked about it. The individual and interpersonal impact of these conditions is considerable, ranging from excruciating pain to ruined and unconsummated relationships.

Unfortunately, the established classification of dyspareunia and vaginismus as sexual pain disorders fails to capture the crucial clinical characteristics of these conditions. The term *sexual pain* suggests that these disorders are characterized by discomfort unique to sexual activities; however, this assumption is contradicted by research and clinical experience. In the case of dyspareunia, the pain is not confined to sexual situations but rather is manifested in a variety of nonsexual contexts, including gynecological examinations, bike riding, tampon insertion, and even walking. In the case of vaginismus, the presenting complaint is not pain but instead a difficulty in experiencing vaginal penetration. Furthermore, a large percentage of women diagnosed with vaginismus also meet the criteria for dyspareunia, which further complicates the distinction between these disorders (Reissing et al. 2004). The traditional clinical approach to dyspareunia is to first exclude physical pathology and then to interpret remaining pain psychogenically. This dualistic approach ignores recent advances in the multidimensional experience of pain and exposes women with dyspareunia to physically and psychologically invasive examinations and interventions. This approach also ignores the inherently social/interpersonal dimension of dyspareunia, in which one member of a couple inflicts the pain on the other.

The traditional Masters and Johnson (1970) conceptualization of vaginismus as muscle spasm is also problematic. Vaginal spasm cannot be directly assessed by a psychiatrist, and thus he or she must rely on a gynecologist to confirm spasm. Unfortunately, women with vaginismus are notoriously fearful of gynecological examinations, and gynecologists understandably often give the diagnosis based on a woman's phobic reaction to the threat of penetration rather than on a direct gynecological assessment of spasm or physical pathology. Equally important, more recent research suggests that only a minority of women with vaginismus who are able to undergo an examination show evidence of vaginal muscle spasm. Furthermore, many of these women meet the criteria for dyspareunia (Reissing et al. 2004).

Conceptualizing so-called sexual pain as a family of pain- and fear-related conditions rather than as sexual dysfunction has resulted in the advancement of research and clinical treatment in recent years. For dyspareunia, this approach assumes that the sensory processing of pain is modulated by physiological, cognitive, and emotional factors. With the prolonged experience of genital pain, these psychological factors focus attention on pain and perpetuate mood disturbances and maladaptive cognitions that ultimately maintain the altered sensation, thereby creating a vicious cycle of psychological and physiological reinforcement of pain. For vaginismus, this approach focuses on the fear of pain and penetration and its consequences, including heightened pelvic floor tension that is symptomatic of anxiety rather than muscle spasm. Furthermore, empirical evidence is mounting that vaginismus and dyspareunia are more similar than not, because women with these conditions appear to overlap on a number of dimensions, including pain, physical pathology, muscle tension, fear of pain or sexual intercourse, and behavioral avoidance of painful activities. The traditional conceptualization of dyspareunia and vaginismus may impose an artificial distinction between the two disorders, which ultimately preoccupies a clinician with the task of differential diagnosis rather than with focusing on the common dimensions that define these disorders.

Definitions

Dyspareunia and vaginismus are currently classified as sexual dysfunctions in DSM-IV-TR (American Psychiatric Association 2000). However, they are unlike other sexual dysfunctions in that they do not reflect impairments in one of the phases of the traditional sexual response cycle (i.e., desire, arousal, orgasm, resolution). Intuitively, dyspareunia should be classified in DSM-IV-TR as a pain disorder (307.80), because it is described as clinically distressing pain with important psychological components. Curiously, however, dyspareunia is the only pain condition excluded from the DSM-IV-TR pain disorders.

Although dyspareunia and vaginismus can be divided into subtypes based on duration (i.e., lifelong vs. acquired) and extent (i.e., generalized vs. situational), no standard nomenclature exists for pain-related subtypes of these disorders. In fact, DSM-IV-TR does not recognize that subtypes of pain quality or location exist. Although little work has been reported recently concerning upper vaginal, cervical, and pelvic pains associated with intercourse, all of which are commonly undifferentiated in the catchall term "deep" dyspareunia, much interest has been shown in "superficial," or vulvar, pain (see classification guidelines put forth by the International Society for the Study of Vulvovaginal Disease; Haefner 2007). Provoked vestibulodynia (previously known as vulvar vestibulitis syndrome) is of particular interest because of its high prevalence in premenopausal women and increasing research attention. This condition is defined by pain localized in the vulvar vestibule and elicited by touch or pressure. In contrast to dyspareunia, no known subtypes of vaginismus are currently recognized.

The traditional diagnostic criteria for dyspareunia and vaginismus, as well as limitations for these criteria, are outlined in Table 11–1. The validity of these diagnostic criteria has been the subject of continuing debate (e.g., Binik 2005).

Etiological Theories

No etiological theory of dyspareunia or vaginismus has received strong empirical support. This lack of knowledge may be partially explained by the problematic definitions of dyspareunia and vaginismus (Table 11–1). However, the crux of the difficulty with previous etiological investigations of women with genital pain is that these women show a remarkable diversity in physiological and psychological characteristics. This diversity suggests that the symptoms used to diagnose these disorders may be the product of multiple disease states, chronic abnormal pelvic floor function, and/or complex psychosocial antecedents and consequences of an intensely personal pain. To further complicate the search for etiology, medical diagnoses may not reflect the cause of pain. The factors that originally produced the pain may not be responsible for the maintenance of pain, and the successful treatment of these factors may still leave a woman with unexplained pain. The biomedical and psychosocial predisposing factors that are thought to contribute to dyspareunia and vaginismus are based on correlational data, and to date, no evidence supports a causal role of these factors.

Biomedically oriented causal theories of dyspareunia have focused on a variety of factors—hormonal (e.g., vaginal atrophy, oral contraceptive use, estrogen deficiency), infectious (e.g., recurrent yeast infections, bacterial vaginosis, human papilloma virus, herpes simplex virus), and dermatological (e.g., lichen sclerosis, lichen simplex chronicus, lichen planus, allergic contact dermatitis, vulvar psoriasis)—that may predispose a woman to develop pelvic or genital pain. Only a small percentage of women who experience these conditions will develop chronic dyspareunia. Therefore, chronic pelvic or genital pain of a physiological origin is likely to require a threshold of pathology that cannot be overcome by the body's adaptive immune system. Increasing evidence in women with provoked vestibulodynia suggests that genetic polymorphisms that alter the body's ability to mount a normal immune response,

Table 11–1.   Evaluation of diagnostic criteria for dyspareunia and vaginismus

DSM-IV-TR criteria	Limitations
Dyspareunia	
Recurrent or persistent genital pain associated with sexual intercourse in either a male or female	• Genital pain may occur in nonsexual situations (e.g., gynecological exam, tampon insertion, bicycle riding, walking, standing). • Genital pain may occur "presexually" during first tampon insertion. • Dyspareunia is classified by the major activity with which it interferes. • It is unclear what constitutes "recurrent or persistent" pain (e.g., situational pain may impact few or many sexual encounters). • Dyspareunia may be comorbid with reduced sexual desire and arousal, thereby reducing vaginal lubrication. • Comorbid medical conditions may not be identifiable due to poorly understood pathophysiological causes of pain.
Vaginismus	
Recurrent or persistent involuntary spasm of the musculature of the outer third of the vagina that interferes with sexual intercourse	• The presence of vaginal spasm has not been empirically supported. • Women who are too fearful to undergo gynecological examinations to verify vaginal spasm are typically given the diagnosis anyway. • The nature of the "interference" with sexual intercourse is not specified (i.e., physical, psychological, interpersonal). For example, interference defined as fear of sexual intercourse indicates sexual phobia or sexual aversion. • Despite its classification as a sexual pain disorder, criteria do not specify presence of pain. • Diagnosis of vaginal spasm can be made only by a health professional with experience in pelvic examinations (not typically a psychiatrist).

such as altered interleukin-1, mannose-binding lectin, and melanocortin-1 receptor function, may predispose some women to develop recalcitrant pathological inflammatory conditions more easily. This may be a reason underlying the presumed association of dyspareunia onset and urogenital pathology. Similarly, dyspareunia has been hypothesized to be a symptom of other chronic pain syndromes, including fibromyalgia (Pukall et al. 2006) and neuropathic pain due to pudendal neuralgia or complex regional pain syndrome.

Psychosocial etiological theories of dyspareunia point to the role of impaired sexual function (e.g., disturbances in sexual desire, arousal, orgasm, and satisfaction), maladaptive pain cognitions (e.g., fear of pain, catastrophizing, hypervigilance to pain), a history of sexual or physical abuse, and couple factors (e.g., partner solicitousness and hostility). Although past research has found that compared with healthy control subjects, women with dyspareunia have a variety of psychological differences, including increased anxiety, depression, hostility, and somatization, no empirical evidence has supported an etiological role of these factors in this condition (Desrochers et al. 2008). The proposed causes of vaginismus have spanned physical explanations (e.g., genital abnormalities, pelvic floor dysfunction), psychological factors (e.g., religious orthodoxy, personality), sexual difficulties (e.g., fear of sexual intercourse, sexual phobia, sexual aversion, negative sexual attitudes/guilt, childhood sexual interference), and sexual partner factors (e.g., lack of sexual knowledge or skill, concurrent sexual dysfunction). Some of these etiological theories have persisted since the work of Masters and Johnson (1970), despite a uniform lack of empirical support.

Assessment

Comprehensive assessment and diagnosis of dyspareunia and vaginismus require a multidimensional approach that necessitates concurrent evaluation by a multidisciplinary team, including a mental health professional, gynecologist, and physical therapist. Given the difficulty of organizing simultaneous assessments, communication among these health care professionals is of primary importance. Considering that knowledge concerning both medical and psychosocial factors is required, a psychiatrist is an ideal professional to coordinate a woman's evaluation and treatment. This task would include tracking referrals; maintaining communication between the health care professionals about assessment, treatment, and progress; and providing concurrent support, psychotherapy, and pain management.

The need for a proper multidisciplinary assessment must be balanced with a woman's previous history of experiences with other health care professionals, which is often protracted and a major cause of distress. Certainly, general medical conditions need to be addressed and ruled out. However, even if a medical explanation is found, it is unlikely to fully account for the current pain. Simply referring a woman to yet another gynecologist without offering follow-up may have a profoundly negative impact on the therapeutic alliance if the woman believes the psychiatrist is trying to "get rid" of her. The possibility remains that additional referrals may not result in an improved understanding of the patient's pain or its causes. In such a case, the psychiatrist is faced with evaluating whether the potential psychological fallout of continuing the referral process (i.e., escalated anxiety, feelings of hopelessness, defining herself through her "disease") is manageable for the patient and deciding whether this risk outweighs the potential benefits of continued treatment in the absence of a clear diagnosis. The woman may become frustrated that no one will be able to treat her pain; that the referrals constitute yet another set of hurdles to face; or, worse, that her treatment providers do not believe her pain is real. These feelings are common in chronic pain patients, and exploring the motivations behind a woman's desire for more referrals (or her reluctance to seek additional help) can help to validate her experience.

Differential Diagnosis

Differentially diagnosing the sexual pain disorders is complicated by the considerable overlap in the presenting characteristics of dyspareunia and vaginismus (i.e., genital pain, fear/anxiety about pain, elevated pelvic floor muscle tension, avoidance of intercourse) and their frequent co-occurrence (e.g., Engman et al. 2004; Reissing et al. 2004). Therefore, conceptualizing them as on a continuum may be preferable to thinking of them as two distinct disorders. Furthermore, dyspareunia and vaginismus are often comorbid with other sexual dysfunctions (e.g., hypoactive sexual desire, female sexual arousal disorder, anorgasmia, sexual aversion), which are covered in other chapters.

Pain Assessment

In assessing a woman's pain experienced during sexual intercourse or other activities, the clinician not only gains a better understanding of a woman's pain problem and diagnosis but also validates her experience and suffering. This is a necessary first step toward establishing a strong therapeutic alliance. A comprehensive pain evaluation involves gathering a variety of information.

Location

At the most basic level, pain is categorized by the affected area(s): superficial (i.e., clitoris, labia minora, vulvar vestibule, vaginal entrance), midvaginal, and/or deep/pelvic (i.e., abdomen, ovaries, cervix). The pain may vary in location or occur in multiple sites. Showing women an anatomical diagram of the genitals and pelvis may facilitate an accurate assessment. If a woman is not certain about the location of her pain, the examiner should ask her to go home and examine her genitals with a mirror on her own or with a partner's help. For women who express discomfort with self-examination, a collaborating gynecologist can provide information about pain location.

Quality

Descriptors of the sensory quality of pain may facilitate differential diagnosis. For example, neuropathic pain tends to be perceived as "burning," "shooting," or like an "electric shock," but "sore" and "aching" sensations may point to pain of muscular or tissue origin. For example, provoked vestibulodynia pain is most often described as "burning" or "cutting"; generalized vulvodynia elicits " tingling" and "shooting" sensations; and deep dyspareunia frequently manifests as "diffuse" and "tender" pain. The Short-Form McGill Pain Questionnaire (Melzack 1987) provides a pain adjective checklist that is useful to help women describe their pain (Figure 11–1). Pain descriptors include varying intensities of sensory and affective words that characterize the quality of genital pain. This scale can be used to track the quality and intensity of pain over time.

Intensity

Ratings of pain intensity provide insight into the patient's perceived level of unpleasantness and distress. The clinician can ask patients to rate the inten-

Short-Form McGill Pain Questionnaire

Patient's Name:_____   Date: _____

	None	**Mild**	**Moderate**	**Severe**
1. Throbbing	0	1	2	3
2. Shooting	0	1	2	3
3. Stabbing	0	1	2	3
4. Sharp	0	1	2	3
5. Cramping	0	1	2	3
6. Gnawing	0	1	2	3
7. Hot–Burning	0	1	2	3
8. Aching	0	1	2	3
9. Heavy	0	1	2	3
10. Tender	0	1	2	3
11. Splitting	0	1	2	3
12. Tiring–Exhausting	0	1	2	3
13. Sickening	0	1	2	3
14. Fearful	0	1	2	3
15. Punishing–Cruel	0	1	2	3

Present Pain Intensity

No Pain	0
Mild	1
Discomforting	2
Distressing	3
Horrible	4
Excruciating	5

Figure 11–1.   Short-Form McGill Pain Questionnaire.

The short form of the McGill Pain Questionnaire includes sensory pain descriptors (items 1–11) and affective pain descriptors (items 12–15), with each descriptor rated on a pain intensity scale from *none* (0) to *severe* (3). Sensory and affective domain scores are obtained by summing the values of items 1–11 and 12–15, respectively. The Present Pain Intensity scale measures total pain intensity using a scale range of *no pain* (0) to *excruciating* pain (5).

Source.   Reprinted from Melzack R: "The Short-Form McGill Pain Questionnaire." *Pain* 30:191–197, 1987. Copyright 1987, R. Melzack. Used with permission.

sity of their pain and associated distress on a scale from 0 (*no pain/distress*) to 10 (*worst pain/distress ever experienced*) for each pain-inducing activity.

Elicitation and Duration

Pain may be provoked by the application of pressure, or it may be unprovoked (i.e., spontaneous pain). For example, spontaneously occurring vulvar pain is indicative of generalized vulvodynia, whereas vulvar pain that is elicited by mechanical stimulation (e.g., touch, friction, contact with clothing) is suggestive of provoked vestibulodynia. The clinician should 1) assess the range of activities that evoke pain, including sexual activities and nonsexual situations (e.g., tampon insertion or removal, aerobic activity, urinating, bicycling); 2) note the duration of elicited pain; and 3) record the factors that exacerbate pain (e.g., phase of the menstrual cycle, stress, lack of sexual arousal) and improve pain (e.g., cold or hot compress, physical relaxation, distraction).

Interference

Pain and associated fear and avoidance may interfere with both sexual and nonsexual activities. This information may indicate why the woman is presenting to the clinician and her motivations for seeking treatment. For example, is the woman or couple avoiding sexual activity altogether in response to the pain? Has the presence of vaginismus interfered with the couple's desire to conceive?

History

The onset of pain, including any precipitating events, should be noted. Have there been any changes to the pain since it began (including location, sensory quality, time course)? Note whether the pain is chronic (lasting more than 6 months).

Meaning

The woman's personal attributions and theories about the causes of her dyspareunia mediate her subjective pain experience and provide useful information for treatment formulation. Compared with physical causal attributions, psychosocial causal attributions have been associated with higher pain intensity, increased psychological distress, more marital problems, and sexual aversion (Meana et al. 1999). Therefore, a woman's personal conceptualizations may cue the assessor to her distress level and the possible factors that contribute to and maintain her pain.

Psychosexual Assessment

An in-depth sexual history, involving both partners whenever possible and appropriate, provides important information for case conceptualization and treatment. Furthermore, the woman's motivations for seeking treatment are important to assess and address within the therapeutic process.

Sexual Functioning

The interference with sexual desire, arousal, and orgasm that is caused by dyspareunia or vaginismus is nonspecific. As a result, the clinician needs to assess the impact of pain on each phase of the sexual response cycle to determine comorbid sexual dysfunction. The patient or couple should be questioned about previous experiences with vaginal penetration (e.g., tampon use, finger insertion), masturbation, the couple's typical sexual routine (i.e., initiation, foreplay, intercourse positions, afterplay, and the emotions associated with sexual activities), and past and current frequency of sexual activity and satisfaction. Partners may also develop sexual dysfunction as a consequence of their reaction to the woman's pain.

Sexual History

The woman or couple should be asked about parental, familial, religious, and cultural attitudes toward sexuality that form the framework for their sexual identities. They also should be asked about their first and early sexual experiences, as well as sexual or physical abuse and trauma.

Relationship History

The clinician should discuss with the woman or couple the quality of and satisfaction with past and present relationships, including the impact of sexual difficulties on distress, couple dynamics, and couple factors that may influence genital pain. Dyspareunia and vaginismus are often associated with an avoidance of physical contact, decreased intimacy, interpersonal conflict, guilt, and compromised sexual functioning in the partner. Genital pain developing within a long-established and happy couple may have less impact on overall couple satisfaction and cause less distress than in new or younger couples. Particular attention should be paid to the assessment of relationship adjustment, approach-withdrawal behaviors, sexual avoidance within the relationship, and partner solicitousness and hostility that are frequently correlated with increased pain intensity (Desrosiers et al. 2007). The clinician should assess whether dyspareunia or vaginismus has occurred in previous sexual relationships, whether the occurrence is partner specific, or whether the dysfunction has varied over time with the same partner.

Psychosocial Impact of Dyspareunia/Vaginismus

A thorough assessment of mood, comorbid psychiatric disturbances, and pain coping style provides valuable information for clinical management. As with other pain conditions, sexual pain is associated with depressive and anxious affect (Payne et al. 2005). Because vaginismus is characterized by an intense phobia-like fear of vaginal penetration or associated pain and avoidance of sexual contact, the clinician should assess comorbid fear and aversion toward sexual contact. Similarly, but to a somewhat lesser degree, fear and behavioral avoidance are also frequent results of recurrent dyspareunia. Furthermore, when a woman's genitals become a source of pain and suffering, she may experience a sense of loss, a decreased sense of femininity, low self-esteem, and impaired body image.

Practice Point

Ask the patient to provide a detailed description of her and her partner's reactions immediately following the experience of pain during sexual activity. Her description will provide valuable information about how the couple has learned to cope with the dyspareunia. Do they continue engaging in less painful sexual activity? Do they stop sexual activity altogether and not talk about what has happened?

Medical Assessment

Painful intercourse may be a symptom of physical pathology, and the patient should be referred for appropriate medical assessment(s) if she has not already received adequate medical treatment and pain management. Medical examination procedures often vary from one specialist to another, even within the same field; however, we present an overview of common examination procedures to familiarize the reader with the patient's experience.

Women with dyspareunia or vaginismus typically seek initial assessment and treatment from gynecologists. A thorough gynecological examination might include a speculum examination; a cotton-swab test; internal palpation to locate dyspareunic pain; vaginal and cervical cultures; and, when deemed necessary, hysteroscopy, colposcopy, or transvaginal ultrasound. For women suffering from vaginismus, a gynecological examination is often highly anxiety provoking and sometimes traumatic. An examination is important to exclude the contribution of physical obstructions to penetration (i.e., imperforate hymen, vaginal septum), but the procedure may be impossible for a woman to endure due to fear, withdrawal reactions, and involuntary vaginal contractions.

Women with genital pain may also seek treatment from dermatologists or urologists, because dyspareunia may be associated with several dermatological and urological conditions (e.g., lichen sclerosis, interstitial cystitis, descended bladder). Appropriate evaluation may include cell cultures or samples, urine assays, or cystoscopy.

A pelvic floor physical therapist may assess and treat women with dyspareunia or vaginismus, because pelvic floor muscle tension, weakness, and instability are frequent components of these conditions (Reissing et al. 2005). Pelvic muscle tension may also develop involuntarily as a protective response to dyspareunia, which in turn exacerbates pain. A pelvic floor examination by an experienced physiotherapist involving external and internal (when possible) vaginal palpation to assess pelvic floor muscle tone, contractility, reactivity, and stability is highly recommended to determine whether rehabilitation is necessary.

Case Example

Elania, age 28, was referred to our clinic with a diagnosis of provoked vestibulodynia after having consulted with a family doctor and two gynecologists.

She brought her partner Alexander, age 31, to the initial psychosexual pain assessment. Elania described sharp burning sensations at the vaginal entrance during intercourse that had lasted for 2 years. She reported that the onset of her pain coincided with a string of yeast infections that started while she and Alexander were on a beach vacation. Upon their return, she was treated with topical and oral antifungal medications, which resolved her infections but did not alleviate her vulvar symptoms. The pain from penile penetration gradually became more intense and persisted for several hours after intercourse. Elania described their most recent attempt at sexual intercourse: "As soon as Alex entered me and I felt that miserable pain, it was as if my muscles down there just clenched up. My entire pelvis was like a machine going into lockdown; all of the muscles just tightened around his penis and pushed him out." Her pain was slightly relieved with the application of a cold compress to her vulva or a cool bath immediately following sex. In the previous 6 months, Elania also felt increased genital sensitivity and irritation prior to menstruation that precluded her from wearing tight-fitting clothes at this time.

Elania and Alexander had been living together for 4 years and had been engaged for 1 year. Both partners were insistent that their relationship was very strong and supportive. However, a comprehensive psychosexual assessment revealed that both were feeling increasingly detached and insecure about their relationship. As Elania's dyspareunia intensified, she no longer enjoyed sex and rarely felt desire. Her sexual arousal and lubrication during intercourse were diminished, thereby further exacerbating her pain. Alexander was often fearful of inflicting pain on Elania but also felt rejected when his occasional advances were rebuffed. They began to avoid sexual intercourse and all intimate contact for fear that it might lead to pain. Her pain had been a source of frustration and guilt for both partners, and they found themselves growing apart as their intimacy dwindled.

Treatment

Psychosocial Treatment

Psychosocial treatment may enhance a patient's ability to develop effective coping strategies for living with vaginismus or dyspareunia. Due to the role of cognitive and emotional factors in the modulation of pain, the psychological component of chronic pain is a primary focus of psychosocial treatments. Psychotherapeutic (and pharmacological if required) mood regulation should be initiated as soon as possible, because the restoration of normal mood may enhance a patient's response to other forms of biomedical and psychosocial treatment.

Cognitive-Behavioral and Sex Therapy

Based on the clinical and empirical evidence that rather than being sexual disorders, dyspareunia and vaginismus are essentially pain conditions that negatively impact sex, the combination of cognitive-behavioral pain management and sex therapy can be used to promote the alleviation of pain and help to restore interpersonal and sexual functioning. The broad goals of this treatment approach include 1) a psychoeducational component wherein genital pain is reconceptualized as physical pain that is impacted by thoughts, emotions, and behaviors; 2) the cognitive restructuring of maladaptive pain-related thoughts; and 3) the development of useful coping strategies to reduce the negative impact of pain. A cyclical relationship between negative affect from performance anxiety, increased attention on threat cues, sexual dysfunction, and sexual avoidance may maintain anxiety-related sexual dysfunction (van den Hout and Barlow 2000). Accordingly, pain is discussed in its relation to the avoidance of sexual intercourse, the loss of sexual desire, and difficulties with sexual arousal. Strategies for increasing nonpainful sexual activity and enhancing sexual desire and arousal are generated so that the woman begins to envision pleasurable sexual activity with minimal or no pain.

Individual or group cognitive-behavioral therapy (CBT) is effective in reducing pain in women with dyspareunia and in enabling sexual intercourse in women with vaginismus. The landmark randomized controlled trial (RCT) of Bergeron et al. (2001) supported the use of a pain-focused treatment approach that draws on principles of sex therapy. Group CBT included psychoeducation about pain and genital anatomy, relaxation and deep breathing, vaginal dilatation and Kegel exercises, cognitive restructuring, and coping strategies specific to pain. Using this paradigm, 39% of group CBT participants reported great or complete pain relief, and these women continued to experience improvements in pain at the 2.5-year follow-up (Bergeron et al. 2008).

Although vaginismus is widely believed to be an easily treatable condition, the existing psychotherapy literature does not support this assumption (van Lankveld et al. 2006). Of the studies that have claimed high "cure" rates for vaginismus (see Heiman and Meston 1998), the definition of successful treatment as a single act of penile-vaginal intercourse is clinically problematic. This outcome measure completely disregards the putative diagnostic criterion of the disorder, which is muscle spasm (Reissing et al. 1999), and some "cured" women may not attempt additional sexual intercourse and are rarely questioned as to whether they found sexual intercourse pleasurable. A single RCT has been conducted on CBT treatments for women with lifelong vaginismus (van Lankveld et al. 2006). This study evaluated a CBT-based program in a group versus individual bibliotherapy format, compared to waitlist controls. The therapy included sexual education, relaxation, rational emotive cognitive therapy, sensate focus, and gradual behavioral exposure to finger and penile penetration, or treatment self-administered at home with support phone consultations. At the 12-month follow-up, success rates in achieving penetrative intercourse reported by group and bibliotherapy participants were 21% and 15%, respectively, and both groups reported higher rates of nonintercourse penetration compared to baseline. Importantly, fear of coitus and nonintercourse penetration behavior mediated treatment success in women who reported engaging in vaginal intercourse during the study (ter Kuile et al. 2007).

Although CBT and sex therapy are equally applicable to women with dyspareunia and vaginismus, the psychological treatment of vaginismus includes a central behavior therapy component that is more intensive than that needed for the treatment of dyspareunia. This therapeutic approach assumes that vaginismus is a conditioned phobic response to anxiety-provoking stimuli (i.e., sexual and/or nonsexual penetration), and treatment is preferentially aimed at interrupting the learned association between fear, penetration, and sexual avoidance (via a hierarchy of imagined and in vivo exposure to the feared stimuli). This process may begin with sensate focus, in which couples are instructed to engage in nonsexual touch and massage with a concurrent ban on sexual intercourse. Similar to manual therapy used by physiotherapists, sensate focus allows a woman to become reaccustomed to physical touch and pressure while being physically relaxed, and this exercise functions as a form of tactile desensitization. The intercourse ban removes her anxiety about penetration and allows her to open herself to a sensual experience with her partner without fear of pain. At more advanced levels of her personal hierarchy, the woman attempts finger and then dilator self-insertion. She should be in complete control of the stimulus application, and insertion should not be terminated until her anxiety level has reduced so that fear avoidance is not reinforced. If possible, the presence and encouragement of the woman's partner can facilitate the exposure process.

Pain Management

Based on empirical evidence that sensory pain can be strongly modulated by cognition and affect, pain management is central to the treatment of women with dyspareunia and vaginismus. This approach is based on psychoeducation regarding how the pain experience is intensified by attention to the pain, negative mood, and increased muscle tension secondary to anxiety. Pain management focuses on the utility of cognitive distraction in reducing the intensity and unpleasantness of pain, the moderation of the negative impact of anxiety and depression on the perception and consequences of pain, and the practice of muscle relaxation to reduce pain due to tense pelvic floor musculature. A clinical manual on cognitive therapy for chronic pain can provide theoretical and practical guidance in pain management (e.g., Thorn 2004).

Practice Point

Show the patient a diagram of how distorted thoughts about pain reinforce negative emotional reactions and avoidance behaviors (see Figure 11–2 for example). Have the patient note the thoughts and feelings that precede and follow painful behavior to help her understand how her experience of the pain may be augmented by negative thoughts and emotions.

Medical Treatment

Dyspareunia

No medical treatments for dyspareunia are consistently supported by controlled empirical data, and only a few treatments have been evaluated with RCTs. The majority of data on the treatment of dyspareunia has been collected on women with provoked vestibulodynia and postmenopausal dyspareunia, although medical treatment of deep dyspareunia and generalized vulvodynia are also briefly addressed.

Provoked vestibulodynia.   Medical treatments for provoked vestibulodynia may include topical estrogen, lidocaine, capsaicin, corticosteroids, botulinum toxin, and interferon-α injections, yet results are variable and few of these

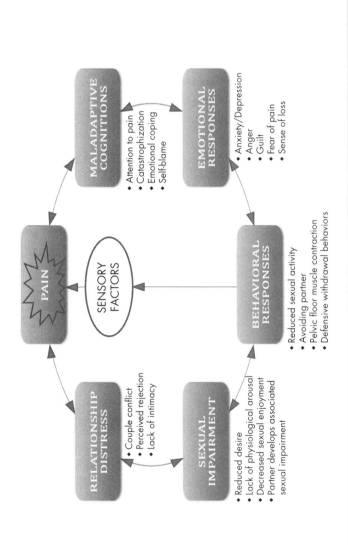

Figure 11–2.   Example diagram of how distorted thoughts about pain reinforce negative emotional reactions and avoidance behaviors.

treatments are empirically supported (see Landry et al. 2008). Topical preparations and oral antifungal medications do not improve provoked vestibulodynia (see Table 11–2). Preliminary results from a randomized comparison of 1% corticosteroid cream and CBT have indicated comparable improvements in vulvar pain between treatment groups.

Postmenopausal dyspareunia.   Perimenopausal or postmenopausal women presenting with pain during intercourse may have developed vaginal atrophy (i.e., atrophic vaginitis), which is associated with a variety of symptoms that may result in dyspareunia, including vaginal dryness, irritation or burning sensations, tissue thinning and fragility, bleeding during intercourse, diminished physiological arousal to sexual stimulation, and a lack of lubrication (Bachmann and Nevadunsky 2000). Local estrogen replacement therapy is widely considered the intervention of choice for postmenopausal dyspareunia associated with vaginal atrophy. Current treatment guidelines advise that postmenopausal women experiencing dyspareunia secondary to vaginal atrophy can be prescribed a conjugated estrogen cream, a sustained-release intravaginal estradiol ring, or a low-dose estradiol vaginal tablet (North American Menopause Society 2007; Suckling et al. 2006). Despite the beneficial effects of estrogen supplementation for pain during intercourse associated with vaginal atrophy, between 10% and 27% of women with dyspareunia do not report improvements in pain (Kao et al. 2008). Hormone replacement therapy is recommended for postmenopausal dyspareunia with vaginal atrophy. When local estrogen supplementation is contraindicated, Replens, a vaginal moisturizing gel, is the only recommended nonhormonal treatment.

Deep dyspareunia.   Pelvic or abdominal dyspareunic pain may occur with deep thrusting in the absence of pathophysiology. Watchful waiting and regular monitoring is a common treatment option for patients diagnosed with deep dyspareunia due to small ovarian cysts or mild endometriosis. Pharmacological interventions to treat deep dyspareunia include antibiotics, nonsteroidal anti-inflammatory drugs, oral contraceptive pills, or other forms of hormonal therapy such as progesterone supplementation and gonadotropin-releasing hormone agonists. Excellent discussions on differential diagnosis and treatment of deep dyspareunia (Reid and Lininger 1993) and medical management for deep dyspareunia associated with endometriosis (Davis and McMillan 2003) are available.

Table 11–2.   Randomized trials of medical treatments for provoked vestibulodynia

Study	Sample characteristics	Diagnostic criteria	Groups	Outcome	Limitations
Bornstein et al. 2000 (*N*=40, age range= 18–70)	No data on symptom duration	• Friedrich criteria • Symptom duration ≥ 6 months • No oral or topical treatment 1 month before study	Fluconazole (150 mg/week) and low-oxalate diet vs. low-oxalate diet	No significant group differences	• No true placebo group • Dichotomous outcome variable • Not double-blind • No long-term follow-up
Nyirjesy et al. 2001 (*N*=26, mean age=26.5)	Cromolyn group (*n*=13): average symptom duration= 2.3 years Placebo group (*n*=13): Mean symptom duration = 2.0 years	• Self-reported vulvar pain • Vulvar tenderness • Vulvar redness • No other diagnoses • Symptom duration ≥ 6 months	Cromolyn (4%) in acid mantle cream vs. vehicle	No significant group differences	• Outcome variable applicable to sexually active participants only • Cromolyn group used amitriptyline without benefit • Side effect of cromolyn (stinging) • Concurrent fluconazole use (*n*=12) • Not double-blind • No long-term follow-up

Table 11–2. Randomized trials of medical treatments for provoked vestibulodynia (*continued*)

Study	Sample characteristics	Diagnostic criteria	Groups	Outcome	Limitations
Munday et al. 2004 (*N*=14)	Not available	• Introital pain • Vulvar tenderness • Vulvar redness	Clobetasol propionate (0.05%) vs. hydrocortisone (0.5%)	Most participants improved	• Minimal patient information • Unclear if diagnostic criteria were self-reported • Hydrocortisone not a true placebo • No statistical tests • No long-term follow-up
Danielsson et al. 2006 (*N*=37, mean age=24.5)	Mean symptom duration= 37 months; 22% and 43% primary PVD in sEMG and lidocaine groups, respectively	• Introital pain • Vulvar tenderness • "Moderate to pronounced" pain with intercourse • Symptom duration≥ 6 months	Lidocaine gel (2%) and lidocaine ointment (5%) vs. biofeedback training	No significant group differences	• Pooled primary/secondary PVD • Poor compliance in sEMG group • Improved pain sensitivity did not coincide with self-reported pain intensity

Note.   PVD=provoked vestibulodynia; sEMG=surface electromyography.

Generalized vulvodynia. Traditional pharmacological management of unprovoked vulvar pain includes a wide repertoire of treatment strategies, including acetaminophen, nonsteroidal anti-inflammatory drugs, corticosteroids, tricyclic antidepressants, anticonvulsants, narcotics, and cannabinoids (Fischer 2004). No RCTs support the use of specific pain medications in the treatment of dyspareunia.

Vaginismus

No efficacious medical treatments are available for vaginismus (Crowley et al. 2006). A handful of case reports have described the potential utility of topical and localized systemic treatments for vaginismus, including botulinum toxin injections, topical anesthetics, topical glyceryl trinitrate, and local injection of acetylcholine antagonists. However, controlled evaluations of these treatments have not been conducted.

Physical Therapy

Dyspareunia and vaginismus are associated with abnormalities in the stability, strength, and relaxation of the pelvic floor muscles (Rosenbaum 2007). A secondary consequence to pain induced by muscle tension is a woman's learned fear response to this pain. Women who chronically experience genital pain may avoid using pelvic muscles for fear of pain, and the muscles weaken from disuse. Chronic genital pain (or fear of pain) may encourage the avoidance of any form of potentially painful genital contact. Pelvic floor physical therapy rehabituates the pelvic muscles to touch and pressure so that stimulation is perceived as normal rather than excessive and harmful, acting as in vivo exposure to genital touch and vaginal penetration.

A single RCT has evaluated electromyographic (EMG) biofeedback as a treatment for provoked vestibulodynia. In a comparison of vestibulectomy, EMG biofeedback, and CBT, Bergeron et al. (2001) found that 36% of the biofeedback group reported substantial or complete relief of vulvar pain by the 6-month follow-up (roughly equivalent to levels obtained in the CBT group and less than the robust improvements seen in the surgery group). A previous study on self-administered biofeedback in women with provoked vestibulodynia reported a greater success rate, with 83% of participants reporting an improvement in self-reported pain (Glazer et al. 1995).

A combination of biofeedback, physical therapy techniques (i.e., massage, myofascial release, trigger-point pressure), psychoeducation, home dilatation, and Kegel exercises produced substantial reductions in gynecological (cotton-swab test) and intercourse pain in women with provoked vestibulodynia (Bergeron et al. 2002). At follow-up, the authors concluded that the treatment was successful in 51.5% of their sample, and 82% of these participants attributed their improvement to physical therapy.

Pelvic floor physical therapy is thought to play a prominent role in the treatment of vaginismus (Rosenbaum 2007), yet no RCTs of physical therapy have been conducted in women with vaginismus. Every vaginismus treatment study that uses Masters and Johnson–type sex therapy incorporates crude physical therapy techniques, including Kegel exercises, finger self-insertion, vaginal dilatation, and progressive muscle relaxation (for a review of treatment studies, see Wijma et al. 2007). However, the effectiveness of these techniques in treating vaginismus has not been established.

Surgical Treatment

Provoked Vestibulodynia

The surgical treatment of provoked vestibulodynia has received consistent empirical support for the alleviation of provoked vulvar pain (Bergeron et al. 2001; Bornstein and Abramovici 1997; Weijmar Schultz et al. 1996). Perineoplasty consists of excision of painful vulvar vestibule tissue extending down to the perineum, with vaginal advancement to cover the removed tissue. The more common surgery is vestibulectomy, which involves the excision of only the posterior and anterior vestibular tissue and hymen, with vaginal advancement when needed. In the first RCT that demonstrated the efficacy of surgical treatment of provoked vestibulodynia, both behavior therapy alone (including physical therapy, patient education, and sex therapy) and perineoplasty followed by behavior therapy resulted in comparable reductions in pain (Weijmar Schultz et al. 1996). No treatment differences have been found in total versus partial perineoplasty plus vulvar vestibule interferon-α injections in an RCT of women with provoked vestibulodynia, with both groups exhibiting response rates of 67%–70% (Bornstein and Abramovici 1997). Bergeron et al. (2001, 2008) found that surgical treatment of provoked vestibulodynia resulted in a robust decrease in clinically assessed and intercourse vulvar pain after initial treatment and at 2.5-year follow-up. Interestingly, these improvements were not significantly different at 2.5-year follow-up from those in women who received group CBT. The vestibulectomy and CBT groups did not differ in frequency of intercourse, indicating that a greater reduction in vestibular pain did not result in a concurrent improvement of intercourse frequency.

Deep Dyspareunia

The available prospective evidence suggests that dyspareunia and pelvic pain significantly decrease after hysterectomy for the majority of women, although a substantial minority of women reported worsened pain following hysterectomy (Flory et al. 2005). In an RCT, Flory et al. (2006) found that total hysterectomy significantly decreased deep dyspareunic pain intensity, whereas subtotal hysterectomy yielded improvement to a lesser degree. High levels of preoperative sexual functioning and intercourse frequency were positive predictors of psychosexual improvement with hysterectomy, whereas menopausal hormonal changes, low physical or emotional well-being, stress, anxiety, and depression were negatively predictive (Flory et al. 2005).

Vaginismus

No evidence is available regarding the surgical treatment of vaginismus. In case reports, women with vaginismus have been described as having hymenal abnormalities, including an imperforate hymen, which have been corrected with hymenectomy. Whether anatomical abnormalities constitute a causal factor in the development of vaginismus is unclear, and no empirical evidence supports the effectiveness of surgical treatment in this population.

Other Treatments

Many medical professionals and women consider treatments such as hypnotherapy, low-oxalate diet, changes in vulvar hygiene, or acupuncture to be viable alternatives to empirically supported treatments, but few controlled studies and no RCTs have evaluated the effectiveness of these treatments. Hypnotherapy has received some support from an uncontrolled study on eight women with provoked vestibulodynia, in which women reported enhanced sexual function and a reduction in gynecological, intercourse, and vulvar pain following hypnotherapy treatment (Pukall et al. 2007). A low-oxalate diet has received minimal support in producing a satisfactory treatment response (e.g., Harlow et al. 2008). Changes in vulvar hygiene may help to remove factors that exacerbate genital pain; these changes include the avoidance of potential irritants (e.g., personal care products, scented soaps, laundry detergent, dryer sheets, restrictive underwear and panty hose) and the use of protective creams (e.g., silicone barrier creams, Vaseline). Acupuncture was found to improve quality of life in women with provoked vestibulodynia (Danielsson et al. 2001), but the authors did not discuss whether this improvement corresponded with an alleviation of vulvar pain.

Case Example *(continued)*

Over a period of 8 months, Elania and Alexander (introduced in the earlier case example) were treated weekly as a couple, and Elania had sporadic individual sessions. The primary goals of psychotherapy were to help Elania reduce her pain, to reinstate sexual desire and arousal, and to improve the couple's intimacy and communication about their sexual difficulties and relationship issues. Elania was also referred to a pelvic floor physical therapist to receive treatment concurrent with psychotherapy. Therapy began by validating Elania's pain and providing psychoeducation about provoked vestibulodynia. The clinician focused on cognitive, affective, behavioral, and environmental factors that maintained and exacerbated the pain. Coping skills were evaluated and enhanced to help with the couple's anxiety, catastrophization, and avoidance of pain and sexual activity. The couple learned to identify each other's sexual needs, and their sexual repertoire was expanded beyond intercourse to improve arousal and enjoyment. Additionally, the couple focused on nonsexual ways of increasing their intimacy. Throughout psychotherapy, Elania faithfully completed her daily homework of dilation and desensitization exercises.

At the end of 8 months, Elania's pain still fluctuated with her menstrual cycle but was reduced by about 70%. She was able to enjoy intercourse most of the time, and when Elania experienced pain, the couple engaged in mutually enjoyable nonpenetrative sexual activities. The couple had learned to communicate about the impact of pain on their sexual intimacy and relationship satisfaction. Elania experienced an improvement in sexual desire, and Alexander's fear of causing pain was no longer an issue. With a combined pain management and physical therapy approach, the couple did not feel it was necessary to pursue vulvar vestibular surgery to further alleviate pain because their increased communication had significantly improved their physical intimacy and sexual satisfaction.

Conclusion

A pain-focused approach to the assessment and management of dyspareunia and vaginismus is currently a clinically useful strategy. If this approach fails, then a more general therapeutic intervention or surgery may be considered. In the majority of cases, the differential diagnosis of dyspareunia and vaginismus is difficult if not impossible, and we are not convinced that this is important for treating women with genital pain. By focusing on the factors that can maintain dyspareunia or vaginismus, including pain, muscle tension, fear of pain or sexual intercourse, behavioral avoidance of painful activities, and physical pathology, a multidisciplinary treatment plan can aim to maximize pain relief, increase daily functioning, and enhance sexual enjoyment and satisfaction.

Key Points

- The clinician should legitimize the patient's experience of pain.
- A thorough pain assessment, including pain location, quality, intensity, history, and duration, is critical for gathering important clues to guide diagnosis and treatment.
- The clinician needs to identify the impact of pain on sexual functioning, as it relates to sexual and relationship history.
- A combined pain- and sexuality-oriented approach to treatment includes an emphasis on the quality and location of pain, physical pathology, muscle tension, fear of pain and sexual intercourse, behavioral avoidance of pain, and psychosexual impact of pain.
- Multidimensional treatment incorporates a pain management approach (targeting the maladaptive cognitive and affective factors that augment the physical sensation of pain) and sex therapy techniques (including sexual education, sensate focus, Kegel exercises, and behavior desensitization using vaginal dilatation).
- The clinician should communicate with collaborating treatment providers about patient progress, treatment success, and psychotherapy as appropriate.

References

American Psychiatric Association: Diagnostic and Statistical Manual of Mental Disorders, 4th Edition, Text Revision. Washington, DC, American Psychiatric Association, 2000

Bachmann GA, Nevadunsky NS: Diagnosis and treatment of atrophic vaginitis. Am Fam Physician 61:3090–3096, 2000

Bergeron S, Binik YM, Khalifé S, et al: A randomized comparison of group cognitive-behavioral therapy, surface electromyographic biofeedback, and vestibulectomy in the treatment of dyspareunia resulting from vulvar vestibulitis. Pain 91:297–306, 2001

Bergeron S, Brown C, Lord M, et al: Physical therapy for vulvar vestibulitis syndrome: a retrospective study. J Sex Marital Ther 28:183–192, 2002

Bergeron S, Khalifé S, Glazer HI, et al: Surgical and behavioral treatments for vestibulodynia. Obstet Gynecol 111:159–166, 2008

Binik YM: Should dyspareunia be retained as a sexual dysfunction in DSM V? A painful classification decision. Arch Sex Behav 34:11–21, 2005

Bornstein J, Abramovici H: Vulvar vestibulitis. Am J Obstet Gynecol 176:953–954, 1997

Bornstein J, Livnat G, Stolar Z, et al: Pure versus complicated vulvar vestibulitis: a randomized trial of fluconazole treatment. Gynecol Obstet Invest 50:194–197, 2000

Crowley T, Richardson D, Goldmeier D: Recommendations for the management of vaginismus: BASHH Special Interest Group for Sexual Dysfunction. Int J STD AIDS 17:14–18, 2006

Danielsson I, Sjoberg I, Ostman C: Acupuncture for the treatment of vulvar vestibulitis: a pilot study. Acta Obstet Gynecol Scand 80:437–441, 2001

Danielsson I, Torstensson T, Brodda-Jansen G, et al: EMG biofeedback versus topical lidocaine gel: a randomized study for the treatment of women with vulvar vestibulitis. Acta Obstet Gynecol Scand 85:1360–1367, 2006

Davis CJ, McMillan L: Pain in endometriosis: effectiveness of medical and surgical management. Curr Opin Obstet Gynecol 15:507–512, 2003

Desrochers G, Bergeron S, Landry T, et al: Do psychosexual factors play a role in the etiology of provoked vestibulodynia? A critical review. J Sex Marital Ther 34:198–226, 2008

Desrosiers M, Bergeron S, Meana M, et al: Psychosexual characteristics of vestibulodynia couples: partner solicitousness and hostility are associated with pain. J Sex Med 5:418–427, 2007

Engman M, Lindehammar H, Wijma B: Surface electromyography diagnostics in women with partial vaginismus with or without vulvar vestibulitis and in asymptomatic women. J Psychosom Obstet Gynaecol 25:281–294, 2004

Fischer G: Management of vulvar pain. Dermatol Ther 17:134–149, 2004

Flory N, Bissonnette F, Binik YM: Psychosocial effects of hysterectomy: literature review. J Psychosom Res 59:117–129, 2005

Flory N, Bissonnette F, Amsel RT, et al: The psychosocial outcomes of total and subtotal hysterectomy: a randomized controlled trial. J Sex Med 3:483–491, 2006

Glazer HI, Rodke G, Swencionis C, et al: Treatment of vulvar vestibulitis syndrome with electromyographic biofeedback of pelvic floor musculature. Obstet Gynecol Surv 50:658–659, 1995

Haefner HK: Report of the International Society for the Study of Vulvovaginal Disease terminology and classification of vulvodynia. J Low Genit Tract Dis 11:48–49, 2007

Harlow BL, Stewart EG: A population-based assessment of chronic unexplained vulvar pain: have we underestimated the prevalence of vulvodynia? J Am Med Womens Assoc 58:82–88, 2003

Harlow BL, Abenhaim HA, Vitonis AF, et al: Influence of dietary oxalates on the risk of adult-onset vulvodynia. J Reprod Med 53:171–178, 2008

Heiman JR, Meston CM: Empirically validated treatments for sexual dysfunction, in Empirically Supported Therapies: Best Practice in Professional Psychology. Edited by Dobson KS, Craig KD. New York, Sage, 1998, pp 259–303

Kao A, Binik YM, Kapuscinski A, et al: Dyspareunia in postmenopausal women: a critical review. Pain Res Manag 13:243–254, 2008

Landry T, Bergeron S, Dupuis MJ, et al: The treatment of provoked vestibulodynia: a critical review. Clin J Pain 24:155–171, 2008

Laumann EO, Paik A, Rosen RC: Sexual dysfunction in the United States: prevalence and predictors. JAMA 281:537–544, 1999

Masters WH, Johnson, VE: Human Sexual Inadequacy. Boston, MA, Little, Brown, 1970

Meana M, Binik YM, Khalifé S, et al: Psychosocial correlates of pain attributions in women with dyspareunia. Psychosomatics 40:497–502, 1999

Melzack R: The Short-Form McGill Pain Questionnaire. Pain 30:191–197, 1987

Munday PE: Treatment of vulval vestibulitis with a potent topical steroid. Sex Transm Infect 80:154–155, 2004

North American Menopause Society: The role of estrogen for the treatment of vaginal atrophy in postmenopausal women: 2007 position statement of the North American Menopause Society. Menopause 14:357–369, 2007

Nyirjesy P, Sobel JD, Weitz MV, et al: Cromolyn cream for recalcitrant idiopathic vulvar vestibulitis: results of a placebo controlled study. Sex Transm Infect 77:53–57, 2001

Payne KA, Binik YM, Amsel R, et al: When sex hurts, anxiety and fear orient attention towards pain. Eur J Pain 9:427–436, 2005

Pukall CF, Baron M, Amsel R, et al: Tender point examination in women with vulvar vestibulitis syndrome. Clin J Pain 22:601–609, 2006

Pukall CF, Kandyba K, Amsel R, et al: Efficacy of hypnosis for the treatment of vulvar vestibulitis syndrome: a preliminary investigation. J Sex Med 4:417–425, 2007

Reid R, Lininger T: Sexual pain disorders in the female, in Handbook of Sexual Dysfunctions: Assessment and Treatment. Edited by O'Donohue W, Geer JH. Boston, MA, Allyn & Bacon, 1993, pp 344–354

Reissing ED, Binik YM, Khalifé S: Does vaginismus exist? A critical review of the literature. J Nerv Ment Dis 187:261–274, 1999

Reissing ED, Binik YM, Khalifé S, et al: Vaginal spasm, pain, and behavior: an empirical investigation of the diagnosis of vaginismus. Arch Sex Behav 33:5–17, 2004

Reissing ED, Brown CL, Lord MJ, et al: Pelvic floor functioning in women with vulvar vestibulitis syndrome. J Psychosom Obstet Gynaecol 26:107–113, 2005

Rosenbaum TY: Physical therapy management and treatment of sexual pain disorders, in Principles and Practice of Sex Therapy, 4th Edition. Edited by Leiblum S. New York, Guilford, 2007, pp 157–180

Stewart EG, Spencer P: The V Book: A Doctor's Guide. New York: Bantam Books, 2002

Suckling JA, Kennedy R, Lethaby A, et al: Local oestrogen for vaginal atrophy in postmenopausal women. Cochrane Database of Systematic Reviews, Issue 4, Art. No.: CD001500. DOI: 10.1002/14651858.CD001500.pub2, 2006

ter Kuile MM, van Lankveld JJDM, de Groot E, et al: Cognitive-behavioral therapy for women with lifelong vaginismus: process and prognostic factors. Behav Res Ther 45:359–373, 2007

Thorn BE: Cognitive Therapy for Chronic Pain: A Step-by-Step Guide. New York, Guilford, 2004

van den Hout M, Barlow D: Attention, arousal, and expectancies in anxiety and sexual disorders. J Affect Disord 61:241–256, 2000

van Lankveld JJDM, ter Kuile MM, de Groot E, et al: Cognitive-behavioral therapy for women with lifelong vaginismus: a randomized waiting-list controlled trial of efficacy. J Consult Clin Psychol 74:168–178, 2006

Weijmar Schultz WCM, Gianotten WL, van der Meijden WI, et al: Behavioral approach with or without surgical intervention for vulvar vestibulitis syndrome: a prospective randomized and non-randomized study. J Psychosom Obstet Gynaecol 17:143–148, 1996

Wijma B, Engman M, Wijma K: A model for critical review of literature—with vaginismus as an example. J Psychosom Obstet Gynaecol 28:21–36, 2007

Recommended Readings

Binik YM, Bergeron S, Khalifé S: Dyspareunia and vaginismus, in Principles and Practice of Sex Therapy, 4th Edition. Edited by Leiblum SR. New York, Guilford, 2007

Landry T, Bergeron S, Dupuis, MJ, et al: The treatment of provoked vestibulodynia: a critical review. Clin J Pain 24:155–171, 2008

Rosenbaum TY: Physical therapy management and treatment of sexual pain disorders, in Principles and Practice of Sex Therapy, 4th Edition. Edited by Leiblum SR. New York, Guilford, 2007

Stewart EG, Spencer P: The V Book: A Doctor's Guide. New York, Bantam Books, 2002

Thorn BE: Cognitive Therapy for Chronic Pain: A Step-by-Step Guide. New York, Guilford, 2004

12

Paraphilic Disorders

Jeanne M. Lackamp, M.D.

Cynthia Osborne, M.S.W.

Thomas N. Wise, M.D.

Paraphilic disorders are defined as recurrent and preferred sexually arousing fantasies or behaviors involving nonhuman objects, sadomasochistic behaviors, or children or other nonconsenting persons. The duration of such behaviors and urges must be for at least 6 months and must not be due to another disorder. Individuals with paraphilic disorders often lack motivation for change or treatment and therefore do not come to clinical attention without external motivating factors, whether personal or legal (Krueger and Kaplan 2001). Thus, data regarding paraphilic phenomena and treatments are limited due to the ego-syntonic nature of these recurrent erotic interests (Lehne et al. 2000). Clinical reports are from patients who seek mental health evaluations and who may have comorbid states, such as affective disorders, anxiety disorders, or substance use disorders, that lead to such evaluations. Additionally,

335

paraphilic behaviors that involve cruelty, illegality, or inappropriately coercive sexual behavior often are studied in the forensic population of patients who have been apprehended by legal authorities. Although management or reduction of paraphilic behaviors is possible, treatment with the goal of eliminating or "curing" these behaviors may not be realistic, and many clinicians feel that patients may be at risk of acting on paraphilic urges regardless of psychological or biological treatments (Hall and Hall 2007; Saleh 2005). Despite such challenges, in this chapter, we review what is known about the conceptualization, assessment, management, and treatment of paraphilic disorders.

General Considerations

Paraphilic fantasies and urges often begin in childhood or adolescence and may vary in frequency and intensity over time (American Psychiatric Association 2000; Grant 2005; Krueger and Kaplan 2001; Shiah et al. 2006). Some patients may have a vague awareness of an unusual interest earlier in their lives and find their interest potentiated by triggers, other comorbid issues, or increased opportunity (e.g., exposure to Internet-related stimulation). After such a trigger, the fantasies, urges, and behaviors can escalate to problematic levels (Bradford 2006; Osborne and Wise 2005). The paraphilic fantasy or behavior may be obligatory (required for arousal) or nonobligatory (wherein the individual experiences arousal with other erotic stimuli as well). Many individuals report a nonobligatory paraphilic pattern in early life, with the pattern becoming increasingly obligatory over time and with increased exposure to the stimulus (American Psychiatric Association 2000; Osborne and Wise 2005).

Paraphilic fantasies and behaviors exist along a continuum of expression (Sadock and Sadock 2007). At one end of the continuum, an individual may simply experience variant thoughts or behaviors on an occasional basis. The paraphilic fantasy is not obligatory, and its behavioral expression is but one in a repertoire of sexual expressions for the individual. At the other end of the continuum, an individual engages in thoughts, fantasies, and behaviors related to the sexual variation as an exclusive, required, or obligate means of achieving sexual arousal and satisfaction. Individuals also may integrate the sexual variation into their social or lifestyle identity. Problematic expressions may occur at any point on the continuum if an individual's attitude about the fantasy or behavior is ego-dystonic, if it causes impairment in a significant life domain, if it is associated with loss of ability to manage sexual urges, or if it leads to illegal or socially unacceptable acts (American Psychiatric Association 2000).

DSM-IV-TR (American Psychiatric Association 2000) defines paraphilias based on the particular focus of the paraphilic fantasy: exhibitionism, fetishism, frotteurism, pedophilia, sexual masochism, sexual sadism, transvestic fetishism, and voyeurism. Unfortunately, categorizing paraphilias according to their specific foci implies that each paraphilia represents a distinct disease process. Difficulties arise because individuals with one paraphilia may be prone to develop others, and individuals with multiple paraphilias present with relatively high frequency (Abel and Osborn 1992; Bradford et al. 1992). As when distinguishing one specific phobia from another or one compulsive behavior from another, a more clinically useful approach might be to conceptualize the many paraphilic variations as reflections of an underlying phenomenon. Lehne and Money (2003) proposed the term *multiplex paraphilia* to describe variations of paraphilic content being expressed in one individual. Bancroft (1989) proposed that paraphilias may develop in response to individual differences in the nervous system and that, therefore, the same conditions that allow the development of one paraphilia may invite the development of others.

Legal Issues

Clinicians should remain mindful that "paraphilic patients" are not necessarily "sex offenders" (Hall and Hall 2007; Krueger and Kaplan 2001; Lehne et al. 2000). Not only are these terms taken from different contexts (medical vs. legal), but not all sex offenders have paraphilias, and not all patients with paraphilic disorders commit sexual offenses because their arousal patterns may not necessarily involve sadomasochistic fantasies or coercive behaviors. Comorbidities may include various Axis I diagnoses, such as major depressive disorder, social phobia, or various issues of substance abuse, and Axis II diagnoses, such as antisocial personality disorder or paranoid personality disorder (Dunsieth et al. 2004). Comorbidities are addressed later in the chapter.

Historically, regulatory efforts regarding individuals' sexual behaviors were often related to consensual homosexual activities, which are now recognized to be neither illegal nor related to mental disability (Ridinger 2006). Sadomasochism is another realm in which legal regulation has been attempted. As noted by Ridinger (2006), numerous legal cases highlight the blurred lines between consensual sexual acts (with sadomasochistic overtones) and sexual assault. Issues such as sexual freedom, discrimination, and right to privacy further complicate the legal issues related to sadomasochism in particular and paraphilias in general. Furthermore, some variance still exists in state-specific laws governing issues including sadomasochism, sodomy, and other intimate interactions (Ridinger 2006).

The DSM-IV-TR definition of paraphilias has potential legal ramifications. As noted recently by First and Frances (2008), Criterion A of the paraphilia section includes "fantasies, sexual urges, or behaviors"; the inclusion of "behaviors" may pose diagnostic and legal problems. The "behaviors" criterion, newly added as of DSM-IV (American Psychiatric Association 1994), may lead some to believe that people with recurrent sexually exploitative behaviors have a mental condition (paraphilia), which would then necessitate indefinite civil commitment for mental health problems after incarceration. In fact, this may not be the case for individuals who participate in recurrent sexually exploitative behaviors with nonparaphilic motivation (First and Frances 2008). As we mention throughout this chapter, clinicians need to remain cognizant of the distinction between paraphilia and sexual offense, and to review issues of safety (both of patients and of others in the community) during evaluations.

Prevalence

Paraphilic *behaviors* may differ from paraphilic *disorders* as defined in DSM-IV-TR. Individuals with paraphilias rarely present in general mental health or medical facilities, and prevalence rates in patient samples from sexual disorder clinics or psychiatric inpatient units cannot be viewed as representative of prevalence rates in the general population (Lehne et al. 2000). Additionally, prevalence data often are drawn from legal records in cases of sexual offense. These data do not distinguish between those individuals whose offense is due to a paraphilia and those individuals with antisocial behavior, and drawing conclusions for the general population based on this population with legal records is problematic. Finally, with the advent of Internet technology, more individuals may be exposed to paraphilia-related stimuli and be participating in paraphilic behaviors (Bradford 2006). Therefore, prevalence rates remain unknown.

Gender

Males are much more likely than females to have paraphilic disorders, although some exceptions in females include sadomasochism and certain paraphilias not otherwise specified, such as autoerotic asphyxia (Behrendt et al. 2002; Shields et al. 2005). Other exceptions include case reports of female exhibitionism and fetishism (Hollender et al. 1977; Zavitzianos 1982). Although historically pedophilia in females was attributed to a sexually obligate proclivity for underage sexual partners or another psychiatric issue such as psychotic disorder, some researchers suggest that females do have the capacity for pedophilic behaviors (Hall and Hall 2007).

Comorbidities

As noted above, multiple paraphilias often co-occur in patients with paraphilic disorders, including patients whose primary diagnosis is fetishism, pedophilia, or exhibitionism (Abel and Osborn 1992; Bancroft 1989; Crepault and Couture 1980; Dunsieth et al. 2004; Gosselin and Wilson 1980; Grant 2005; Langevin 1983, 1985; Raymond et al. 1999). Per DSM-IV-TR criteria, paraphilias cannot be diagnosed without clinical impairment or distress (Criterion B); this can be problematic in paraphilias that are ego-syntonic. That being said, as currently defined in DSM-IV-TR, patients may be diagnosed with multiple paraphilias if they meet full criteria for each.

Various researchers have attempted to describe nonparaphilic Axis I comorbidities in paraphilic patients. These comorbidities include mood disorders, anxiety disorders, retrospectively diagnosed childhood attention-deficit/hyperactivity disorder, substance use disorders, and impulse control disorders, among others (Allnutt et al. 1996; Fagan et al. 1988; Grant 2005; Kafka and Hennen 2002; Kafka and Prentky 1998; Krueger and Kaplan 2001; Raymond et al. 1999). Remaining cognizant of possible comorbidities is crucial in evaluating and treating patients, particularly because sexual acting-out behaviors can be components of nonparaphilic disorders. Furthermore, in many patients with paraphilia, the comorbid condition of an anxiety or affective disorder is secondary to relationship difficulties caused by the paraphilia. In such situations, the paraphilia still is ego-syntonic.

Clinicians may conceptualize personality disorders, particularly antisocial personality disorder, as being related to or necessary for paraphilic fantasies or behaviors. However, they may fail to differentiate behaviors that reflect a paraphilia from behaviors that reflect antisocial traits *not* related to a paraphilia. Some individuals with pedophilia never act on their urges and may express the wish that their sexual desires trended toward more typical patterns of sexual engagement. Conversely, patients with antisocial personality disorder may engage in pedophilic acts as part of a wider repertoire of harming others without empathy, remorse, or consideration of consequences. The authors of several widely cited studies noted that antisocial personality disorder was diagnosed in a relative minority of patients with paraphilias, particularly if the patients were not currently incarcerated (Grant 2005; Raymond et al. 1999). However, in one study of 47 incarcerated sexual offenders, 72% of the sample had at least one personality disorder, and the most prevalent was antisocial personality disorder (Borchard et al. 2003). In another study of 113 convicted male sexual offenders, 55.8% met criteria for antisocial personality disorder, the highest frequency of any of the personality disorders in this sample (Dunsieth et al. 2004). Again, the correlation between legal offense and antisocial personality disorder may be more significant than the correlation between sexual deviancy and antisocial personality disorder.

Other Axis II conditions, such as borderline intellectual functioning or mental retardation, may play a role in *paraphilic-type* behaviors, although patients technically are not paraphilic. Patients may participate in such behaviors by virtue of intellectual limitations, stimulus availability, or lack of social skills training or sex education (Cantor et al. 2004; Coleman et al. 1993). Other research has noted paraphilic-type behaviors in patients with neurological limitations or injuries, including serious head injuries (Blanchard et al. 2002, 2003). Again, DSM-IV-TR exclusion criteria apply.

Assessment Issues

The evidence for treatment of paraphilic disorders is limited primarily to case reports and a few open medication trials. Nevertheless, clinical experience allows general comments on the assessment and treatment of such sexual disorders, and the most current recommended treatment incorporates both biological and psychological modalities (Osborne and Wise 2005). For assessment and treatment purposes, paraphilias can be partitioned into two types: coercive and noncoercive. Noncoercive paraphilias are more likely to consist of solo and/or consensual activities; these include sadism, masochism, fetishism, and transvestic fetishism. Coercive paraphilias, for which patients may be apprehended by legal authorities for imposition of their paraphilic drives onto others, consist of nonconsensual activities such as voyeurism, exhibitionism, frotteurism, and pedophilia. Not only are behaviors different in these two groups—indeed, some patients with paraphilias never act on their urges or fantasies, and many never come to the attention of the medical or law enforcement communities—but motivations for treatment can be quite diverse as well. For patients with either category of disorder, the clinician needs to first understand why the patient entered treatment at this time.

Patients may present to a clinician because of legal problems resulting from coercive paraphilic behaviors. When evaluating a patient as part of legal or criminal proceedings, the clinician needs to understand his or her role—as a clinician treating the patient, as a witness in court (for either the prosecution or the defense, as a fact or expert witness), or as provider of a second opinion. If the patient was forced into the evaluation because of legal difficulties, this may limit his or her honesty or disclosure to the clinician (Krueger and Kaplan 2002). Clinicians should be aware of the circumstances surrounding the evaluation from the beginning so they can undertake their assessment in the appropriate context.

Treatment considerations for individuals who present on their own, without legal problems, are highly dependent on circumstance and context. Did spousal discovery lead to a marital crisis? Did the behaviors or fantasies provoke anxiety or lead to a particularly frightening experience? Did a significant other reach a new level of intolerance or frustration in trying to satisfy the partner's sexual demands? Does the patient have a comorbid affective disorder or substance abuse condition? Does an association exist between the paraphilia and the concomitant condition, such that exacerbation of one follows or triggers a worsening of the other? Did family members reach a breaking point in their ability to tolerate the patient's paraphilic behaviors? These questions may help illuminate the treatment context so that the clinician and patient both are able to freely discuss the reasons for presentation. Some patients may present individually, whereas other patients may be accompanied by family members or significant others. These additional informants may provide valuable collateral information (Coleman et al. 1993; Lehne et al. 2000).

An important issue to examine during the initial assessment is whether the individual truly desires treatment. This is a key consideration because paraphilias are often ego-syntonic and patients rarely seek treatment merely for insight into their behavior. Does the patient with transvestic fetishism wish to assuage his spouse rather than truly limit his cross-dressing? Does the patient with pedophilia accept the damage that he is doing to his victims and desire treatment, or just hope to avoid incarceration? Fetishism typifies a disorder in which the aberrant behaviors are gratifying and may cause only subtle problems. Some patients begin treatment in earnest after a life event or after worsening of fetishistic behaviors increases their motivation (Wise and Goldberg 1995). Some patients seek treatment based on their own desires, whereas others seek treatment based on pressure from significant others or family members (Coleman et al. 1993; Shiah et al. 2006). If the patient succeeds in identifying problems caused by the fetish at more than a cerebral level, a treatment alliance may be forged. Unfortunately, some patients with fetishism may discover the potency of their ambivalence as treatment proceeds, and may drop out of treatment rather than relinquish the pleasure or comfort associated with the behavior (Sadock and Sadock 2007). These patients may prove exceptionally difficult to engage in treatment.

Interview

Prior to initiating therapy, the clinician must perform a comprehensive evaluation of patients presenting for paraphilia-related treatment. Krueger and Kaplan (2002) noted many challenging aspects of this process. The first step involves getting informed consent from the patient, alerting the patient that the evaluative process may prove stressful, and advising the patient of the necessary limits of confidentiality regarding current or potential abuse situations. Patients should know that clinicians will be obligated to report information disclosed during clinical interviews if "mandatory reporting" requirements apply (Gellerman and Suddath 2005). Although this warning may have an impact on the completeness of patients' disclosures to their clinicians during treatment, knowing the state's law and communicating it clearly to patients during the initial evaluation is essential.

   The clinician must indicate willingness to discuss patients' sexual issues openly. Although an important goal in working with every patient is that the clinician establish rapport and be receptive to sensitive material (particularly because many general psychiatric patients have sexual concerns and/or experience sexual side effects from medications), doing so is pivotal in working with this patient population. Also, the clinician needs to remember that patients may habitually minimize or deny problematic behaviors and may have significant cognitive distortions upon which they rely for rationalizing their behavior (Bradford 2006; Hall and Hall 2007).

The clinician might begin the interview by inquiring, "Tell me about the circumstances that led to this evaluation." This opening allows the patient to focus on the current situation rather than immediate details of the paraphilic fantasies and behaviors. In coercive situations, the patient may first focus on use of the Internet or actual legal issues. Patients with other paraphilic disorders might focus on discovery by the spouse. The clinician can then review the patient's life history and ask questions about the individual's initial learning about sexuality. "Tell me when you first discovered your own sexual arousal" is a neutral entry request that should lead into more focused details about currently preferred arousal stimuli. The clinician should inquire about the patient's complete sexual history—paraphilic issues, nonparaphilic issues, childhood sexual experiences or activities, adult sexual experiences or activities, or lack thereof. This approach will help provide the clinician with appropriate background instead of targeting paraphilic issues in isolation (Krueger and Kaplan 2002).

As noted earlier, patients' paraphilias may evolve over time in intensity, frequency, and area of desire. For example, although exhibitionistic behaviors may be conceptualized by some in the general public as lighthearted pranks, the fact remains that exhibitionism is neither humorous nor harmless (Firestone et al. 2006). Patients who engage in these behaviors may go on to re-offend and may develop more serious sexually offensive behaviors, including hands-on offenses. This possibility emphasizes the importance of getting a full chronological history. The clinician also needs to maintain a sense of nonjudgmental inquiry as the therapeutic alliance continues over time, so that any broadening of the patient's paraphilic repertoire is discovered and addressed in a timely and appropriate manner. Patients may deny fetishistic arousal patterns due to shame or fear of legal issues. For example, cross-dressing men often deny any erotic stimuli when they present with gender dysphoria. However, when asked, "In the past have there been any occasions of sexual excitement, even during adolescence?" many will admit that such excitement did occur in the past (Wise and Meyer 1980).

Once a discussion of actual paraphilic activities has commenced, the clinician must ascertain the level of danger or risk related to the paraphilic behaviors. Certain behaviors, such as autoerotic asphyxiation and some cases of sexual sadism or masochism, may or may not pose an immediate danger. In sadism and masochism, the thrill associated with power differential and potential danger is often central to both the masochist's and the sadist's experience (Osborne and Wise 2005). The danger may be benign and symbolic, but could be potentially lethal in actuality. In extreme cases of sadomasochism, in which loss of control or confusion occurs regarding the boundary between consent and coercion, behaviors can cause physical harm. The clinician's task is to accurately decipher what is occurring in the sexual experience, on both overt and covert levels. What appears insignificant may hold key details of subtle sexual, intrapsychic, and relational processes that comprise sadomasochistic interactions that have gone awry. Only a detailed deconstruction of the partners' moment-to-moment interactions permits meaningful decoding of complex sadomasochistic experiences. Evaluation of danger applies to the other paraphilias as well. Once imminent risk has been explored and addressed if necessary, goals of treatment and various treatment modalities can be discussed.

Assessment Tools

Although some instruments have been developed to assess patients' sexual behaviors or levels of psychopathy (including the Derogatis Sexual Functioning Inventory and the Psychopathy Checklist—Revised; Derogatis 2008), no reliable or valid psychometric inventories have been developed specifically for assessment of paraphilic sexual disorders (Firestone et al. 2006; Krueger and Kaplan 2002). Thus, careful interviewing is the essential "tool" for assessing and diagnosing paraphilias (Derogatis 2008; Lehne et al. 2000). Checking hormone levels and other laboratory test results is generally not useful in the assessment of subjects with paraphilia, because patients can experience paraphilic thoughts and engage in paraphilic behaviors even if their hormone levels are altered by treatment (Hall and Hall 2007; Saleh 2005). Objective measures, such as penile plethysmography and polygraphy, have been reported to assist in the evaluation of patients with paraphilia (Hall and Hall 2007; Krueger and Kaplan 2002). These techniques have been most widely used in research and with sexual offender populations, so their generalizability is unknown.

Penile plethysmography, also called *phallometry,* involves measuring the patient's penile response to sexually stimulating material (audiotapes, still photos or slides, or videotapes or DVDs). The age of depicted persons and coercive versus noncoercive content may vary in stimuli. During stimulus presentation, measurements are taken of either changes in penile circumference or changes in penile volume. Changes in circumference are recorded via a mechanical device that the patient places on his own penis. Changes in penile volume are more complicated and are measured with the assistance of a technician who helps the patient with proper device placement (Krueger and Kaplan 2002). Although some professionals think that plethysmography is a valid measurement of male sexual arousal, others have found that patients' sexual desires are not consistently correlated with plethysmographic findings (Firestone et al. 2006). In fact, one study of sexual offenders revealed no significant relationship between the apparent age of persons depicted in the stimulus and the patient's arousal. Arousal during testing was thought to be more a function of general arousability than of predicting or confirming offending behavior (G.C. Hall 1989). Confounders may include patient anxiety or intentional "faking good," which may alter test results. Additionally, no validated or standardized stimulus sets exist against which to compare patient responses (due, in part, to the fact that certain stimuli—such as pornographic pictures of children—are illegal in the United States). Also, variance in procedures may cause differences at various research centers. Finally, this method clearly is inappropriate and impossible to use with the population of female paraphiliacs (Hall and Hall 2007; Krueger and Kaplan 2002).

Other assessment tools include polygraphy and measures of viewing time. Although not typically used in legal settings to prove innocence or guilt, polygraphy is sometimes used to determine if sexual offenders have violated parole or probation (Krueger and Kaplan 2002). Viewing time measurements attempt to draw conclusions between viewing time and specific areas of sexual interest (Krueger and Kaplan 2002). Patients are shown various sexually interesting stimuli (typically via slides), and a recording is made of how long the patient views each stimulus. Patients also are asked to rate how attractive each stimulus is (Krueger and Kaplan 2002). This assessment practice has been in existence for many years, but the Abel Assessment for Sexual Interest (Abel 1992) is a more modern and sophisticated version of viewing time assessments (Hall and Hall 2007; Lehne et al. 2000). This instrument combines a self-report survey with measurements of visual reaction times to nonpornographic pictures of people of various ages. Because patients often minimize or deny problematic behaviors, such as paraphilic behaviors or desires, subjective variables such as self-report surveys must be considered cautiously.

Despite advances, the use of diagnostic instruments remains an imperfect undertaking. In some research studies involving patients with paraphilias, structured clinical interviews are used for standardized diagnosing of Axis I and II disorders (Grant 2005). Although these scales can be extremely useful in research settings, their utility in general clinical settings is unknown. As noted in Lehne et al.'s (2000) article on treatment, "There are still no reliable and valid substitutes for a good clinical history and interview accompanied by a thorough review of any independent collateral information that may be available in arriving at a diagnosis" (p. 570).

Comorbidities

Identifying and treating comorbid psychiatric issues may resolve paraphilic-type behaviors. As noted earlier, patients with paraphilias often have other clinically significant comorbidities, including additional paraphilias, affective disorders, substance use disorders, personality disorders, anxiety disorders, and impulse control disorders. Furthermore, although paraphilias occupy their own diagnostic category, some clinicians conceptualize these disorders as belonging to a spectrum of other psychiatric constructs, such as impulse control disorders, anxiety disorders (with obsessive-compulsive–type symptoms), affective disorders (with behavioral dysregulation during extreme phases of mood disturbances), substance use disorders, or personality disorders (Krueger and Kaplan 2001; Lehne et al. 2000). Even if paraphilic disorders belong in their own category, evidence suggests that symptoms such as worsening anxiety may escalate paraphilic wishes and activities, and extreme affective distress also may contribute to exacerbations of paraphilic behaviors (Osborne and Wise 2005). Therefore, clinicians must be thorough in their patient assessments and cognizant of possible symptom overlap or comorbidities, so the best patient outcomes can be realized.

Treatment Issues

As in any therapeutic population, individual patients with paraphilia may vary widely in their personal therapeutic goals and in the treatment modalities they wish to consider. Modalities typically include various forms of psychotherapy and/or medication therapy. Along with serotonin reuptake inhibitor antidepressants, other psychiatric medications and hormonally active agents will be reviewed as we describe management and treatment options in patients with either noncoercive or coercive paraphilias. Emphasis is placed on transvestic fetishism and pedophilia, the two diagnostic categories about which the most research and writing have been done. Additionally, sexual sadism and masochism are reviewed briefly.

Although psychodynamic psychotherapy has been reported as an intervention for various fetishistic behaviors and transvestism, limited evidence supports its efficacy (Bemporad et al. 1976; Hunter 1976). Unfortunately, diagnostic categorization in such case reports often is imprecise, and outcome measurements verified by external or corroborative methods such as penile plethysmography have been limited (Greenacre 1970). This criticism can be made for most treatment interventions in patients with paraphilia. Psychodynamic interventions can help the patient better understand issues in his development that led to his present situation, and can potentially allow understanding of the conflicts that fostered paraphilic symptoms (McHugh and Slavney 1982; Wise 1979). The validity of such conclusions depends on the therapist's theoretical stance (McHugh and Slavney 1998). For instance, does the patient fear women due to castration anxiety or separation from maternal figures, as is found in Freudian theory that has evolved over the decades (Bak 1974; Freud 1988)? Does the patient have issues that Jungian analytic psychology can illuminate (Springer 1996)? Such theoretical approaches may help the therapist organize the data that the patient presents, but formal psychodynamic outcome studies are lacking in this patient population (Frank and Frank 1991). In the following discussion, we do not discount psychodynamic methods but aim to present the most empirically based data.

Case Example

A 47-year-old government employee sought evaluation for urges to ingest his feces, a behavior that he occasionally acted upon. He noted that this behavior began in early adolescence when he would become genitally aroused as he defecated. The arousal pattern evolved into a routine wherein he would go in a shower and defecate while masturbating and thinking of ingesting the material. There were no other associated fantasies. He reported that visceral sensations of a bowel movement were stimulating. Further history revealed that the behavior began shortly after he began masturbating. He linked this period in his life to his parents' divorce and his mother's beginning to date men. In retrospect, he wonders whether he was curious about her sexual behavior with these "boyfriends." The paraphilic pattern would ebb and flow depending on the stressors that the patient experienced. He eventually married, but his wife was an alcoholic. When he sought evaluation, he lamented her chronic substance abuse that resulted in an early dementing process and liver disease. He was emotionally dependent on her and feared her demise. He was not psychotic and was actually ashamed to be admitting such a behavior. He also demonstrated a major mood disorder.

Treatment involved reviewing the patient's feelings of loss and abandonment by his wife due to her alcoholism and dementia. He was able to link this to his earlier sense of abandonment by his mother when she turned her attention to dating following the divorce from his father. Concurrent treatment of his major depression with an antidepressant improved his mood and other symptoms of depression. During this time, his coprophagic proclivities diminished. Although he occasionally had fleeting thoughts of his paraphilic arousal pattern, he was able to consciously override the tendency to act it out.

In this case, the patient's paraphilic behavior was clearly disgusting. The clinician had to make an effort not to immediately react to the paraphilic content, but rather to try to learn about the circumstances in which the behavior occurred and its connection to other situations. Identification of comorbidity was also necessary. Treatment actually modified the patient's urges and limited the behaviors but probably did not "cure" the preferred fantasy. This is the usual outcome for a paraphilia, which rarely can be completely abolished for a more normative arousal pattern.

General Education

Reviewing the treatment of paraphilias without addressing the basics of patient and family education would be an unfortunate omission. Whether or not a patient has presented voluntarily for treatment—unlikely in many cases, because of the ego-syntonic nature of most paraphilias—education of the patient and spouse or family members, as well as the debunking of any myths, can be helpful in the initial phase of treatment. For instance, one of the most common presentations of transvestic fetishism is that of a patient who has been discovered by a spouse, partner, or family member. In these cases, the clinician needs to understand the other (nonparaphilic) party's perception of the behavior, so that correction of misperceptions and education can take place (Wise et al. 1991). A spouse, for example, may report that she entered the relationship with knowledge of the behavior, while naively assuming that her partner would no longer feel the need to engage in it once he had a sexually satisfying marriage. Another may report that she had no knowledge of the behavior until years later when her partner's carelessness led to her accidental discovery; she may even misread the behavior as implying homosexuality. Yet another spouse may report that she knew of the behavior and found it painfully intolerable, but coped with those feelings by a mutual unspoken agreement to ignore it and avoid discussing it. She may have wrongly assumed that she could hold such a stance for the long term, while simultaneously maintaining satisfying emotional and sexual intimacy. These are only some of the common misperceptions that family members or spouses may have when attempting to understand their loved one's apparently aberrant sexual behaviors. Education can be beneficial for all involved (Coleman et al. 1993; Wise et al. 1991).

Social skills training, sex education, and even vocational rehabilitation should be considered as other possible treatment modalities (Brunette and Mueser 2006; Coleman et al. 1993; Krueger and Kaplan 2002; Sadock and Sadock 2007). These all have educational components inherent to them and are potentially valuable additions to the educational and therapeutic process for patients with paraphilia or paraphilic-type behaviors.

Therapeutic Strategies

Cognitive-Behavioral Therapy

At present, cognitive-behavioral therapy (CBT) is considered the mainstay of treatment for patients with paraphilia. CBT not only is cited in numerous papers on paraphilias but also is reported by the Safer Society Foundation and the Association for the Treatment of Sexual Abusers as a widely accepted and effective treatment modality (Krueger and Kaplan 2002). CBT focuses on the interaction of thoughts, affects, and behaviors. This treatment strategy has been found effective in psychiatric disorders as variable as affective disorders, anxiety disorders, eating disorders, and impulse control disorders (Reinecke and Freeman 2003). As with pharmacotherapeutic treatments, the majority of literature on CBT in paraphilias focuses on sexual offender populations. The applicability of this literature may be questionable in the case of a patient with paraphilia who has not committed sexual offenses, as well as in the case of an individual who has committed a sexual offense but may not have a paraphilia (Lehne et al. 2000).

Literature on sexual offenders indicates that the use of CBT modalities reduces recidivism (Lehne et al. 2000; Studer and Aylwin 2006). The critical aspects of cognitive therapy include identifying and challenging cognitive distortions and breaking through patients' denial (Hall and Hall 2007; Krueger and Kaplan 2002; Studer and Aylwin 2006). *Thought substitution, redirection,* and *distractions* are taught as ways to replace maladaptive thoughts and redirect thinking toward more healthy topics (Osborne and Wise 2005). This cognitive restructuring is pivotal, as patients learn to challenge and eliminate maladaptive rationalizations that they use to justify their harmful behaviors (Sadock and Sadock 2007). Advanced features of cognitive therapy include *victim empathy training,* which is particularly important for patients with coercive paraphilias (Hall and Hall 2007; Krueger and Kaplan 2002). According to Studer and Aylwin (2006), creating and maintaining rapport in the therapeutic relationship during the course of CBT is as important for the paraphilic population as for any psychiatric patient population. This poignant observation is conspicuously absent from much of the psychiatric literature on patients with paraphilias.

Several behavioral methods are specific to patients with paraphilias who want to focus on decreasing aberrant sexual urges. These include *satiation,* or changing the patient's behavioral response to previously sexually exciting stimuli by overuse of the stimuli until response ceases; *covert sensitization,* or sensitizing the patient to the stimuli by associating negative outcomes with the stimulus; *fading,* or teaching the patient to mentally transition from aberrant stimuli to more normative stimuli; and *aversive stimulation,* or making the stimulus frankly unappealing by pairing it with an unpleasant stimulus (Krueger and Kaplan 2002). Other methods include *behavioral rehearsal, behavioral abstinence,* and *positive conditioning* (Osborne and Wise 2005). These techniques help patients enhance behavioral control along with cognitive control, so that patients can resist urges and make cognitively active choices, instead of automatically thinking and responding in habitual and harmful ways.

Relapse Prevention

Although relapse prevention modalities are better known from the field of substance abuse treatment (Brunette and Mueser 2006; Osborne and Wise

2005), because paraphilias share some features with addictive disorders, some researchers have noted the utility of relapse prevention with this patient population. Similar to patients who abuse substances, patients with paraphilia must learn to navigate a world in which the subjects of their preoccupation (whether people of specific ages, particular circumstances, or inanimate objects) are all around them. Identifying risks, learning to deal with urges, and developing a plan of action if faced with a trigger are imperative for this patient population (Brunette and Mueser 2006; Krueger and Kaplan 2002; Osborne and Wise 2005; Studer and Aylwin 2006).

Medications

Patients may require multiple medications to adequately manage paraphilic fantasies and curb paraphilic behaviors. Although some clinicians think of paraphilias as "driven" behaviors instead of frankly compulsive behaviors (Lehne et al. 2000), antidepressant medications—particularly selective serotonin reuptake inhibitors (SSRIs)—are used for paraphilias, just as for anxiety disorders such as obsessive-compulsive disorder. Other commonly used medications include hormonal compounds. However, the literature regarding treatment of paraphilias is extremely limited, as is the active research on such disorders. Much of the literature consists of case reports, letters to editors, or small studies that focus mainly on sexual offenders. The general psychiatric literature would benefit from more investigation of medication use in this patient population, particularly in patients with noncoercive and/or nonoffending paraphilias.

Selective Serotonin Reuptake Inhibitors

Even though no double-blind, randomized, placebo-controlled trials of SSRIs have been reported in patients with paraphilias, these medications are widely prescribed in this patient population (Briken and Kafka 2007; Hall and Hall 2007). In fact, Briken and Kafka (2007; Greenberg and Bradford 1997) named SSRIs as the most prescribed medications for populations of sexual offenders in nonresidential settings. The reason for SSRI effectiveness remains somewhat theoretical, based on debates regarding whether paraphilias are related to obsessive-compulsive or impulse control problems and whether serotonin dysregulation is the key to paraphilia development or exacerbation

(Kafka 1997). SSRIs may be helpful in treating paraphilias at least in part because they lower sex drive by increasing serotonin (Osborne and Wise 2005). Their side effects are known to include erectile dysfunction, ejaculatory difficulties, and/or reduced libido. However, some researchers remind clinicians that erectile dysfunction is not sufficient for reduction in paraphilic behaviors, and some patients may continue to partake in paraphilic behaviors despite chemical or even physical castration (Hall and Hall 2007; Saleh 2005). Additionally, temporary benefit from these medications should not necessarily imply sustained benefit, and some authors warn against conceptualizing SSRIs as pharmacological agents specifically for treatment of paraphilias (Lehne et al. 2000). Despite these conflicting views, SSRIs will likely continue to be used as one among the limited selection of medications for treatment of paraphilias. In addition to SSRI medications, the tricyclic compound clomipramine has been used with some success (Clayton 1993), and its efficacy also has been attributed to its significant serotonin reuptake inhibition (Osborne and Wise 2005).

Dosing of SSRI medications should be within recognized guidelines for the treatment of anxiety or affective disorders, but can go to the upper levels recommended (Schatzberg and Nemeroff 2006). As in any psychiatric disorder, the choice of SSRI medication is specific to the clinician and patient. One must consider the patient's other comorbid conditions when initiating and titrating the medication, particularly as related to affective or anxiety spectrum disorders. This strategy, along with close and frequent follow-up, will help ensure that optimal benefit can be achieved with maximum patient adherence to the treatment regimen.

Hormonally Active Medications

With the decreasing popularity of physical castration for patients with sexually deviant behaviors, the use of medications to elicit so-called chemical castration has increased. Among the several types of hormonally active medications are a competitive testosterone inhibitor cyproterone acetate (not available in the United States), progestogen, medroxyprogesterone acetate, and luteinizing hormone–releasing hormone or gonadotropin-releasing hormone analogues such as leuprolide acetate or triptorelin (Briken et al. 2003; Hall and Hall 2007; Krueger and Kaplan 2002; Rösler and Witztum 1998;

Sadock and Sadock 2007). These compounds work via reduction of testosterone levels, thereby reducing sexual desire and arousal response, and can be administered either orally or via depot injection (Hall and Hall 2007; Krueger and Kaplan 2002). Readers are directed to Krueger and Kaplan (2002), Osborne and Wise (2005), and Briken et al. (2003) for thorough reviews of biochemical details. Although some authors wonder if hormonal treatments are more punitive than therapeutic, and if the requisite regular appointments for medication administration and side effect monitoring may contribute to poor compliance (Briken and Kafka 2007), these medications are becoming more widely used with time. Notably, some authors suggest that regular follow-up appointments are beneficial for close patient monitoring (Hall and Hall 2007), something that is key in paraphilic disorders.

Side effects of hormonal treatments are not incidental. They may include weight gain; alterations in liver functions; decreased calcium and bone density; hypertension; diabetes; thromboembolic events; hormonal effects including hot flashes, erectile dysfunction, and gynecomastia; and mood problems such as depression (Briken et al. 2003; Hall and Hall 2007; Krueger and Kaplan 2002; Rösler and Witztum 1998). Of note, some research has found that supplemental "add-back" therapy, wherein small doses of testosterone are given back to the patient, can remedy osteoporosis and erectile dysfunction without reactivating paraphilic thoughts (Briken et al. 2003). Other supplemental medications for bone demineralization can include calcium, vitamin D, and the bisphosphonate alendronate (Krueger and Kaplan 2002).

Other Medications

In addition to antidepressant and hormonal medications, other medications may be helpful in some patients with paraphilias. Historically, antipsychotic medications were used with some success, although it is unclear if these medications were targeting the paraphilia itself or an associated psychotic or affective disorder (Osborne and Wise 2005).

Antiepileptic medications (e.g., topiramate) may be beneficial in the treatment of paraphilias such as fetishism (Shiah et al. 2006), as well as other nonparaphilic sexual addictions or compulsions (Fong et al. 2005; Khazaal and Zullino 2006). The hypothesized mechanism of action involves blockage of voltage-gated ion channels, potentiation of gamma-aminobutyric acid (an inhibitory neurotransmitter), and blockage of kainite/AMPA (α-amino-3-hydroxyl-5-methyl-4-isoxazole-propionate) glutamate (excitatory) receptors. Also, Varela and Black (2002) reported successful treatment of a patient with pedophilia using a combination of the antiepileptic medication carbamazepine and clonazepam. This patient had significant anxiety and dysphoria associated with his pedophilic behaviors, but otherwise had no comorbid psychiatric diagnoses. Once started on these medications, his unwanted thoughts and behaviors ceased, and his success was noted to have lasted 1 year (at the time of case report publication). Use of the anxiolytic buspirone also has been cited as helpful in patients with paraphilia; however, some case reports involved patients with separate and comorbid anxiety disorders (Balon 1998; Federoff 1988, 1992).

In another interesting case report, Rubenstein and Engel (1996) reported using lithium and a serotonin reuptake inhibitor in combination to treat a patient's transvestic fetishism, after antidepressant therapies alone were unsuccessful. This patient also had tried other medications, including anxiolytics and an antipsychotic. He was not diagnosed with bipolar disorder; rather, lithium was used to augment the antidepressant effect. Not only was the combination of lithium and an SSRI effective in eliminating the patient's behaviors, but he did not suffer orgasmic dysfunction as he had with unopposed antidepressant medications. The authors posited that lithium acted as an "antiparaphilic augmenter" to the serotonin reuptake inhibitor because of presynaptic serotonin system enhancement (Rubenstein and Engel 1996), again highlighting the importance of serotonin in the manifestation of paraphilias.

Sympathomimetic medications have been cited as helpful for patients with paraphilias (or those with paraphilia-related behaviors) who have comorbid attention-deficit/hyperactivity disorder (Kafka and Hennen 2000). Ryback (2004) reported that naltrexone, an opiate antagonist, was helpful in a group of adolescent sexual offenders. Effectiveness was by measured by reduction in frequency of sexual fantasies and masturbatory activity. Finally, the use of the H_2-receptor antagonist cimetidine has been proposed as beneficial in paraphilias, although the literature is limited to a single study using cimetidine in patients with dementia and sexual acting-out behaviors (Wiseman et al. 2000).

Although the above-mentioned reports focus on individual patients or small groups of patients, they serve as evidence that these challenging psychiatric disorders may require therapeutic and pharmacological creativity on the part of treating clinicians. Given the multiple approaches for treatment, developing an individual treatment plan for patients with paraphilias may be confusing. Bradford (2001) developed a treatment algorithm based on severity of the disorder, from mild to catastrophic. He advocated various levels of treatment, beginning with CBT and relapse prevention for all patients with paraphilias, and proceeding to institution of medication as the disorder becomes more severe. For the most severe paraphilias, the use of hormonally active medications is advised (Bradford 2001). In another algorithm, Briken et al. (2003) identified the need for concurrent psychotherapeutic interventions along with medications if needed. As in Bradford's algorithm, use of SSRIs is recommended initially, with the addition of hormonal agents with worsening symptoms. Although more research needs to be done, the potential for successful treatment using these and other medications should be noted and pursued.

Special Issues

Although the biopsychosociocultural debate surrounding paraphilias is beyond the scope of this chapter, a brief mention seems warranted here. According to DSM-IV-TR criteria, paraphilic preferences must include personal distress, or social or occupational dysfunction, to qualify as a disorder and to warrant treatment. This criterion leads to debate from those who feel that engaging in paraphilic behaviors without experiencing distress does not qualify as a disorder, and perhaps should not be deemed "abnormal" or "pathological." The line blurs further when one considers nonparaphilic issues such as gender identity disorder. Some current schools of thought incorporate a continuum-based view of sexuality and gender, and consider a more encompassing view of gender identity. This is not something to ignore in the current social climate (Burdge 2007). However, as currently defined, paraphilias stand apart from gender issues. The impact of one's paraphilic sexual behaviors on another person, particularly if the other party is nonconsenting or underage, cannot be minimized merely because the patient was not sufficiently "distressed" to fit criteria. In the following subsections, we describe current conceptualization of three complex paraphilias and the challenges associated with treatment.

Pedophilia

Both psychological and biological interventions are used in the psychiatric assessment and treatment of patients with pedophilia (Berlin 1997; Berlin and Coyle 1981; Berlin and Meinecke 1981). Because individuals with pedophilia represent a heterogeneous group, treatment must be individualized (Fagan et al. 2002). Assessment and treatment for those who have been charged with a crime involve collaboration with the legal system and place the clinician in a complicated and difficult position. This position contrasts significantly from the traditional clinician-patient alliance in which confidentiality and patient rights are primary. While acting as an advocate for the patient's rehabilitation, the clinician also is mandated to report abuse and ethically is obligated to consider the greater good of the community (Gellerman and Suddath 2005). Clinicians considering this work should be clear and comfortable with this role and should clarify their responsibility to the patient and to the community in the initial phase of treatment. Although doing so increases the risk that the patient may limit disclosure, the therapist must actively inquire into such abusive activity to avoid the impression of collusion and rationalization of illegal behavior.

For patients with pedophilia, cognitive-behavioral–based group psychotherapy has been deemed the "treatment of choice" (Studer and Aylwin 2006). Through this modality, the defenses of denial and minimization can be confronted, as can the associated cognitive distortions that permit the individuals to rationalize and justify their behavior. Self-deceptions—minimizing the harmful effects of the offender's behaviors on children and minimizing responsibility for the behavior—are common cognitive distortions that can be challenged and corrected in the context of group psychotherapy with other offenders (Fagan et al. 2002). Another aspect of treatment that lends itself to group methods is the deconstruction of the pedophilic "seduction," or "grooming," of a child. This process often takes place over time and may involve both subtle and overt behaviors intended to isolate the child, persuade the child to comply with sexual requests, indoctrinate the child with a sense of shared responsibility for the behaviors, and instill in the child fear of the consequences of noncompliance or disclosure. Identifying the precise behaviors utilized to accomplish the seduction, and then assuming full personal responsibility for it, is central to correction of the offending adult's cognitions.

The offender's recovery depends in part on the assumption of responsibility for the impact of his actions. His confusion, often fueled by denial or by his or her distorted interpretations of his victim's responses, must be corrected (Hall and Hall 2007; Krueger and Kaplan 2002; Studer and Aylwin 2006). For many offenders, individual psychotherapy may be a necessary adjunct to reinforce and deepen learning that takes place in group treatment.

Although some nonoffending patients with pedophilia may find group treatment with offenders a useful learning experience, they do not necessarily exhibit the same cognitive distortions as do offenders. In fact, they may present with profound shame and anxiety regarding their sexuality (Osborne and Wise 2005). Additionally, they are less likely to minimize the potential harm of behavioral manifestations of their urges than are their offender counterparts, and may be grateful and relieved to have an opportunity for treatment. The nonoffending patients may demonstrate no imminent risk of acting on their urges. Instead, defining features of their clinical presentation often include shame, anxiety, and distress about the inability to function or fully experience a peer-age sexual relationship. Central aspects of treatment incorporate acceptance of their sexual "difference," expression of grief, resolution of shame by breaking social isolation and secrecy, experience of support from other like-minded individuals, and, especially in cases where the pedophilic orientation is exclusive, development of a realistic and meaningful life plan without adult romantic relationships (Osborne and Wise 2005). Although nonoffending persons with pedophilia need to develop concrete strategies for future behavioral control and the ability to identify risk factors for escalation of their fantasies and urges, the urgency of these themes is not equivalent to that of offenders.

As in treating the other paraphilias, pharmacological interventions to lower libidinal urges are frequently used in the treatment of pedophilia (Lehne et al. 2000). SSRIs may lower drive by increasing levels of serotonin. SSRIs also may be helpful in reducing intrusive sexual obsession and preoccupation. In cases where the risk of offending is marked, medications that have a direct suppressing effect on testosterone levels, and therefore on sexual drive, are used. Antiandrogenic medications commonly used are medroxyprogesterone acetate and leuprolide acetate (Berlin and Meinecke 1981; Briken et al. 2003; Krueger and Kaplan 2002). Although these medications may result in erectile dysfunction, many individuals maintain adequate sexual functioning. The goal of such medications is to augment the individual's ability to achieve be-havioral self-control (Fagan et al. 2002). Without such pharmacological sup-port, some patients with paraphilias are unable to effectively respond to psychotherapeutic interventions aimed at developing self-control.

Transvestic Fetishism

The two most common presentations of transvestic fetishism are patients who have been discovered by a spouse, partner, or family member, or patients who have become sufficiently gender dysphoric to seek consultation regarding sex-ual reassignment surgery. In cases of transvestic fetishism, individual therapy is often the best initial approach, with conjoint couple therapy as a subse-quent or concurrent intervention. However, if the couple is in crisis, conjoint treatment is critical. An inherent bind complicates conjoint therapy. For the transvestic partner, the challenge to stop the cross-dressing behavior may be an unrealistic goal because transvestic fetishism is often quite intractable. At the same time, the female partner is challenged toward greater acceptance, an equally difficult challenge given the destructive impact she perceives the fe-tishism to have on herself and the marriage. The focus of conjoint psycho-therapy in transvestic fetishism is to help the couple face the bind in their relationship (Osborne and Wise 2005).

The clinician must ask patients with transvestic fetishism about self-mutilating behaviors and gender dysphoria. Gender-dysphoric patients have been reported to consider and attempt autocastration by various methods, and in relation to varying psychiatric diagnoses (Greilsheimer and Groves 1979; Martin and Gattaz 1991; Russell et al. 2005). Such genital mutilation may signify intense gender dysphoria and requires thorough yet delicate in-vestigation into the patient's status. Special treatment considerations are war-ranted. Although directly challenging the patient about the authenticity of the dysphoria is countertherapeutic, the clinician needs to remember that in-tensely dysphoric states may be transient "state phenomena" related to a co-morbid affective state and may respond to aggressive antidepressant treatment (Wise and Meyer 1980). However, not all gender dysphoria is attributable to comorbid issues. Some patients who desire sexual reassignment based on gen-der dysphoria may meet criteria for gender identity disorder. The DSM-IV-TR diagnostic elements of this disorder include persistent cross-gender identification; discomfort with one's sex or sense of inappropriateness in the gender role of that sex; and significant distress or impairment. Patients who meet full criteria for gender identity disorder as well as transvestic fetishism should be given both diagnoses. If a patient displays cross-dressing behavior and gender dysphoria but does not meet full criteria for gender identity disorder, the diagnosis of transvestic fetishism with gender dysphoria is more appropriate (American Psychiatric Association 2000). In any event, patients presenting with gender dysphoria should be questioned for thoughts about autocastration and self-mutilation as part of the initial evaluation, because these thoughts or behaviors could significantly alter the course of treatment.

In working with an individual who is gender dysphoric and requests sexual reassignment surgery, the clinician needs to help the patient recognize the pros and cons of such a drastic undertaking. Helping the patient face the potential consequences of reassignment, including loss of family, spouse, children, and/or occupation, is of utmost importance as the clinician establishes the therapeutic relationship (Kockott and Fahrner 1987; Levine and Shumaker 1983). Although societal acceptance is greater and the risks are lower than in the past, a deliberate and realistic assessment of potential consequences and consideration of less extreme alternatives is imperative. For some transvestites, initial optimism is displaced by depression when issues of loss emerge (Osborne and Wise 2005). As in working with patients with any paraphilias, clinicians are advised to avoid simplistic short-term solutions and to remain cognizant of the possible emergence of worsening dysphoria, along with self-destructive thoughts and behaviors, as treatment progresses (Sadock and Sadock 2007). The clinician must maintain a long-term perspective and exercise restraint in judgment regarding the ultimate diagnosis and appropriate course of treatment.

Complex underlying themes and comorbid conditions may become more apparent as treatment progresses and suggest the need to pursue a long-term treatment approach (often combining psychotherapy with medication). Many patients with complex presentations of transvestism and gender dysphoria utilize psychiatric treatment as a long-term resource in their lives. Much like patients with other psychiatric illnesses, these patients may return for reevaluation at regular intervals to assess for changes in manifestation of their disorder, to assess the degree of dysphoria, and to reassess the appropriateness of the current therapeutic regimen.

Sexual Sadism and Masochism

As noted earlier, to reach the level of a psychiatric diagnosis, paraphilic preferences must confer personal distress and/or social or occupational dysfunction. Like transvestic fetishism, sadism and masochism are paraphilias in which unusual sexual behaviors are preferred, and patients rarely seek psychiatric evaluation. These behaviors often involve role-playing and fantasy gratification without inflicting real physical pain or humiliation (Weinberg and Kamel 1983), although the power differential is often arousing to all participants. Involvement in these paraphilic activities may lead to distress or impairment in other realms of life, even if the patient denies personal distress as a result of the paraphilia. The following two examples show the different ways that ego-syntonic sexual activities may be interpreted.

> A governmental intelligence agency requested a psychiatric evaluation for a 28-year-old married woman, after a security evaluation revealed that she preferred sadomasochistic role-playing with her husband, who also enjoyed this form of sexual gratification. She and her husband took pleasure in these activities equally and consensually, and the patient exhibited no formal psychiatric disorder. She was able to pass the security evaluation because her preference for this behavior was not secret to her employer (thereby not deeming her a security risk) and involved no coercive elements.

> A 34-year-old female attorney frequented sadomasochistic clubs and engaged in fantasy role-playing with strangers. Although she had not yet experienced any physical harm, she began to fear that she was at risk of assault or rape if she met someone at a club who was a sadistic rapist. Her situation merited a psychiatric categorization as paraphilic, because her preferred sexual repertoire both exposed her to clear physical risk and became distressing to her. She entered therapy because of this, and benefited from having a psychotherapeutic forum in which to explore the underlying reasons for her drive to participate in such activities.

These two examples, as well as the entire "Special Issues" section, highlight the challenges of treating patients with paraphilias—from their initial motivation for treatment, to their interpersonal struggles, to the wide impact that these disorders can have on their lives. Clinicians can begin to help these patients through sensitive and thorough initial evaluations, corroborating information, and treatment (both psychotherapeutic and psychopharmacological if needed).

Conclusion

As demonstrated amply in this chapter, the effort to assess, manage, and treat paraphilias is among the least evidence-based undertakings in all of psychiatric practice today. The task is daunting due to the limited number of publications, the lack of randomized control trials of medications, and the intricacies inherent in such a diverse patient population. Additionally, the division and fragmentation of paraphilias into discrete entities make them even more difficult to analyze in a cohesive way. These issues are further complicated by the fact that the vast majority of patients with paraphilias do not voluntarily seek treatment. Understandably, in the present social climate, much of the current psychiatric literature concerns the sexual offender population, which is not necessarily synonymous with the paraphilic population in general. However, even if behaviors are not remotely illegal, and therefore do not place the patient in contact with the forensic system, the patient's presentation for treatment often follows external motivation by someone in his or her social network.

Assessment tools, psychotherapeutic techniques, and medications (ranging from psychiatric medications to hormonally active medications) are useful for the clinicians who endeavor to treat such a varied and complex population. This patient population requires future research, via intensive investigation, formalized research, and well-reasoned therapeutic trials, for conceptualizing the most appropriate treatment modalities for this population in need of care.

Key Points

- Paraphilias are divided into three categories according to triggering stimuli:
  - Excitement stimulated by nonhuman objects (fetishism);
  - Excitement stimulated by real or imagined suffering or humiliation of oneself or another person who is the sexual partner (masochism and sadism); and
  - Excitement from preferred sexual attraction toward children (pedophilia).

- Paraphilias are predominant in males.
  - Other aspects of demographics and epidemiology are not well defined.
  - Difficulties arise in evaluation and diagnosis because patients hesitate to get treatment.
- Specific populations may be quite different from general paraphilic populations.
  - Findings on forensic populations may not generalize to nonforensic patient populations.
  - Also, sexually deviant or opportunistic behaviors as related to personality disorders, such as antisocial personality disorder, may not represent paraphilias per se.
- Treatment begins with a thorough assessment of the patient.
  - The clinician determines why the patient presented at the current time and whether the individual truly desires treatment.
  - Evaluation and treatment of psychiatric comorbidities is essential.
  - Comorbid issues, such as mood or anxiety disorders, may be secondary to paraphilic behaviors or stresses (interpersonal problems, threat of discovery).
- Cognitive-behavioral therapy is the mainstay of psychotherapeutic treatment.
  - Other behavioral therapies, such as social skills training, sex education, and vocational rehabilitation, also may be helpful for specific patients.
  - Relapse prevention techniques may be relevant as well.
- Psychiatric medications are commonly used in this patient population.
  - Selective serotonin reuptake inhibitors are most widely used.

- Antipsychotics, antiepileptics, anxiolytics, psychostimulants, and the opiate antagonist naltrexone may prove beneficial as well.
- Hormonal agents may act by decreasing testosterone, desire, and arousal response.
  - Side effects include weight gain, hypertension, gynecomastia, hot flashes, erectile dysfunction, depression, and bone demineralization, among others.
  - Routine follow-up appointments and monitoring of side effects is crucial with any medication.

References

Abel GG, Osborn C: The paraphilias: the extent and nature of sexually deviant and criminal behavior. Psychiatr Clin North Am 15:675–687, 1992

Allnutt SH, Bradford JM, Greenberg DM, et al: Co-morbidity of alcoholism and the paraphilias. J Forensic Sci 41:234–239, 1996

American Psychiatric Association: Diagnostic and Statistical Manual of Mental Disorders, 4th Edition. Washington, DC, American Psychiatric Association, 1994

American Psychiatric Association: Diagnostic and Statistical Manual of Mental Disorders, 4th Edition, Text Revision. Washington, DC, American Psychiatric Association, 2000

Bak RC: Distortions of the concept of fetishism. Psychoanal Study Child 29:191–214, 1974

Balon R: Pharmacological treatment of paraphilias with a focus on antidepressants. J Sex Marital Ther 24:241–254, 1998

Bancroft J: Human Sexuality and Its Problems, 2nd Edition. London, Churchill Livingstone, 1989

Behrendt N, Buhl N, Seidl S: The lethal paraphilic syndrome: accidental autoerotic deaths in four women and a review of the literature. Int J Legal Med 116:148–152, 2002

Bemporad JR, Dunton HD, Spady FH: Case reports of the treatment of a child foot fetishist. Am J Psychiatry 30:303–316, 1976

Berlin FS: "Chemical castration" for sex offenders. N Engl J Med 336:1030, 1997

Berlin FS, Coyle GS: Sexual deviation syndromes. Johns Hopkins Med J 149:119–125, 1981

Berlin FS, Meinecke CF: Treatment of sex offenders with antiandrogenic medication: conceptualization, review of treatment modalities and preliminary findings. Am J Psychiatry 138:601–607, 1981

Blanchard R, Christensen BK, Strong SM, et al: Retrospective self-reports of childhood accidents causing unconsciousness in phallometrically diagnosed pedophiles. Arch Sex Behav 31:511–526, 2002

Blanchard R, Kuban ME, Klassen P, et al: Self-reported head injuries before and after age 13 in pedophilic and non-pedophilic men referred for clinical assessment. Arch Sex Behav 32:573–581, 2003

Borchard B, Gnoth A, Schulz W: Personality disorders and "psychopathy" in sex offenders imprisoned in forensic-psychiatric hospitals: SKID-II and PCL-R results in patients with impulse control disorder and paraphilia. Psychiatr Prax 30:133–138, 2003

Bradford JM: The neurobiology, neuropharmacology, and pharmacological treatment of the paraphilias and compulsive sexual behavior. Can J Psychiatry 46:26–34, 2001

Bradford JM: On sexual violence. Curr Opin Psychiatry 19:527–532, 2006

Bradford JM, Boulet J, Pawlak A: The paraphilias: a multiplicity of deviant behaviors. Can J Psychiatry 37:104–108, 1992

Briken P, Kafka MP: Pharmacological treatments for paraphilic patients and sexual offenders. Curr Opin Psychiatry 20:609–613, 2007

Briken P, Hill A, Berner W: Pharmacotherapy of paraphilias with long-acting agonists of luteinizing hormone-releasing agents: a systematic review. J Clin Psychiatry 64:890–897, 2003

Brunette MF, Mueser KT: Psychosocial interventions for the long-term management of patients with severe mental illness and co-occurring substance use disorder. J Clin Psychiatry 67(suppl):10–17, 2006

Burdge BJ: Bending gender, ending gender: theoretical foundations for social work practice with the transgender community. Soc Work 52:243–250, 2007

Cantor JM, Blanchard R, Christensen BK, et al: Intelligence, memory, and handedness in pedophilia. Neuropsychology 18:3–14, 2004

Clayton AH: Fetishism and clomipramine (letter). Am J Psychiatry 150:673–674, 1993

Coleman E, Siributr P, Leelamanit V, et al: The treatment of fetishism and socially inappropriate sexual behavior in a young male with dull normal intelligence. J Med Assoc Thai 76:531–534, 1993

Crepault C, Couture M: Men's erotic fantasies. Arch Sex Behav 9:565–581, 1980

Derogatis LR: Measures of sexual dysfunction and disorders, in Handbook of Psychiatric Measures, 2nd Edition. Edited by Rush AJ, First MB, Blacker D. Washington, DC, American Psychiatric Publishing, 2008, pp 601–602

Dunsieth NW Jr, Nelson EB, Brusman-Lovins LA, et al: Psychiatric and legal features of 113 men convicted of sexual offenses. J Clin Psychiatry 65:293–300, 2004

Fagan PJ, Wise TN, Derogatis LR, et al: Distressed transvestites. J Nerv Ment Dis 176:626–632, 1988

Fagan PJ, Wise TN, Schmidt CW, et al: Pedophilia. JAMA 288:2458–2465, 2002

Federoff JP: Buspirone hydrochloride in the treatment of transvestic fetishism. J Clin Psychiatry 49:408–409, 1988

Federoff JP: Buspirone hydrochloride in the treatment of an atypical paraphilia. Arch Sex Behav 21:401–406, 1992

Firestone P, Kingston DA, Wexler A, et al: Long-term follow-up of exhibitionists: psychological, phallometric, and offense characteristics. J Am Acad Psychiatry Law 34:349–359, 2006

First MB, Frances A: Issues for DSM-V: unintended consequences of small changes: the case of paraphilias. Am J Psychiatry 165:1240–1241, 2008

Fong TW, De La Garza R II, Newton TF: A case report of topiramate in the treatment of nonparaphilic sexual addiction (letter). J Clin Psychopharmacol 21:512–514, 2005

Frank JD, Frank JB: Persuasion and Healing: A Comparative Study of Psychotherapy, 3rd Edition. Baltimore, MD, Johns Hopkins University Press, 1991

Freud S: Freud and fetishism: previously unpublished minutes of the Vienna Psychoanalytic Society. Psychoanal Q 57:147–166, 1988

Gellerman DM, Suddath R: Violent fantasy, dangerousness, and the duty to warn and protect. J Am Acad Psychiatry Law 33:484–495, 2005

Gosselin C, Wilson G: Sexual variations. New York: Simon & Schuster, 1980

Grant JE: Clinical characteristics and psychiatric comorbidity in males with exhibitionism. J Clin Psychiatry 66:1367–1371, 2005

Greenacre P: The transitional object and the fetish with special reference to the role of illusion. Int J Psychoanal 51:447–456, 1970

Greenberg DM, Bradford JM: Treatment of the paraphilic disorders: a review of the role of the selective serotonin reuptake inhibitors. Sex Abuse 9:349–361, 1997

Greilsheimer H, Groves JE: Male genital self-mutilation. Arch Gen Psychiatry 36:441–446, 1979

Hall GC: Sexual arousal and arousability in a sexual offender population. J Abnorm Psychol 98:145–149, 1989

Hall RC, Hall RC: A profile of pedophilia: definition, characteristics of offenders, recidivism, treatment outcomes, and forensic issues. Mayo Clin Proc 82:457–471, 2007

Hollender MH, Brown CW, Roback HB: Genital exhibitionism in women. Am J Psychiatry 134:436–438, 1977

Hunter D: Case reports: the treatment of a child food fetishist. Am J Psychiatry 30:303–316, 1976

Kafka MP: A monoamine hypothesis for the pathophysiology of paraphilic disorders. Arch Sex Behav 26:343–358, 1997

Kafka MP, Hennen J: Psychostimulant augmentation during treatment with selective serotonin reuptake inhibitors in men with paraphilias and paraphilia-related disorders: a case series. J Clin Psychiatry 61:664–670, 2000

Kafka MP, Hennen J: A DSM-IV Axis I comorbidity study of males (N=120) with paraphilias and paraphilia-related disorders. Sex Abuse 14:349–366, 2002

Kafka MP, Prentky RA: Attention-deficit/hyperactivity disorder in males with paraphilias and paraphilia-related disorders: a comorbidity study. J Clin Psychiatry 59:388–396, 1998

Khazaal Y, Zullino DF: Topiramate in the treatment of compulsive sexual behavior: case report. BMC Psychiatry 6:22, 2006

Kockott MP, Fahrner E: Transsexuals who have not undergone surgery: a follow-up study. Arch Sex Behav 16:511–522, 1987

Krueger RB, Kaplan MS: The paraphilic and hypersexual disorders: an overview. J Psychiatr Pract 7:391–403, 2001

Krueger RB, Kaplan MS: Behavioral and psychopharmacological treatment of the paraphilic and hypersexual disorders. J Psychiatr Pract 8:21–32, 2002

Langevin R: Sexual Strands. Hillsdale, NJ, Erlbaum, 1983

Langevin R: Erotic Preference, Gender Identity, and Aggression in Men: New Research Studies. Hillsdale, NJ, Erlbaum, 1985

Lehne GK, Money J: Multiplex versus multiple taxonomy of paraphilia: case example. Sex Abuse 15:61–72, 2003

Lehne GK, Thomas K, Berlin FS: Treatment of sexual paraphilias: a review of the 1999–2000 literature. Curr Opin Psychiatry 13:569–573, 2000

Levine SB, Shumaker RE: Increasingly Ruth: toward understanding sex reassignment. Arch Sex Behav 12:247–261, 1983

Martin T, Gattaz WF: Psychiatric aspects of male genital self-mutilation. Psychopathology 24:170–178, 1991

McHugh PR, Slavney PR: Methods of reasoning in psychopathology: conflict and resolution. Compr Psychiatry 23:197–215, 1982

McHugh PR, Slavney PR: Perspectives in Psychiatry, 2nd Edition. Baltimore, MD, Johns Hopkins University Press, 1998

Osborne CS, Wise TN: Paraphilias, in Handbook of Sexual Dysfunction. Edited by Balon R, Segraves RT. Boca Raton, FL, Taylor & Francis, 2005, pp 293–330

Raymond NC, Coleman E, Ohlerking F, et al: Psychiatric comorbidity in pedophilic sex offenders (comment). Am J Psychiatry 156:786–788, 1999

Reinecke MA, Freeman A: Cognitive therapy, in Essential Psychotherapies: Theory and Practice, 2nd Edition. Edited by Gurman AS, Messer SB. New York, Guilford, 2003, pp 224–271

Ridinger RB: Negotiating limits: the legal status of SM in the United States, in Sadomasochism: Powerful Pleasures. Edited by Kleinplatz PJ, Moser C. Philadelphia, PA, Harrington Park Press, 2006, pp 189–216

Rösler A, Witztum E: Treatment of men with paraphilia with a long-acting analogue of gonadotropin-releasing hormone. N Engl J Med 338:416–422, 1998

Rubenstein EB, Engel NL: Successful treatment of transvestic fetishism with sertraline and lithium (letter). J Clin Psychiatry 57:92, 1996

Russell DB, McGovern G, Harte FB: Genital self-mutilation by radio-frequency in a male-to-female transsexual. Sex Health 2:203–204, 2005

Ryback RS: Naltrexone in the treatment of adolescent sexual offenders. J Clin Psychiatry 65:982–986, 2004

Sadock BJ, Sadock VA: Paraphilias and sexual disorder not otherwise specified, in Kaplan and Sadock's Synopsis of Psychiatry, 10th Edition. Edited by Sadock BJ, Sadock VA. Philadelphia, PA, Lippincott Williams & Wilkins, 2007, pp 705–717

Saleh F: Issues to consider in the assessment and treatment of paraphilic patients (letter). J Clin Psychiatry 66:802–803, 2005

Schatzberg AF, Nemeroff CB: Essentials of Clinical Psychopharmacology, 2nd Edition. Washington, DC, American Psychiatric Publishing, 2006

Shiah I, Chao C, Mao W, et al: Treatment of paraphilic sexual disorder: the use of topiramate in fetishism. Int Clin Psychopharmacol 21:241–243, 2006

Shields LB, Hunsaker DM, Hunsaker JC 3rd, et al: Atypical autoerotic death, part II. Am J Forensic Med Pathol 26:53–62, 2005

Springer A: Female perversion: scenes and strategies in analysis and culture. J Anal Psychol 41:325–338, 1996

Studer LH, Aylwin AS: Pedophilia: the problem with diagnosis and limitations of CBT in treatment. Med Hypotheses 67:774–781, 2006

Varela D, Black DW: Pedophilia treated with carbamazepine and clonazepam (letter). Am J Psychiatry 159:1245–1246, 2002

Weinberg T, Kamel GWL: S and M: Studies in Sadomasochism. New York, Prometheus Books, 1983

Wise TN: Psychotherapy of an aging transvestite. J Sex Marital Ther 5:368–373, 1979

Wise TN, Goldberg RL: Escalation of a fetish: coprophagia in a nonpsychotic adult of normal intelligence. J Sex Marital Ther 21:272–275, 1995

Wise TN, Meyer JK: The border area between transvestism and gender dysphoria: transvestic applicant for sex reassignment. Arch Sex Behav 9:327–340, 1980

Wise TN, Fagan PJ, Schmidt CW, et al: Personality and sexual functioning of transvestic fetishists and other paraphilics. J Nerv Ment Dis 179:694–698, 1991

Wiseman SV, McAuley JW, Freidenberg GR, et al: Hypersexuality in patients with dementia: possible response to cimetidine. Neurology 54:2024, 2000

Zavitzianos G: The perversion of fetishism in women. Psychoanal Q 51:405–425, 1982

Recommended Readings

Briken P, Kafka MP: Pharmacological treatments for paraphilic patients and sexual offenders. Curr Opin Psychiatry 20:609–613, 2007

Briken P, Hill A, Berner W: Pharmacotherapy of paraphilias with long-acting agonists of luteinizing hormone-releasing agents: a systematic review. J Clin Psychiatry 64:890–897, 2003

Fagan PJ, Wise TN, Schmidt CW, et al: Pedophilia. JAMA 288:2458–2465, 2002

Hall RC, Hall RC: A profile of pedophilia: definition, characteristics of offenders, recidivism, treatment outcomes, and forensic issues. Mayo Clin Proc 82:457–471, 2007

Kafka MP, Hennen J: A DSM-IV Axis I comorbidity study of males ($N=120$) with paraphilias and paraphilia-related disorders. Sex Abuse 14:349–366, 2002

Krueger RB, Kaplan MS: The paraphilic and hypersexual disorders: an overview. J Psychiatr Pract 7:391–403, 2001

Krueger RB, Kaplan MS: Behavioral and psychopharmacological treatment of the paraphilic and hypersexual disorders. J Psychiatr Pract 8:21–32, 2002

Lehne GK, Thomas K, Berlin FS: Treatment of sexual paraphilias: a review of the 1999–2000 literature. Curr Opin Psychiatry 13:569–573, 2000

PART III

Age-Related Sexual Issues

13

Counseling Children, Adolescents, and Their Families About Sexual Issues

Derek C. Polonsky, M.D.

For many psychiatrists, talking directly and practically about sexual issues does not come easily, especially with children and adolescents. Theories about genital phases of development and about sexual fantasies and wishes in childhood, as well as their attendant conflicts, do little to help clinicians address the real-life concerns of patients and their families. Most psychiatric training programs provide some information regarding sexuality and sexual dysfunction but include no practical training and education that assist clinicians in talking about and helping patients with their sexual development. The consequence is that few psychiatrists are prepared to inquire about specific sexual thoughts and activities or to offer information and help with patients' sexual growth and problems. For psychiatrists, particularly those treating children and adolescents, dealing directly with sexuality and relationships provides a unique opportunity to be part of their patients' sexual and emotional growth, which may be central to the patients' future relationships.

Laumann et al. (1994) reviewed the spectrum of adult sexual functioning in the United States. Their findings indicated that 43% of women and 37% of men experienced some long-standing sexual issue. However, the literature sheds little light on the frequency of sexual difficulties in adolescents. What children do sexually is chronicled quite well (Mosher et al. 2005), but inquiry into difficulties they may encounter has been sparse. Given that sexual experiences begin in early adolescence, often with little guidance or practical information, the sexual problems with which so many couples struggle may frequently begin at this time.

Masters and Johnson (1970) were pioneers in developing a novel treatment approach to sexual dysfunctions for adult couples. Kaplan (1974), a psychoanalyst and couples therapist, integrated the Masters and Johnson model into a dynamic therapy for individuals and couples. Although treatment can be helpful in many instances, a long-standing sense of defectiveness and shame regarding sex has often become an internalized part of a patient's identity. The emotional cost for the individual and couple is considerable, and the challenge of therapy is increased by having to deal with the impact of many years of perceived defect. An adolescent, however, is just beginning his or her sexual journey and is struggling to figure out what that means and how to manage the physical uncertainty at the same time he or she is in unknown terrain regarding forming meaningful love attachments.

In this chapter, I review some of the cultural and social factors related to the "sexual incompetence" of patients, of their families, and of therapists. Patients are reluctant to bring up sexual difficulties they have been unable to discuss with anyone and do not know how to manage. Therapists mirror this discomfort and are similarly reluctant to ask about sex, in large part because training programs provide little guidance or education regarding human sexuality.

When a clinician treats a child or adolescent, a triadic relationship exists between parents, child, and therapist. The parents are looking for guidance and help, the child often is the unwilling participant, and the therapist tries his or her best to read between the lines, understand and translate, and use his or her skills to help the group manage better.

Although the clinician has many opportunities to confront sexual issues head on and openly, most training programs provide little encouragement to discuss sexuality. This occurs either directly (by teaching that this is intrusive, overstimulating, or problematic countertransference) or indirectly (by providing no integrated, in-depth course on human sexuality). Many texts contain information about sexual history taking and treatment approaches, yet details are alluded to indirectly, and the reader does not learn what therapists do, say, and think in the office with their patients. The clinical material in this chapter aims to fill this void. Any discussion about sex has to be seen in the context of the individual's emotional development, and in adolescents who are dealing with separation, sexuality, and new attachments, the richness of the therapy is remarkable, and the changes are dramatic.

Developing Sexuality of Children and Adolescents

Fonseca and Greydanus (2007) have described in detail sexuality from birth through adolescence. For the newborn, sucking and cuddling, being held, and being fed provide the foundations for trust and the later development of attachments. Sucking is essential for survival, and the mouth and tongue are richly supplied with sensory inputs. The adult equivalent of this "orality" is the pleasure that can be associated with kissing, touching, and affection. Within 6–9 months, infants randomly discover their genitals, and given the children's interest from that point on, touching and rubbing their genitals must be associated with a good feeling. As children develop, the genital play becomes more purposeful. As Lamb (2006) pointed out, masturbation is a means of self-soothing, and for some children who have high energy levels, it may be used as a way of calming themselves.

Sexual development constantly involves interplay between a child and parents; by their actions, parents may facilitate a sense of goodness and well-being associated with discovery of genitals and the pleasurable feelings associated with touching them. If the parents are conflicted about sexuality and have strong negative feelings associated with genital exploration and play, their prohibitions and reprimands may have repercussions in the child's comfort in investing positively in his or her sexual feelings. At one end of the spectrum are parents who respond in a calm and accepting way. As their children become more verbal, these parents might say, "Touching your penis or clitoris feels really good and also enjoyable. It is fine for you to do, but you need to do it in your own room and not at the dining room table." At the other extreme are parents who abhor any such contact and have intensely negative reactions, which may include constant "correction" of the child's attempts to play with his or her genitals. As the child gets older, more direct admonitions, such as "Don't touch yourself down there," are common. The positive or negative introjection of the parental attitudes can have an impact on the child's later ability to experience pleasure with sexual feelings.

As children become more verbal, the parents have an opportunity to introduce the words for penis, scrotum, testicles, vagina, labia, and clitoris into the list of body parts. Children have a natural curiosity to explore and amass information about themselves and the world around them. Genitals are no exception. The absence of a vocabulary for parts above the knees and below the waist is remarkable, and "privates" and "down there" are poor substitutes for the correct words.

Lamb (2001) described the almost universal children's "doctor" game with the "I'll show you mine if you show me yours" theme. In most situations, this game represents a normal, healthy development. Some parents, when they discover their children in this game, simply talk about it in a positive way, making sure that no one is being forced to do something uncomfortable and framing the need for boundaries. At the other extreme are parents who have a rageful outburst, filled with recriminations and negative consequences. In some instances, older siblings or their friends are being coercive with a younger child, and these games or preoccupying masturbation may be an indication of behavior that should raise parents' concern.

An obvious difference between boys and girls is that the penis is "out there" and easily seen. For boys, the penis is often viewed as a prized possession, which he might display proudly, much to the consternation of those around him. A boy can easily explore his penis, feel his scrotum and testicles, and talk more openly about them.

For girls, more effort is required to view their genitals and know what they look like. Lamb (2001) described games girls play with friends in which they explore each others' genitals and engage in looking and touching. Most parents, if they discover this activity, are uncomfortable, but it can be a "teaching

moment" for girls that has enormous potential in fostering a positive invest-
ment in their genitals.

As they begin to reach puberty, girls and boys experience some divergence
of paths. Girls have to deal with a unique and unkind competitiveness with
each other, being faced with "in groups" and "out groups"; appearance becomes extremely important, and the influence of the media in terms of female
sexiness and attractiveness assumes burdensome and destructive proportions.
Although more public discussion about masturbation occurs, it has usually
centered on boys doing it, and masturbatory pleasure for girls has only relatively recently become recognized. One of the goals for clinicians is to help
girls discover their own desire despite the conflicting messages about being
sexy and staying pure (Lamb 2001). In 1953, Kinsey et al. described the difference in the masturbation rates between men and women: although 62% of
women masturbated and 58% masturbated to orgasm, the figures for men were
in the high 90s. Anecdotally, I have given an anonymous questionnaire to
first-year medical students for the past 25 years and have consistently found
that between 90% and 95% of the men reported masturbating, whereas the
figures for women range between 55% and 60%.

When asked about her sexual experiences, a 19-year-old college woman
reported, "When I first started masturbating, I felt like I was doing something
wrong, something 'unnatural.' It was as if I was ashamed of what I was doing,
even though I enjoyed it tremendously in the moment. None of my girl-
friends talked about it, and everyone made it seem like girls didn't masturbate.
I thought I was the only girl doing it."

Although adolescents are told that masturbation is not harmful, they rarely
hear it described as fun, pleasurable, or exciting in their sex education classes.
Given the silence that usually surrounds female sexuality, a therapist talking
openly about sexuality with a teenage girl, including an open discussion about
masturbation, can be affirming and validating, and the matter-of-fact manner
disarms the taboo. Male therapists may worry that they would be crossing a
boundary or appear too suggestive in broaching this topic, believing that girls
would prefer working with a woman therapist. Lamb (2006, p. 156) addressed
this topic: "A female suggesting to a teenage girl to masturbate is akin to presenting her with a role model. Could a male therapist suggest to a teenage girl
to masturbate? This is trickier. But if he comes from the perspective that she
has a right and an obligation to know her own body, and he expresses this in a

caring voice, he can get around her suspicions that he's got a fantasy or two on this very subject." I would go one step further and suggest that the respectful discussion of sex and her body with a male clinician might provide the girl with a model she can emulate in her own intimate relationships.

We should not assume that boys need no guidance or education regarding masturbation. As Lamb (2006) noted,

> While we may assume that kids in this culture today know that masturbation is fine and will not cause disease or blindness, kids may still need to know how frequently is fine, what fantasies are fine, how hard is fine, what objects are fine, and what length of time it takes to reach orgasm is fine. It's incredibly difficult to find that information in books, and not many teen boys seek out book information. It's also difficult to find this information on the Internet without wading through a lot of pornography sites to figure out which ones give real information for teens. Those that do offer sex education often merely say that masturbation is fine and normal and don't go into specifics a teen really needs. There is way too much vague reassurance out there with very little information for the nervous kid about specifics. (p. 165)

Brown and Brown (2006) discussed four important factors that have an impact on sexual development: biology, family, culture, and society. *Biology* refers to the child's awareness of maleness or femaleness and the subsequent hormonal influences during puberty. *Family* relates to the values and expectations in which the child grew up. These may be communicated overtly, covertly, or ambivalently. *Culture* refers to the assignment of roles between the sexes. For some groups, whether directly or indirectly, sex is seen as mutual and pleasurable. Other cultural and ethnic groups may have a more restrictively defined role of gender and sex. There is a challenge in integrating these differences into the expectations that are so constantly presented in the media. The impact of *society* refers to multicultural influences seen in the United States. Messages may be confusing—that is, media often promote sexual images, whereas the culture itself may have a more constrained view. The mixed signals can be confusing for children. Meanwhile, many parents, by not discussing their own sexual beliefs with their children, abdicate their roles, while being distressed at what their children may be taught at school. The parents often have limited guidance or resources from which to get advice. As noted by Brown and Brown (2006), in Western society, boys learn from an early age that dominance, aggression, and achievement are defining characteristics of masculinity. For girls, despite the significant changes that have developed over many years, becoming more prominent with the start of the women's movement in the 1960s, society still approaches women's sexuality with ambivalence and negativity. These mixed messages add to the challenges that many girls face in developing their sexual selves.

In most instances, I believe that some discussion about sex is an important part of the relationship a therapist has with a patient. When dealing with adolescents from different cultural or ethnic backgrounds, care should be taken to assess the degree to which the adolescent has assimilated the culture and to learn what the teenager understands regarding his or her parents' sexual values and expectations. Although society has moved beyond the days of John Harvey Kellogg and Sylvester Graham, who in the nineteenth century developed foods that were specifically designed to dampen the impulses to masturbate, the culture is still ambivalent about its practice. In 1994, the surgeon general of the United States, Joycelyn Elders, was fired by President Clinton after she responded to a question about masturbation. At a United Nations meeting, she was asked, "What do you think are the prospects of a more explicit discussion and promotion of masturbation?" She replied, "As to your specific question in regard to masturbation, I think that is something that is part of human sexuality, and it is part of something that perhaps should be taught. But we've not even taught our children the very basics. I feel that we have tried ignorance for a very long time, and it is time we try education" (Cornog 2004).

For adolescents, masturbation serves a very important function; through this activity, the individual realizes that there is something special about that part of the body that is associated with unique (sexual) feelings. The sense of ownership and control of his or her sexuality is valuable. Masturbation is an opportunity to learn about one's body: what feels good sexually, how one's genitals respond to touch, and what one does to have an orgasm. By so doing, the adolescent is able to enter into a sexual relationship with some self-awareness about his or her sexuality. Rather than relying on the boy to "give" her an orgasm, a girl can think of her sexual responses as her own, and she can guide a partner to do what she likes. For boys, masturbation provides an opportunity to learn about their sexual responses. Having some encouragement to think about the "journey to orgasm" rather than simply the orgasm itself can set the stage for a more interactive sexual sharing with a partner. Landolphi (1994) astutely observed that if the adolescent cannot talk about sexual feelings, then he or she is not ready to have a sexual relationship. The therapist is an important guide when it comes to "relationships 101," and encouraging a teenager to talk with a partner about what he or she wants or likes sexually is a skill that most couples with sexual difficulties never received. Calderone and Johnson (1981) opined that one of the main reasons that adults fail to achieve sexual satisfaction is the interference with the discovery of the pleasure of their own bodies in early life. Moglia and Knowles (1997) noted that boys and girls often receive confusing information about masturbation from peers, parents, and other sources and may need help seeing masturbation as positive sexual behavior. When discussing sex with teens, I joke that masturbation is an "underrated activity and is a cheap, renewable resource." I point out that it provides them with an opportunity to learn about their sexual feelings and responses in a private, unpressured way.

The sample script below is intended as a general guide for the therapist who decides to inquire about masturbation. The individual therapist needs to decide how much to ask and how much advice to give. In my practice, I have found that adolescents (and also adult patients) actually welcome the discussion. The clinician should begin by acknowledging that the topic might initially be uncomfortable, but ultimately talking about masturbation provides a model for open, respectful, and helpful discussions dealing with sex.

> For most individuals there is very little serious talk about masturbation. When people tell me about their experiences in sex education, they never report having been told, "Masturbation feels good and is fun to do." I think of masturbation as a great way of getting to know what kinds of sexual feelings your own body can produce. How did you discover masturbation?

For boys:

> I'd like to offer a few suggestions: Take your time and don't rush to have an orgasm. Get to know the range of feelings you experience on the way. I know that pornography is easy to find, and most guys use it to get turned on. Try to get turned on using your imagination. Using pornography all the time sometimes makes it harder to get aroused when you are with a partner. Guys masturbate in different ways: Some use a dry fist, and some use lubrication, which they say feels better. Others just hump the bed or pillow. Remember, it is your body; see what you can learn about how it works.

For girls:

Learning about your body is important because it is your sexuality and not someone else's. Looking at your vagina, labia, and clitoris helps you to know your genitals. Touching your genitals and paying attention to the feelings lets you know what is enjoyable and feels good. Make sure you are relaxed and comfortable and have privacy, and think of the experience as your special time to feel your own body. I hope it is OK for me to ask if you masturbate. What has it been like for you? Do you have orgasms? Can you let yourself get out of your head and pay attention to what you are feeling?

As boys approach puberty, their physical and sexual changes are prominent, without the same growth in psychological maturity. To parents (and therapists), the child might look like a young adult; he might be bigger and taller than the adult, and certainly has developed a verbal ability that resembles that of a legal scholar. However, the adolescent is fundamentally a little boy in many ways, struggling to separate from his parents (mother in particular) and beginning to think of attachments that begin to involve sexual feelings. Some boys manage their anxiety with bravado, sounding tough and confident sexually, bragging about conquests, and often talking about girls in an objectified way. As Thompson and Kindlon (2000, p. 193) stated, "Boys want to be loved and to love, only it feels too complicated. Many need help making the journey from the simplicity of sex to the complexity of relationships, from aggression and competition to love and caring." The therapist can be helpful as a guide, providing information and coaching, and validating the apprehension a boy feels at beginning to do something that is personal and, although associated with excitement and pleasure, not without fear and anxiety. Many boys who are socially uncomfortable have the added task of wondering how to approach a girl and feeling even less competent physically.

Girls focus more on the "romantic" aspect of a relationship and are often emotionally more mature than boys. However, the pressure around appearance and being accepted is considerable, and for many, sex may become the vehicle to attain acceptance, at a cost to their own sexual growth. A therapist can provide helpful and encouraging support for girls navigating this part of their lives.

Sexual Education for Children and Adolescents

For many children, sexual information is acquired in a random and unstructured manner. Parents may talk about the "facts of life," a term that is itself revealing for its indirect allusion to the topic of sexual facts. Often information is obtained from friends or siblings, with all the inaccuracies such hearsay may entail.

Sex education in schools has been a contentious issue for a very long time. Parents have strong feelings about who will provide their children with sexual information, in many instances insisting that it is the parents' responsibility to educate their children and to decide what information is appropriate and what moral position they hold. Although this position is legitimate, parents seldom follow through. Brown and Brown (2006) noted that parents often abdicate their role in this endeavor, and their children are left open to the influence of the societal culture as viewed through the media. Parents usually have had no models themselves as to how to talk about sex; they have not clearly articulated their own sexual values; they focus on disease and pregnancy prevention while leaving out the fact that sex is exciting and a part of a close attachment to another person. Again, given the lack of sexual information provided to the parents themselves and the high incidence of sexual difficulties among adults, this situation is no surprise. To have "the talk" when children are 12 or 13 achieves very little. The parents feel anxious and tongue-tied, and given that no previous discussions have occurred, both parties want to get it over as quickly as possible with just enough time to raise the specter of sexually transmitted diseases (STDs) and the admonition to participate in safe sex. Some parents are direct in their prohibitions regarding sex of any kind with a variety of dire consequences, which may cause the children to have an internalized sense of badness regarding sexual feelings or result in a compliant sexual constriction that is lifelong.

During George W. Bush's presidency, the U.S. government supported abstinence-only education programs, although studies have shown that these programs are ineffective and probably harmful. Little difference has been found in rates of sexual intercourse between those who took the course a year earlier and those who did not. The program stresses abstinence but provides little information regarding the range of sexual activities, safe sexual practices, condom use, STDs, and realistic approaches to decision making regarding sex. Adolescents who are gay, lesbian, bisexual, or transgender have little with which to identify, and even less guidance.

McGee (2006) suggested that the abstinence only programs did not serve our youth well, and the absence of information about sexual practices, risky behavior, and contraception options and decision making was, in his view, harmful. At this time in their lives, young people have a great need for reliable and concrete information and guidance from interested and supportive adults. Parents, teachers, and physicians most often let them down either through their own ignorance about sex or their reluctance to broach the subject deeply. Kirby (2002) reported that greater evidence supports the effectiveness of comprehensive sex education than of abstinence-only programs, with findings indicating that a comprehensive sex education leads to a delay of first sexual intercourse, high rates of condom use, and learning to make choices based on risk.

The Sexuality Information and Education Council of the United States (1996) proposed four primary goals for comprehensive sex education:

1. To provide young people with accurate information about human sexuality
2. To provide an opportunity for young people to question, explore, and assess their sexual attitudes
3. To help young people develop interpersonal skills, including communication, decision-making, assertiveness, and peer-refusal skills, as well as the ability to create satisfying relationships
4. To help young people exercise responsibility regarding sexual relationships, by addressing abstinence, resisting pressure to become prematurely involved in sexual behaviors, and the use of contraception and other sexual health measures

In many schools, despite their best attempts, the core message is to emphasize the dangers of sex: HIV, STDs, and pregnancy. The obligatory biological discussion usually includes the statement that masturbation under most circumstances is not harmful, the assumption of course being that boys always do it, whereas girls do not. The fact that masturbation is pleasurable or fun and is the first experience with learning the sexual feelings one can derive from one's body is never addressed. I have noticed with dismay that the concept of sex as fun, playful, exciting, and enjoyable rarely finds its way into teaching programs at schools or teaching moments at home. In a peculiar way, the awareness of AIDS and STDs has provided some justification for parents and teachers to talk to children about sex. Doing so could be viewed as protecting them from the dangers lurking "down there," and the more personal and intimate aspects of sex could once again be avoided. As Tiefer (2002) wrote, "The neglect of pleasure as a subject in current writings is the legacy of a puritanical and naturalistic sex as function, sex for reproduction model that is still popular in medicine." According to McGee (2006), "Sensuality is, after all, one of the primary components of sexuality. Denying this can lessen our credibility. We need to be talking with our kids about appreciating their bodies, what their bodies can do, how they feel…This pleasurable aspect of sexuality is critical to normal and healthy development."

An important goal, as McGee (2006) proposed, would be that when individuals "are mature enough to act on their feelings, they will talk with a partner about sexual activity before it occurs, including sexual limits (theirs and their partner's), contraceptive and condom use, and the meaning of the relationship and of relationships in general.…Teenagers benefit from conversations that identify the differences between love and lust and the self-esteem that comes from responsibly managing these feelings. Part of this conversation is about the positive feeling of intimacy that people can have without sexual intercourse."

For adolescents, sex is often a preoccupying theme. They are curious about the many changes they experience, and they need good information. The therapist who has the information and chooses to engage with adolescent and preadolescent patients as a wise and guiding coach will soon be convinced that young patients appreciate and value this opportunity. An approach I have found valuable is to simply talk about various sexual topics, often using anecdotes as illustrations. This invariably leads to questions, and soon an active dialogue develops. This dialogue, which serves as a model for talking about sex directly and respectfully, becomes an experience the adolescent usually incorporates into his or her own relationships. The clinician also serves as a resource for more information, and someone with whom the adolescent can raise real concerns (e.g., "I have a small penis" or "I don't think I have a clitoris"). Additionally, the discussions lead the adolescent to develop an attachment to and trust for the therapist, which benefits the approach to any nonsexual issues discussed in the treatment.

Role of the Media

Television and Movies

Given the general reluctance in the culture to deal with sexuality openly, an interesting consideration is the development of sexual fantasy in the media. In the 1950s, the film industry had to conform to rigid guidelines in terms of any kind of sexual allusion. Married couples' bedrooms always contained two twin beds separated by a night table, and any hint of sensuality was usually purged from view. As the constraints weakened, sexuality became more graphic, with Bernardo Bertolucci's *Last Tango in Paris* being a breakthrough film in 1972. Sex has now been co-opted by the advertising and merchandising industries, with appeals to increasingly younger audiences. Children are pushed into a precocious pseudosexuality, often with parents' unwitting complicity.

A Kaiser Family Foundation survey (Kunkel et al. 2005) found that the number of scenes on television with sexual content almost doubled from 1998 to 2004. Sex is portrayed as a power struggle, as a manipulative tool in relationships, and as easy and without much consequence. Sex occurs with no preliminary relevant talking (e.g., "I have a problem," "Tell me if you ever had an STD," "Let's talk about condoms"). Sex results from a rapid rise in passion between people with perfect bodies, who achieve a mutual simultaneous orgasm, which is followed by orchestral music in the background. The shows specifically for children and adolescents are filled with pseudosexual precociousness: skimpy outfits, so-called sexy behavior, jealousy, and the idea that to be hip is to be sexual. Rarely do viewers see someone thoughtfully considering whether or not to have sex or someone feeling anxious or ambivalent about sex. Brown and Brown (2006) pointed out that children are exposed to a dramatically increased amount of sex and sexual innuendo from television and the Internet. The fact that it is uncensored and rarely commented on by responsible adults (parents in particular) leaves children without the guidance they need.

Internet Pornography

Pornography on the Internet is varied and abundant. Unless parents (and therapists) have spent any time surfing sex sites, they will have no understanding about the ease with which these sites can be accessed and the nature of the material their children can see. Parents often raise these concerns with the therapist, in the context of their own therapy or that of their children. The therapist can provide suggestions for talking about the topic and using the opportunity as one of the ways they can engage their children in discussing sexual information.

As boys mature physically, a combination of media and Internet pornography is often their entrée to masturbation. The association between masturbation and viewing online pornography reflects a significant change from the pre-Internet experiences of boys. Although pornography was available, access was limited, and many boys would describe the discovery of their father's *Playboy* magazine, with which they would begin to masturbate. The *Playboy* centerfolds were stimulating, and boys would use their imaginations about what they might do with these women. In addition, they may have felt an unconscious connection with their fathers, who were also viewing these pictures. The Internet has changed the scene, and the pornographic images bear little relation to the *Playboy* images of the past. I believe that, among other things, they limit the development of creative fantasy and imagination. In working with boys who begin to masturbate with online pornography, I have often observed that an unanticipated consequence is that as they get older, they have difficulty getting aroused in a partner sex setting. Most images also objectify women; for many boys, this objectification defends against their anxiety and fears at forming attachments with girls, and the pornography only legitimizes this view. Sex is portrayed in a mechanical and impersonal way. The focus is mainly on genitals; the men usually have abnormally large penises and their erections seem to last forever, and the women invariably have enormous breasts and seem to have developed a "sword-swallowing" ability that portrays oral sex in an unrealistic way. All of this can cause boys to struggle alone with worries about their adequacy and performance, as well as to have unrealistic expectations from their partners.

Sexual Activity in Children and Adolescents

Parents are often not prepared for their children's becoming sexual, and may try to deny its occurrence, hoping to avoid dealing with the experimentation that needs to happen. Many adolescents are active sexually, and the statistics relating to adolescent sex have been fairly consistent over the last 15 years.

Many high schoolers and even middle schoolers are experimenting with oral sex and with anal sex, which they claim is "not sex" because "you can't get pregnant." About half of high school students have had intercourse before graduation, and many have had four or more partners. The Internet represents one of the most significant developments for adolescents' sexuality, with online pornography, chat rooms, and opportunities for contacts that were not previously so readily available.

Teenagers reportedly engage in oral sex at school, on the school bus, in limousines on the way to the prom, or at home. Oral sex appears to be considered an enjoyable recreational activity, with little meaning in terms of relational attachments. In 2005, a private school in the greater Boston area made national headlines when it expelled five male students for receiving oral sex in the locker room from a 15-year-old girl. The "event" was to celebrate one of the boy's birthdays.

In 2005, the Centers for Disease Control and Prevention examined current sexual activities among boys and girls ages 15–17 (Mosher et al. 2005; see Table 13–1). Because adolescents are active sexually and often have little guidance regarding relationships and sex in the context of relationships, I believe the therapist can benefit young patients by venturing into this arena.

Providing Guidance to Parents

When working with parents, either as individuals or couples or as the parents of a child in treatment, the clinician has a valuable opportunity to inform, educate, and reassure them about their children's sexual development, with possible benefits to the entire family. Parents rarely have good models for talking with children about sex. Most parents are uncomfortable, avoid the topic as much as possible, and do not know what to say. Regrettably, the conversation usually becomes the mother's responsibility. Beginning the conversation about sex at adolescence is too late. With no previous discussions, the conversation feels awkward to parent and child, and usually the content revolves around protection and safe sex. Richardson and Schuster (2003) provide a guide for parents, with the goal of helping parents to survive their children's sexual development, to learn how to live comfortably with it, and to play a crucial role in fostering its natural, healthy growth.

Table 13–1.   Sexual activities among boys and girls ages 15–17 (percentages)

	Vaginal intercourse	Girl touched penis	Received oral sex	Gave oral sex	Anal sex	No sexual contact	Same-sex activity
Boys	36.3	42.7	40.3	28.2	11.2	46.1	3.9
Girls	38.7	–	38	30.4	5.6	48.6	8.4

Source.   Data from Mosher et al. 2005.

Suggestions for Parents

- Parents should talk about bodies when a child develops language skills. When naming body parts, the parents should talk about the penis, scrotum, testicles, vagina, clitoris, and labia.
- Parents should keep the conversations simple, providing only the facts, and respond to any questions that arise. One parent described the jolt of anxiety he felt when his child asked, "Where do I come from?" After taking a deep breath, he began the discussion about the sperm and the egg, to which his child responded, "No! Did I come from Boston [the site of the hospital] or Brookline [where they lived]?"
- Children may see women who are pregnant and be curious as to "where babies come from." Parents can begin the process of discussion without the loaded qualities that result when children are older. Preliminary discussions of bodies and sex help to create a climate in which children feel they can approach sexuality as a topic.
- Parents often ignore or discourage masturbation as an activity, without framing what is happening. Many young children begin to fondle their genitals early in life. From a child's perspective, masturbation feels good, but the parental message is that the activity is bad. In a matter-of-fact manner, the parents can say to boys, "It can feel nice to touch your penis. Sometimes it might even get hard and feel good to rub it. This is called masturbation. It is fine for you to do it in the privacy of your room. Just don't do it at the dinner table." Similarly, for girls, the parents can say, "It can feel good to touch your clitoris…"

- When children reach puberty, the parents should think about their own experiences and what might have been helpful for them at that time. Parents can consider these questions: What guidance would you have given yourself about dating from your adult perspective? What advice would you have wanted?

A patient of mine, a psychologist, became concerned about her 12-year-old son, Peter, who was taller and physically more mature than his peers. My patient had discovered some Internet pornography sites on his computer, and was also concerned about a relationship with a 13-year-old girl that appeared to be moving rapidly to becoming more sexual. I suggested that she and her husband discuss their own values and reactions to what he was doing, and we discussed a possible way to talk about it with their son. What follows may seem like a lecture, but it is meant as a rough road map that may be helpful for the parents as they begin a discussion with their son.

> Peter, we want to talk with you about sex. You are probably going to groan at the thought of this conversation. We don't have any practice with discussing sex, so we might all feel self-conscious, but we are going to try to do it anyway because we feel it is important.
>
> You are becoming an adolescent, and of course with that comes a lot of feelings about sex. Sex is a part of us all—the feelings are intense, exciting, and very pleasurable. Sex is to be enjoyed, but it is also something that we take seriously; by that we mean that we do not believe in random hookups, we do not believe in forcing anyone to do anything they don't want, and we don't believe in being forced to do anything.
>
> Learning to be with someone in a more physically intimate way needs to be a slow growing process. We feel that the first thing that needs to happen is to know whether you like the person and whether the person likes you. Knowing someone in a personal way—wanting to be with her, hang out with her, and feel good with her—is the first step.
>
> As this continues, touching—holding hands, being more affectionate, and kissing—is the next phase. Kissing can be very personal, and also very enjoyable, but only if you take the time to learn what you and your partner like.
>
> Touching and learning what each other likes—knowing something about what you like and what your partner says feels good—requires trust and good communication.

Although it does feel good to get a lot more personal with touching sexually, we believe that you are too young for that. Why? Because learning to have a relationship and developing some personal connection come before that. All of this sex stuff is easy to do, but—and you won't believe what we say—in the long run, you are better off waiting.

As for intercourse—yes, we know that lots of kids are having intercourse—again, our feeling is that one should wait. It's very personal and involves some responsibilities beyond being safe. Also, if you can't talk about it directly with a girl, you should not be doing it.

Sex on the Internet is another thing we have feelings about. The images do not represent what happens with real sex at all. There are no relationships, and the focus is mainly on genitals. You may not believe this, but when kids begin to use these pornography sites to get turned on, it creates problems later because it often becomes difficult to feel turned on without them.

Also, as you know, there are risks: first pregnancy, then STDs. Of course you can use condoms, but they are not very effective against herpes and some other STDs. Also, remember that many people who have herpes don't even know they have it.

It is also important to remember that alcohol and fooling around do not mix. People's judgment is not good, and bad things can happen.

If you have a girlfriend, we want to meet her. This relationship cannot interfere with family life—your being on the phone all the time or texting while we are having dinner—and cannot affect your studies at school. If you go to parties, we want to speak with the parents and find out what is happening, who is there, and what kind of supervision there is.

Talking About Sex With Young Patients

If one accepts that sex is a big part of adolescence, not talking about it inadvertently supports the cultural avoidance of the subject, or the idea that it is too private to talk about your "privates." When meeting for the first time, I want to get an idea of the adolescent's understanding of why he or she is in my office, and I want to see how the patient relates to me. Although I may choose not to talk about sex in the first meeting or even the second, at some point I want to have the topic on the table as something we can talk about.

I suggest the following general principles for clinicians discussing sex with adolescents (*Note:* when kids say "sex," they mean intercourse"):

1. Frame the conversation. Say, "I'd like to talk about sex," in a calm, respectful way.

2. Explain the reasons for the questions. Say, for example, "Sex is a big deal for people, and my experience is that there are few opportunities to talk about it."

3. Ask where the individual acquired information about sex. I have found that it is helpful, once a problem has been mentioned, to move into a more general, less charged area. By asking the adolescent about his or her exposure to sex education, the discomfort is lessened.

4. Use humor. It relaxes the individual and conveys the message that this conversation will not be a "heavy," shaming experience, but might even turn out to be enjoyable. For example, when talking about masturbation, I sometimes tell the story of the boy who was found masturbating by his parents. "Don't do that!" they said. "You will go blind!" The son replied, "Well, can I do it until I need glasses?" Or I might say, "How did you discover masturbation? What was it like for you? You know, often people will say 'I invented it!'"

5. Be aware of adolescents' common sexual worries. Concerns often expressed by boys include, "What do I do?" "I don't know what's 'down there.'" "I don't think my penis is big enough." "I came very quickly, and it was embarrassing." For girls, the concerns typically relate to appearance and popularity: "Are my breasts big enough or too big?" "Am I thin enough, too thin, or too fat?" "If I don't 'put out' sexually, I won't be popular." "I've never had an orgasm." "It really hurt."

6. Adolescents are undergoing growth and change at a remarkable rate. The discussion with the therapist may be about sex one week and about parents and teachers the next. Sometimes the adolescent drives the session with an abundance of thoughts and feelings. When the teen is monosyllabic, the therapist needs to be creative and active in guiding a conversation.

The following array of questions is intended as a rough guide for the therapist. Question selection should be based on the individual being seen. In some situations, a more detailed sexual discussion is welcome and helpful; in some, a very brief talk about sex is all that is needed; and in others, the clinician's best judgment is to wait and not broach the subject.

Introducing the topic:

I'd like to talk with you about sex. I'm always curious where people acquire information about sex. Some people learn from friends, some from sex education classes, and a few from parents. What has your experience been?

Have you had any sex education courses at school? What were they like? The ones I've heard about seem to focus on some facts, but the summary is often, "Have sex—you'll die!"

Did anyone ever tell you that the reason people are interested in sex is that it is fun?

What did they say about masturbation? So often, the comment is, "It won't harm you unless you do it too much," whatever that means. I think that masturbation is an undervalued resource. It's a great way of getting to know a special kind of pleasure and enjoyment from your own body.

For girls:

Boys have an easier time in a way. Their penises are out in the open, and they seem to take pride in showing off what a penis can do. Girls have to be a little more resourceful. Looking at "what's down there" with a mirror is a great way of learning about your genitals. Seeing what everything looks like: labia, clitoris, and vagina. Touching the different parts and seeing what they feel like for you really gives you a good knowledge of your body and what touching can feel like.

For boys and girls:

Have you done anything sexual with anyone else? How has it been? So how do you know what the other person likes? Is this a girl or a guy? How does this person know what *you* like? Thinking back to sex ed classes: Was there any talk about the idea of asking and talking with your partner about likes and dislikes? It may feel a bit awkward to do initially, but if you think about it, why should you instinctively know what feels good for another person? And, by asking, you don't have to worry if you are doing it right.

Do you like kissing? What I hear often from girls is they wish the guys would take it slower when kissing.

What about oral sex?

For boys:

Do you reciprocate? Do you enjoy it?

For girls:

Do you enjoy doing it? Does he reciprocate?

For boys and girls:

What about sex? Have you had sex? What has that been like for you?

For boys:

Guys often get macho about this, bragging about all they have done. Most often they exaggerate. Guys, unfortunately, never talk about whether they are scared or worried. They rarely say, "Where is 'it'? How do I get in? I came so fast; I don't know if she enjoyed it." Also, usually the first time you have sex, it may not feel so enjoyable. It's something that requires practice.

For girls:

Did you have any pain? For many girls, the first time is either neutral or a bit uncomfortable. Some say it felt terrific. Usually it takes some time to know what feels right for you. How about the guy? Did he ask you what you like? Did he tell you what he liked?

When it comes to orgasm, there are many ways to have one. For some, intercourse alone will do it; others might like some stimulation of their clitoris, either through oral sex or with some finger rubbing. Having an orgasm with intercourse is not always what happens.

It is important that you don't do anything you don't want to do or are not comfortable with. If a guy says, "I won't use a condom," drop him. If a guy tries to guilt you into sex, say no.

For boys and girls:

I do want to give you some information regarding health and safety. It's a good idea to always use condoms; they are pretty reliable in providing contraception, but when it comes to preventing STDs, condoms are only fair. Even with condoms, you can get herpes. And while talking about condoms, there are different types. The latex condoms provide the best protection from STDs. There are natural membrane condoms that people say feel more like using nothing at all; although they are good for contraception, they do nothing to prevent STDs. If you do have anal intercourse, you need to make sure you use lubrication. Also, if you have vaginal intercourse after anal intercourse, you need to make sure you wash the penis first; bacteria from the rectum can cause nasty vaginal infections. Be aware of your own body, get familiar with how your genitals look, and pay attention to any changes. Genital warts look like little bumps; herpes looks red and blistery. If you see these changes or have any discharge from your vagina or penis, make sure you see a doctor. If you have any vaginal pain, see your doctor. I know that it is probably the last thing you would want to do before having sex, but it is very important to ask your partner about whether he or she has had unsafe sex.

The outline above is intended as a general guide for discussing a range of sexual topics. Whether all topics are dealt with at the same time is a matter of personal judgment. A clinician might move through all topics in one meeting with some adolescents, but approach the issues more cautiously with others. Over time, the therapist accumulates hands-on experience that helps in developing a pattern that works for him or her. Most teenagers do not have access to an adult who will talk expansively about the details that are of most concern to them. To avoid being accused of encouraging children to be sexual, sex education instructors tend to cover topics that are somewhat impersonal and generic. The fact that teenagers welcome and like these discussions with therapists is confirmed by their asking questions and their feelings that the conversation is genuine, with no clichés such as "just say no."

Specific Clinical Situations

Working With Boys

As Thompson and Kindlon (2000) and others have pointed out, dependence and vulnerability in boys are usually discouraged after age 8. At one extreme, boys may behave in a macho manner: "I know what I am doing; girls don't scare me." At the other extreme, the fear and worry may be so close to the surface that the boy retreats from much engagement with girls. Competitiveness for boys adds to the loneliness and isolation they may feel as they go through puberty. If they are gay, bisexual, or transgender, they may have few resources to deal with the confusion around their feelings and impulses.

When it comes to heterosexual engagement, although many boys are able to acquire some skill and confidence, others struggle with their feelings and may manifest impaired sexual functioning. Although most boys feel embarrassed and uncomfortable talking about sex with a therapist, the relief at letting go of all the worry about having to figure it out on their own is dramatic.

Erectile Difficulties

When told of erectile dysfunction by a teenager, I acknowledge how difficult this must be to talk about and reassure him that he is not alone in having this problem. I ask a series of questions:

Do you have morning erections and erections during the day?

How about masturbation? Do you get hard easily, or does it take some time?

Tell me what happened with your partner.

What do the two of you do sexually?

When did you lose your erection?

What did you do or say?

What did she say?

I find that when this happens, the guy can't get this out of his mind, and it only makes the next time worse. What has it been like for you?

I talk about the impact of anxiety on sexual physiology, and how the focus on pleasure and sexy feelings is replaced by a worry about whether his penis will work. Helping an adolescent learn how to talk with his partner about sex provides an important foundation for future relationships.

As part of the treatment for erectile dysfunction, the phosphodiesterase type 5 (PDE5) inhibitors are helpful for several reasons. One can almost certainly predict that a male will have a reliable erection, which helps reduce his anxiety. For the adolescent who has struggled with erectile dysfunction, dread and anxiety are linked to the whole sexual endeavor. My aim is to help the adolescent experience intercourse as pleasurable and not always as associated with a sense of failure. The pills alone are not the cure; the therapist provides guidance and support in terms of what to *do* and, importantly, what to *say* to a partner. For many teenage boys, the idea of one-night stands has a certain symbolic appeal; they think they are doing what guys their age are supposed to be doing. However, for adolescents who are anxious about their sexual functioning, I point out that a one-night stand will only increase anxiety because almost by definition it is an endeavor in which trust and support are absent. I make a case for sex in the context of a relationship with someone the adolescent knows and likes, and with whom he can talk about his sexual worry. I acknowledge that my suggestion probably sounds crazy, but I point out that saying nothing to his partner is a recipe for the problem to continue because he has to pretend that he is confident, when he knows that he is not. The therapist acts as a supportive, informative guide, providing specific sexual information, as well as help with dealing with family and parental struggles and the challenges in developing a close relationship.

Case Example 1

Jason, a 20-year-old college freshman, was having trouble maintaining an erection. He was able to have sex only if he was drunk, and it would usually be a one-night stand followed by months of no sex. Although his concern was centered on his having trouble meeting girls and his worry about his dysfunctional penis, his serious alcohol problem needed to be faced and his difficulties with attachment understood and addressed. The challenge was to engage with Jason around the manifest complaint ("I can't have sex") and the underlying, more germane issue of closeness and attachment. Jason's parents had divorced when he was 2 years old; his father had been unavailable for many years, and his mother had several 2- to 3-year relationships. Jason had become very attached to each of these men, whom he ceased to see once their relationship with his mother ended. It took several years of treatment for Jason to understand the connection between the losses he felt regarding his father (and the subsequent men in his mother's life) and his avoiding a close emotional and sexual attachment with a woman. His "defective penis" served a function in this regard. My therapy with him included many specific discussions about sex, sexual approaches, and sexual functioning. I provided "relationship guiddance" when he would get involved with a woman. It was ultimately with his understanding of the fundamental losses, first as they played out with me in therapy (his disappearing for months at a time) and then as we connected his feelings to the loss he experienced with his father's absence, that he was able to enter into a sober, mutual sexually comfortable relationship with a woman.

The history taking may yield some surprises.

Case Example 2

David was a college freshman who was having trouble with erections. He was upset with the appearance of his penis. He was born with hypospadias, and although it was corrected surgically when he was 2 years old, he felt that his penis never looked right. In addition, he felt that his circumcision was incomplete on one side. He was convinced that this would be obvious to a partner and was obsessed with it. In the context of his therapy, I referred him to a plastic surgeon, who confirmed David's anatomical description and agreed to perform surgery. The results were dramatic. David was delighted with the changes, and within 6 weeks was cured of his erectile dysfunction and began "making up for lost time." His therapy involving relationship issues continued.

Premature Ejaculation

Premature ejaculation is the most common sexual problem for men, and treatment, particularly before the premature ejaculation has become a part of an adolescent's sexual map, can be life changing (Polonsky 2000). The therapist should not assume that the adolescent will bring up this topic himself, due to self-consciousness and shame. As part of the sexual history, I make a statement such as, "Some guys may have a hard time getting it up, or keeping it up. Also, some guys may come very quickly, and there are some guys who just don't feel like having sex. Has any of that happened with you?" In addressing concerns about premature ejaculation, the therapist needs to pose these questions to determine how fast is fast: Do you have an orgasm as soon as your penis is touched, or do you have an orgasm when trying to have intercourse? Does orgasm occur once you have begun thrusting? How soon after beginning thrusting does orgasm occur?

Regardless of the underlying cause, some training exercises using specific masturbation techniques (Polonsky 2000) can be very helpful and reassuring. Although clomipramine (25–50 mg 1 hour before sex) is quite helpful in delaying orgasm, I start off using the behavioral approach with patients. If a patient has followed the training exercises with consistency and experienced no benefit, I then add the drug.

Working With Girls

I do not see many girls whose primary complaint is sexual difficulties; I assume that girls prefer to see a female therapist. In the course of asking girls about sexuality, the concerns I encounter are difficulties having an orgasm, feeling nothing, or having pain associated with sex.

Orgasm Difficulties

If girls say they have difficulties with orgasm, I pursue additional information. The following is a basic outline of the questions I ask.

> I want to ask you some personal questions that will help me understand what you are experiencing. It might feel a bit embarrassing at first This usually passes quite quickly. If there is anything you do not want to discuss, please tell me.
>
> Are you comfortable using your fingers or hand to stimulate yourself?

When you do stimulate yourself, do the feelings begin to rise in intensity? Then what happens? Sometimes people tell me that as the intensity increases, they begin to worry about whether they will be able to come and what it will feel like. As soon as that happens, they become a bit distracted, and then the feelings lessen.

Do you experience vaginal lubrication? If you are having intercourse, how does that feel? Is there any pain? Does it feel good?

Partner technique is also important. Does your partner know what feels good for you?

Dodson has produced a series of videotapes and a book called *Sex for One* (Dodson 1996). Watching Dodson talk to the women she is coaching and hearing her supportive encouragement and instructions is helpful to most teenage girls. The therapist needs to be able to integrate behavioral coaching and relationship guidance as he or she helps an adolescent develop emotionally.

Feeling Nothing

When girls say they feel nothing sexually, the therapist should try to learn more. Sometimes the lack of feelings relates to inadequate sexual education combined with family prohibitions. The girl also may be experiencing a dissociation related to early sexual abuse or trauma, or may have negative feelings about her body, as in eating disorders.

Pain

Girls experience different kinds of pain. They might report knifelike pain when the genitals are touched; pain associated with trying to get a tampon, penis, or dildo into the vagina; a dull rawness associated with thrusting; or a deep ache associated with pressure on the cervix. When a girl has is a history of pain, a consultation with a gynecologist or pelvic physical therapist knowledgeable about vulvodynia is indicated.

Working With Lesbian, Gay, Bisexual, and Transgender Individuals

Adolescents who are lesbian, gay, bisexual, or transgender experience particular challenges in their sexual development. Initially, the adolescent may have a perception of being different from most peers. This feeling is often confusing, and many years may pass before the child is able to name what is happening. The realization of the difference is often very disturbing, accompanied by anxiety about its meaning. These adolescents are understandably worried and anxious about coming out, with all its unknowns, and are apprehensive about the uncharted territory of sexual attachments. The therapist needs to question his or her own beliefs and feelings about sexual orientation and become informed regarding the current understanding. Looking at Web sites provides a way of reading about people who are in various stages of dealing with being gay, bisexual, lesbian, and transgender. Knowing the range of sexual activities is essential for the therapist, who needs to be able to discuss blow jobs and anal sex with the gay teenager, which for the straight therapist might initially be a challenge. In addition to coming to terms with being gay, bisexual, lesbian, or transgender, the adolescent has to deal with the same issues as the straight adolescent regarding sexual competence, forming sexual relationships, and feelings about closeness.

Sexual Abuse

The breach of trust for children who have been sexually abused is monumental, and the impact on their psychological and sexual development can be huge. Kluft (1990) described the adaptive dissociation for these children. When the child is abused, there is little the child can do to protect herself or himself. Dissociation—removing the mind from the body—provides a way of managing an overwhelming situation. Paradoxically, as adults, the children of abuse may be at greater risk for abuse. The dissociation muffles the alarm bells of danger that would normally trigger recognition of a potentially dangerous sexual situation. The impact on the child's sexuality, depending on the nature of the abuse, the age at which it occurred, and the parental responses, can vary from slight to severe. In helping a child deal with the long-term effects of the abuse, the therapist must first develop trust. However, helping a child to reclaim good feelings about his or her body and to invest positively in sexuality needs to be part of the treatment.

Case Example 3

Sam was a 16-year-old high school student who was referred because of generalized anxiety. Many different themes needed to be addressed: his parents' separation and divorce, an unnecessarily punitive reaction of his school to an episode of drinking, and his chronic anxiety. Treatment with a selective serotonin reuptake inhibitor helped considerably with the anxiety, and after a few weeks, Sam began to talk about being repeatedly molested by an athletic coach at a previous school. At another time, he talked about feeling nothing in his penis if he masturbated, and that when he was with his girlfriend, sex was similarly devoid of any pleasure. Learning about this enabled me to link the symptom with his abuse; he felt dirty and slimed, and was ashamed that he actually got aroused with the coach. Kluft (1990) observed that sexual abuse victims often recall the arousal and subsequently feel responsible for the abuse. He observed a reversal of the memories, in which the victim believes that the arousal preceded the abuse. I talked with Sam about this and said that if his penis was totally numb, he did not have to feel so dirty. This exploration resulted in his gradually being able to reinvest in his sexuality, feel pleasure in his penis, and ultimately be more present sexually with his girlfriend. The therapy, which at times focused specifically on his being sexual with his girlfriend, encompassed his issues with his parents, the trauma of his physical abuse, his developing an attachment to a girlfriend, and reclaiming the right to sexual pleasure. Without a discussion about sex, the impact of the abuse in terms of his own sexuality would not have been addressed.

Conclusion

The reader may have the impression that I am stressing the importance of discussing sexuality with adolescents in an insistent, almost dogmatic manner. My approach results from my concern that sex has not been integrated into most psychiatrists' training, and that this results in a loss of opportunities to engage patients in discussions of sex. Although a discussion of sex may not be indicated in many situations, the therapist needs to make the judgment in working with each individual. The therapist should have some knowledge of sexual development, be able to explore the subject with patients, and learn by experience when to approach the topic. A therapist also has to be sensitive to different cultural and ethnic backgrounds; some cultures frown upon open discussions about sex or consider sexual activity by adolescents or before marriage unacceptable. One needs to be creative when dealing with a family of immigrants and be sensitive to the difficulty they have raising an adolescent in the United States, where expectations may be very different from their native countries.

Although I have emphasized the sexual aspect of therapy, discussions of sex cannot occur in a vacuum. The therapist has to be thorough in doing a complete developmental evaluation, and in addressing the whole range of concerns and conflicts with which patients have to deal. Without establishing a solid foundation, any discussion about sex cannot be therapeutic. For the therapist who is willing to face a challenge, there is a richness to be gained in adding sexuality to the treatment process.

Key Points

- When working with children, especially adolescents, a unique opportunity exists to have a major impact on their ability to integrate sexual feelings, sexual competence, and intimate attachments.

- The state of sex education in the United States is cause for great concern. Parents typically are reluctant to have serious, in-depth conversations about sexuality and relationships with their children. Many children are constrained from getting good guidance regarding sex because their parents had little good guidance about the subject themselves. Anecdotally, I have seen the adolescent children of couples I had seen previously for sexual difficulties, and have been impressed by a carryover of similar problems in the children. What is especially important to note, however, is the dramatic shift that occurs for these adolescents in their sexuality with some direct coaching and guidance. Their sexual identity becomes more positive and pleasure focused, which is in stark contrast to the long-term struggles the parents have endured.

- Sex education programs provide little information regarding sexual pleasure, information about sexual activities, and guidance to becoming comfortable lovers. Parents are often left out of their children's sex education program, which perpetuates a "code of silence."

- Therapists receive little training in human sexuality and are therefore reluctant to discuss sex in depth with the people they treat. This is a loss for both therapists and their patients. The adolescent is challenged by a cascade of major changes: physical growth, puberty, sexual feelings, separation from parents, sexual experimentation, and attachments outside of the family. A relationship with a therapist who understands the psychological dynamics in the family and is able to talk directly about the blossoming sexual feelings offers the adolescent something profound and unique.

- Keeping current with cultural trends in terms of what adolescents are doing and talking about sexually and to what they are exposed in the media, music, and the Internet adds to a therapist's effectiveness and credibility.

- The process for the therapist by which he or she gains comfort and expertise in exploring sexuality mirrors the steps the adolescent takes; that is, as the therapist moves into new terrain of talking about sex, he or she will have to deal with unfamiliarity and feelings of anxiety and uncertainty. The therapist will probably feel uncertain and anxious. With practice and guidance, he or she will become more confident and competent and will experience pleasure and enjoyment with this new-found skill.

References

Brown RT, Brown JD: Adolescent sexuality. Prim Care 33:373–390, 2006

Calderone MS, Johnson E: The Family Book About Sexuality. New York, Harper & Row, 1981

Cornog M: The Big Book of Masturbation. San Francisco, CA, Down There Press, 2004

Dodson B: Sex for One: The Joy of Selfloving. New York, Three Rivers Press, 1996

Fonseca H, Greydanus D: Sexuality in the child, teen, and young adult: concepts for the clinician. Primary Care: Clinics in Office Practice 34:275–292, 2007

Kaplan HS: The New Sex Therapy: Active Treatment of Sexual Dysfunctions. New York, Brunner/Mazel, 1974

Kinsey AC, Pomery W, Martin C, et al: Sexual Behavior in the Human Female. Philadelphia, PA, WB Saunders, 1953

Kirby D: Effective approaches to reducing adolescent unprotected sex, pregnancy and childbearing. J Sex Res 39:51–57, 2002

Kluft RP (ed): Incest-Related Syndromes of Adult Psychopathology. Washington, DC, American Psychiatric Press, 1990

Kunkel D, Eyal K, Finnerty K, et al: Sex on TV. Menlo Park, CA, Kaiser Family Foundation, 2005

Lamb S: The Secret Lives of Girls. New York, Free Press, 2001

Lamb S: Sex, Therapy, and Kids. New York, WW Norton, 2006

Landolphi S: Hot, Sexy and Safer. New York, Berkley, 1994

Laumann E, Gagnon J, Michael R, et al: The Social Organization of Sexuality: Sexual Practices in the United States. Chicago, IL, University of Chicago Press, 1994

Masters WH, Johnson VE: Human Sexual Response. Boston, MA, Little Brown, 1970

McGee M: Talking with kids openly and honestly about sexuality. 2006. Available at: http://www.advocatesforyouth.org/parents/experts/mcgee.htm. Accessed March 4, 2009.

Moglia RF, Knowles J (eds): All About Sex: A Family Resource on Sex and Sexuality. New York, Three Rivers Press, 1997

Mosher WD, Chandra A, Jones J: Sexual behavior and selected health measures: men and women 15–44 years of age, United States, 2002. Advance Data From Vital and Health Statistics, September 15, 2005; 362:1–55. Available at http://www.cdc.gov/nchs/data/ad/ad362.pdf. Accessed March 3, 2009.

Polonsky DC: Premature ejaculation, in Principles of Sex Therapy, 3rd Edition. Edited by Leiblum S, Rosen R. New York, Guilford, 2000

Richardson J, Schuster M: Everything You Never Wanted Your Kids to Know About Sex, and Were Afraid They Would Ask. New York, Crown, 2003

Sexuality Information and Education Council of the United States National Guidelines Task Force: Guidelines for comprehensive sexuality education: kindergarten–12th grade, 2nd Edition. New York, Sexuality Information and Education Council of the United States, 1996 [a new (third) edition was published in 2004]

Thompson M, Kindlon D: Raising Cain—Protecting the Emotional Life of Boys. New York, Ballantine Books, 2000

Tiefer L: Pleasure, medicalization, and the tyranny of the natural. SIECUS Report April 1, 2002

14

Sexual Disorders in Elderly Patients

Marc E. Agronin, M.D.

Much of the early research into both human sexuality and sexual dysfunction focused on relatively young, sexually active couples. The terms *sexuality* and *intercourse* were used synonymously, and sexual disorders were assumed to be psychological in origin. Today, however, the average individual seeking help for a sexual problem is likely to be middle-aged or older and to have a number of medical and/or psychiatric problems that are having direct, *organic* effects on sexual function. At the same time, sexuality is playing an increasingly important and vital role for these aging individuals, who are living longer and healthier life spans. This trend is well reflected in popular media advertisements that have moved from featuring one well-known older individual, such as former Senator Bob Dole, to showing scenes of older individuals as physically robust and playfully amorous. Although these media examples may themselves be somewhat ageist in portraying all older individuals as frisky overgrown teenagers, they certainly represent a radical change from previous views of late-life sexuality as nonexistent, inappropriate, or hazardous.

Several large surveys have found that the majority of older individuals continue to be sexually active (typically defined by the rate of sexual intercourse) in late life, men more so than women, but at a rate lower than that of younger cohorts. For example, in a 1999 American Association for Retired Persons (AARP)–commissioned survey of over 1,300 men and women ages 45 years and older, 75% of respondents reported that they remained sexually active and 66% said they were extremely or somewhat satisfied with sex (Jacoby 1999). Approximately 50% of respondents ages 45–59 reported having sex at least once a week, declining to 30% of men and 24% of women ages 60–74 years. A 2004 update of the AARP survey obtained information from more than 3,000 men and women ages 45 years and older (including black, Hispanic, and Asian American minority groups); 84% of the total sample reported being sexually active, with declines in the older age group similar to those in the earlier survey (AARP 2005). Compared with the 1999 AARP survey, the 2004 update found that rates of oral sex and masturbation had increased, and the percentage of men using oral erectogenic agents had doubled from 10% to 22%, with over two-thirds reporting success. Among all racial groups represented in the 2004 survey, white respondents were more likely to oppose sex between unmarried individuals, whereas black respondents were more likely to consider sex a duty to one's spouse or partner. Hispanic respondents reported the greatest degree of sexual satisfaction, and Asian Americans reported the least. Data for older gay and lesbian individuals are more limited and were not collected in the AARP surveys; however, several studies have found that the majority of these individuals continue to be sexually active and report high levels of satisfaction in later life (Adelman 1991; Kimmel 1977; Pope and Schulz 1990).

One concern with the increasing number of sexually active seniors is that rates of sexually transmitted diseases (STDs) will increase as well. However, despite some focus on this concern in the media, 2006 STD surveillance data from the Centers for Disease Control and Prevention (CDC) found that individuals ages 65 years and older had the lowest rates of chlamydia, gonorrhea, and syphilis across age groups, and that these rates had not shown any appreciable change over the last 5 years (CDC 2006). The CDC reported that approximately 15% of all cases of HIV/AIDS are in individuals age 50 years or older, although not all of these cases are related to sexual transmission (CDC

2005). A separate study in Washington State found that the most common STDs in older individuals were nongonococcal urethritis in men and genital herpes in women, representing 1.3% of all reported cases (Xu et al. 2001).

Sexual Function and Dysfunction in Late Life

Clinical work with older individuals who have sexual problems requires an understanding of how sexual function changes over time. For older women, the onset of menopause heralds a 2- to 10-year process of declining levels and eventual cessation of ovarian estrogen production that usually concludes in the early 50s. Although the impact of menopause on sexual behavior is quite variable, all women experience atrophy of urogenital tissue and diminished vaginal lubrication that can negatively impact sexual function (Table 14–1). Concomitant loss of testosterone production may lessen libido in some women (Nappi et al. 2006).

Beginning in their 50s, most men begin to experience a general slowing of sexual response, meaning that erections take longer to achieve, are less rigid, and do not last as long, and orgasm requires greater degrees of stimulation. In addition, the refractory period after orgasm lengthens considerably (Westheimer and Lopater 2002). Although these changes in men may be related to declining levels of testosterone, they are not as predictable as menopausal changes in women and typically occur gradually over years or even decades. By age 80, average levels of male testosterone decline by 35%, with some men developing hypogonadism when levels drop below 200 ng/dL (Morley 2003). Several researchers have proposed the concept of a *male menopause* syndrome or *andropause*, resulting from loss of testosterone and involving not only decreased libido and sexual function but also loss of bone and muscle mass (Morley and Perry 2003). The impact of these age-related physiological changes on sexual function depends on several key physical and psychosocial factors.

Case Example 1

Malcolm, a 62-year-old divorced man, had been sexually active several times a month with his girlfriend. He was a heavy smoker and suffered from hypertension and hypercholesterolemia. He began to notice that achieving an erection was taking longer, and on several occasions he had suffered from erectile dysfunction. In his mind, he initially blamed his girlfriend for his problem, thinking that he no longer found her attractive. Malcolm panicked, however, when the problem occurred when he was with another woman, and he concluded that he had a serious sexual problem. He made an appointment to see his doctor to ask for a prescription for an "erection pill."

Contrary to his own self-diagnosis, Malcolm might not even be suffering from true erectile dysfunction. Instead, he may be overreacting to a normal decline in erectile function and making the problem worse by blaming his girlfriend and seeking another partner to "test" himself, rather than communicating with his girlfriend and adapting their sexual activity (e.g., through more foreplay or the use of a lubricant). His anxiety, in turn, activates his sympathetic nervous system, which then inhibits erectile function. Malcolm is also more susceptible to erectile dysfunction given the likely underlying atherosclerotic disease of his genital vasculature. In addition, his medical regimen likely includes the use of both a statin medication and a beta-blocker, which could be contributing to the erectile dysfunction.

Malcolm's case suggests some more insidious factors that may affect sexual behavior in aging individuals. A decline in sexual function may reinforce fears of aging and cause individuals to silently agree with stereotypes of sexual activity as potentially inappropriate or dangerous. Partners may also misinterpret changes in the other partner as indicating lack of interest or even aversion. Medical illness can further damage a person's sexual self-esteem, especially when physical appearance has been altered by surgery or medication effects. Equally important are psychiatric symptoms such as depression, anxiety, and cognitive impairment that can impair sexual desire and require the use of medications that often have sexual side effects. Many of these factors are listed in Tables 14–2 and 14–3.

In general, rates of sexual dysfunction do increase with age, with erectile dysfunction affecting about one-third of men age 40 and greater than two-thirds of men age 70, and low desire, difficult lubrication, and anorgasmia affecting approximately 40% of older women (Althof and Seftel 1995; Lindau et al. 2007). These rates are higher in older individuals who have debilitating physical or psychiatric illness, especially dementia.

Table 14–1.   Potential sexual impact of menopause

Erotic sensitivity of nipple, clitoral, and vulvar tissue is decreased.

Sexual desire is decreased.

Sexual arousal (e.g., vaginal lubrication and vasocongestion) requires more time.

Sexual intercourse may be uncomfortable due to increased dryness and sensitivity of urogenital tissue.

Orgasms may take longer to achieve and may feel less intense.

Assessment

Although the assessment of sexual problems in older individuals follows the same general guidelines as in younger patients, several unique considerations are important. Many clinicians are not comfortable discussing sexuality with older patients and are stymied by ageist beliefs that sex is not common or appropriate in later life. Clinicians' countertransferential reactions in which they view older patients as parents or grandparents can add to the discomfort about discussing sex. These attitudes not only can prevent important discussions with patients but also can fundamentally disrupt the doctor-patient relationship.

Case Example 2

Simon is an 82-year-old married man with Parkinson's disease and associated depression. His psychiatrist had been treating him for several months with a selective serotonin reuptake inhibitor. Simon's wife Magda often accompanied him to the appointments. At their last meeting, Simon asked whether he could take a medication to help with erectile dysfunction that had started while taking the antidepressant. The clinician was shocked to hear that Simon and Magda were having sex, and had to suppress a smile while looking at Simon and his elderly, rotund wife sitting next to him. "Why do you need such a pill?" he questioned. Simon was upset by the response, and detected an expression of both surprise and disgust on the clinician's face. He wondered to himself whether he was doing something wrong, and felt ashamed and confused. After the appointment, he stopped taking the antidepressant and refused to return to the clinician.

Table 14–2. Medical and psychiatric causes of sexual dysfunction in late life

Alcohol abuse and other substance use disorders

Alzheimer's disease and other dementias

Anxiety disorders

Arthritis

Cancer (especially urological and genital cancers)

Cardiac disease (e.g., congestive heart failure)

Chronic obstructive pulmonary disease

Diabetes mellitus

Major depression and other mood disorders

Multiple sclerosis

Parkinson's disease

Peripheral vascular disease

Schizophrenia and other chronic psychotic disorders

Stroke

Even the most experienced clinician may fail to communicate about sex in a comfortable and appropriate manner. The antidote is for clinicians not only to educate themselves about sexual issues, but also to role-play asking patients about sex and verbalizing sexual terminology repeatedly until they can confidently and fluently ask necessary questions (Agronin and Westheimer 2006).

A basic sexual status examination for the older patient is composed of questions about recent changes in sexual function, attitudes toward these changes, previous history of sexual behaviors and problems, and potential psychological and physical causes. When assessing an older patient, the clinician should ask these questions without any assumptions about what the patient may or may not be doing. Questions should center on several main determining factors of late-life sex: the individual's interpretation of age-related changes in sexual function; medical or medication-related physical comorbidities; psychiatric illness; and the availability, health, and interest of a partner. The last issue is particularly relevant, especially now that many older

Table 14–3. Medications associated with sexual dysfunction in late life

Antiandrogens

Anticonvulsants

Antidepressants (e.g., selective serotonin reuptake inhibitors, tricyclic antidepressants)

Antihistamines

Antihypertensives (e.g., diuretics, α-adrenergic blockers, beta-blockers)

Antipsychotics

Cardiac medications (e.g., digoxin, amiodarone)

Corticosteroids

Source. Agronin 2005; Crenshaw and Goldberg 1996; Thomas 2003.

men assume that a single pill might restore not only their erections but also their sexual relationships. Sometimes the problem is not physical but rather a result of the poor quality of the relationship with the partner or the lack of interest or sexual ability of the partner. Therefore, the clinician should inquire not only about the availability of a partner but also about the state of the relationship. Involving the partner in the assessment process can be useful to obtain more information and begin the process of conjoint treatment.

The medical and psychiatric history and review of systems takes on greater importance in assessing older patients, because their sexual dysfunction likely has an organic cause (see Table 14–2). A combination of factors typically causes the sexual problem, with diabetes, medications, and atherosclerosis being the biggest culprits. Factors that are often overlooked include chronic pain and poor self-image, both of which can lead to loss of libido. During the interview, patients should be asked to review all of their prescribed and over-the-counter medications, including dosages and schedules. Table 14–3 lists medications that are commonly associated with sexual dysfunction in late life. Identification of all these factors helps to provide numerous avenues for therapy with individuals who may present as quite hopeless about restoring their sexual function.

Laboratory and other more invasive diagnostic tests are sometimes helpful when a suspected endocrine, vascular, or neurological problem may be causing the sexual dysfunction. In such a case, the clinician should defer to a consulting urologist, gynecologist, and/or endocrinologist to select the most appropriate diagnostic studies and then evaluate the results. For example, a low testosterone level might seem to be an obvious cause of low libido or erectile dysfunction, but more significant abnormalities, especially in older individuals with multiple comorbid diseases, may require the knowledge of a specialist.

For individuals living in either assisted living or long-term care facilities, the clinician should inquire about sexual interest and barriers to sexuality.

Case Example 3

Charles is an 85-year-old nursing home resident and is dating 78-year-old Sarah, who lives on his floor. They often spend time sitting together in the garden holding hands and kissing, which has resulted in some jealous and nasty comments from other residents. On several occasions, nursing staff have walked into Charles's room and found him engaged in oral sex with Sarah. Charles and Sarah are upset over their lack of privacy, and were extremely embarrassed on one occasion when they heard several nurses giggling outside their doorway. The nursing supervisor even called their children without permission and notified them of their sexual behaviors.

Clinicians should rightly cringe at the invasion of privacy, breaches of confidentiality, and lack of dignity accorded to Charles and Sarah, yet such violations are everyday occurrences at many long-term care facilities. Negative attitudes on the part of both staff and residents toward sexuality, coupled with physical illness and disability, loss of libido, and lack of privacy, are some of the main reasons for low rates of sexual activity among long-term care residents (Hajjar and Kamel 2003; Richardson and Lazur 1995; Wasow and Loeb 1979).

As a matter of procedure, long-term care institutions should include questions about sexuality during the admission process to assess the needs of each resident (Agronin and Westheimer 2006; Richardson and Lazur 1995; Spector et al. 1996). The facility must inform residents about their rights to associate with whomever they wish, including for intimate purposes, as well as provide beauty services (e.g., hairstylists, barbers, manicurists) and sufficient privacy for couples (e.g., locks on doors, "Do not disturb" signs, and reminders to staff and other residents to always knock before entering someone's room). Clinicians should educate staff members about how sexuality is an important part of well-being that does not cease the moment someone is admitted to a facility (White and Catania 1982).

Treatment

Many older individuals approach a clinician with a very specific problem (e.g., erectile dysfunction) and request a specific treatment (e.g., an erectogenic pill). Clinicians must keep in mind, however, that multiple causes are usually involved, and treatment should involve educating both patient and partner (when available and willing to participate) about their sexual concerns, ways to enhance sexual function, communication skills, safe sex, and treatment for the specific problem. This process helps to build trust with the patient so that he or she will feel comfortable returning for follow-up. It can also prevent a patient from engaging in risky sexual behaviors, getting discouraged too quickly when things do not work as expected, and avoiding hazardous situations such as using an erectogenic agent while also taking a nitrate medication. The treatment process involves liaison with other specialists, such as urologists, gynecologists, cardiologists, and primary care physicians, to help select and implement specific strategies.

Never assume that an older patient is necessarily a more experienced and wiser patient when it comes to sex. Certain older cohorts of patients may have been raised in environments or time periods in which sex was not discussed openly or was viewed in a sexist or highly restricted manner, such as only involving sexual intercourse. Negative attitudes toward oral sex, masturbation, sex after divorce or widowhood, foreplay, or homosexuality may limit open discussion, assessment, and treatment. Similarly, many individuals ignore the risks of STDs, assuming that barrier contraceptives are not needed because pregnancy is not a possibility. Finally, patients may be knowledgeable and experienced with sex but feel embarrassed by, unaware of, or overwhelmed by mental or physical issues that are causing the problem.

Psychotherapy and sex therapy for older individuals and couples will be similar in form to those for younger patients. Specific treatment modalities include sensate focus exercises, the use of erectogenic agents for erectile dysfunction, and so forth. These treatments are covered extensively in other chapters in this text. The content of therapy differs, however, given the age- and cohort-specific issues, including the presence of many potential medical, cognitive, and medication-induced limitations.

Education

Educating older patients about normal versus abnormal changes in sexual function is critical. This will enable them to understand what has changed in their bodies and may prompt their own thoughts about underlying causes. Education also informs patients of the basic terminology for sexual function and builds a comfort level to help them discuss it with their clinician and partner. Ideally, education should also help patients feel positive and hopeful about their own sexual functioning.

Several ways to teach the patient to enhance sexuality in late life are listed in Table 14–4. Patients should be taught, first and foremost, that sexuality is normal and expected in later life, regardless of what they perceive others may be thinking or saying. Sexual performance can be enhanced by optimizing physical and mental health, which may involve regular exercise, reduction of stress, dietary changes, minimal use of alcohol, and avoidance of tobacco products.

In terms of sexual activity, patients should know about the use of foreplay to increase sexual arousal, especially in later life when more sustained stimulation may be necessary to achieve orgasm. Numerous water-based lubricants, sold in drugstores, can increase pleasurable stimulation, especially for postmenopausal women whose genital tissue is drier and thinner and tends to lubricate less during sexual activity. Safe sexual practices should also be taught.

Addressing Physical Symptoms and Disabilities

For some patients, the major barrier to sexual activity is a physical symptom, such as pain or shortness of breath, or a disability, such as hemiparesis due to stroke or bradykinesia resulting from Parkinson's disease. Some individuals, such as those who have had a recent myocardial infarction or who have pulmonary disease, may fear that physical exertion will be dangerous. Individuals who have had urological or gynecological surgery or certain treatments for cancer (e.g., radiation) may have diminished or even painful sexual arousal because of nerve or vascular damage, or because of more sensitive and friable

Table 14–4. Maximizing sexual function in late life

Maintain a positive attitude toward sexuality.

Communicate with partner about sexual changes.

Increase sexual foreplay.

Use lubricants to increase comfort.

Recognize that sexual intercourse is not the only means of sexual gratification.

Treat physical symptoms (e.g., shortness of breath, pain) and medical problems that may interfere with sex.

Treat depression or other psychiatric conditions that may interfere with sex.

Reduce psychological stress.

Find creative ways to adapt to physical disabilities.

Identify and address problematic medication side effects.

Participate in physical exercise.

Avoid tobacco use and excessive alcohol intake.

Source. Butler and Lewis 1986; Goodwin and Agronin 1997.

erogenous tissue. Finally, some individuals may be embarrassed by changes in physical appearance due to illness (e.g., having to wear a colostomy bag) or may feel too encumbered by in-dwelling catheters or oxygen tanks to even consider sexual activity.

For each of these situations, the clinician needs to keep in mind that both physical barriers and psychological attitudes have to be addressed. A first step in treatment is to define not only the sexual problem but also the goals. For some individuals, sensual kissing and genital stimulation may be a more realistic goal than sexual intercourse. In other cases, intercourse may be possible but require both time and creativity to account for limitations. For still other couples, just talking about sex or trying to be intimate can be as gratifying as sex itself.

Case Example 4

Edgar and Mary have been married for over 45 years. Edgar has Parkinson's disease and significant bradykinesia. Mary recently had a mastectomy for treatment of breast cancer and is self-conscious about her physical appearance. The last time they attempted intercourse, Edgar was able to get an erection but had a very difficult time maneuvering on the bed to vaginally penetrate Mary. They were eventually able to have intercourse, but it was uncomfortable for Mary, and neither was able to achieve orgasm.

The clinician discovered that the main strength that Edgar and Mary have is a long-standing stable and loving marriage. From the assessment, the clinician needs to ascertain what the couple's sex life was like in previous years, because that information will help establish their overall goals. Partners who have had only intermittent sexual intercourse rarely both want suddenly to have sex all the time, and the pressure for more sex from one partner (such as from a man who begins using an erectogenic agent) could actually be a destabilizing factor. In this case, the clinician learned that Edgar and Mary used to have sexual intercourse about once a month and that their current goal is quite modest. Given their initial limitations, a first step in treatment might be to talk about other ways in which they could be physically intimate in addition to intercourse, such as through physical massage, mutual masturbation, and oral sex. A lubricant would help Mary feel more comfortable with genital stimulation and vaginal penetration.

Because Mary is self-conscious about her appearance, the therapist could initiate some discussion with her alone about her feelings in the wake of surviving breast cancer, and then with the couple together to increase her comfort level. One helpful suggestion to reduce her self-consciousness and increase arousal for both partners might be for her to wear lingerie that helps her feel sexy without being too revealing of surgical scars. For Edgar, a discussion with his neurologist is important to maximize treatment for his Parkinson's disease and improve his bradykinesia. The timing of his medications could potentially be adapted to optimize his physical movements around the usual time of lovemaking. Similarly, some patients can be advised to pretreat their pain with analgesics or their shortness of breath with inhalers prior to sexual exertion. Also, Edgar's lack of motivation and libido may be due to depression, commonly associated with Parkinson's disease, that warrants evaluation and treatment. Finally, even under the best circumstances, Edgar has limitations in the speed and dexterity of his movements, and might be able to perform sexual intercourse better while lying on his back with Mary astride him, or while kneeling on the bed with Mary in front of him. Such simple strategizing about positions during sexual intercourse not only enhances intimate communication but often leads to a solution to the problem.

For Edgar and other men with erectile dysfunction, a phosphodiesterase type 5 (PDE5) inhibitor, such as sildenafil, tadalafil, or vardenafil, is the simplest and most effective treatment. Sildenafil and vardenafil can be taken 30 minutes to 4 hours before anticipated sexual activity, and tadalafil can be taken up to 30 hours earlier. No single agent has been shown to be safer or more efficacious than another in the older patient. Patients who are taking PDE5 inhibitors need to be educated that erections do not occur spontaneously but require physical stimulation. They should also be warned about potential side effects, including headache, skin flushing, dizziness, gastrointestinal discomfort, blurred vision, and the potential for blood pressure decreases when combined with nitrates (e.g., isosorbide, sublingual nitroglycerin). PDE5 inhibitors should be used with caution in men with orthostatic hypotension, severe renal or hepatic disease, abnormal penile shape, and diseases that increase the risk of priapism, such as sickle cell anemia, multiple myeloma, and leukemia, as well as men concomitantly using certain antiviral and antifungal medications (Agronin 2004). A rare but potentially devastating side effect of PDE5 inhibitors is nonarteritic anterior ischemic optic neuropathy, characterized by the rapid onset of visual loss. Changes in visual acuity that occur while taking a PDE5 inhibitor require immediate assessment (Bella et al. 2006).

If low testosterone or hypogonadism is found to be the main cause of erectile dysfunction, treatment will require testosterone replacement therapy in the form of a pill, transdermal gel or patch, intramuscular injection, or subcutaneous implant (Howell and Shalit 2001; Morales et al. 2004). For men who cannot tolerate or have contraindications to the use of either a PDE5 inhibitor or testosterone replacement (e.g., a history of prostate or bladder cancer or bladder outlet obstruction), alternative treatments include penile injections or urethral suppositories of erectogenic agents, such as alprostadil, or the use of a vacuum constriction device (see Chapter 8, "Male Erectile Disorder"). These latter techniques may be less convenient than an erectogenic pill but can still restore erectile function in the majority of men with erectile dysfunction (Althof and Seftel 1995; Dutta and Eid 1999).

When medication-induced side effects are problematic, the clinician should involve the primary care physician and other prescribing physicians to seek dose reductions or alternate medications, when possible. Medication-induced erectile dysfunction can also be treated with oral erectogenic agents. Medication-induced loss of libido, delayed arousal, or anorgasmia can be more difficult to treat and sometimes must be tolerated when the offending medication is critical for survival. Although numerous antidotes are available that can sometimes reverse sexual side effects, they are a strategy of last resort in older individuals who are already on multiple medications.

Although couples may face myriad other situations, the basic principles used to treat Edgar and Mary apply across the board: identify all aspects of the problem and set realistic goals, adapt sexual behaviors and positions to physical limitations, treat interfering medical symptoms and conditions prior to sexual activity, and communicate about creative ways to address concerns about physical appearance.

Sexuality and Dementia

When working with individuals who have Alzheimer's disease or other forms of dementia, clinicians should keep in mind that sexuality often remains an important nonverbal means of communication for couples. However, rates of sexual dysfunction do increase because dementia often impairs the knowledge and mental concentration for proper lovemaking (Duffy 1995; Redinbaugh et al. 1997). One study found that 27% of couples with a partner affected by Alzheimer's disease were sexually active, compared with 82% of couples without dementia (Wright 1991). For individuals with dementia, erectile dysfunction is common in men, occurring in more than 50% of men in one sample (Zeiss et al. 1990), and inhibited orgasm is common in women (Wright 1991). Acetylcholinesterase inhibitors and the N-methyl D-aspartate antagonist memantine, which are used to treat Alzheimer's disease, have not been associated with sexual dysfunction.

Navigating sexual activity can be particularly challenging for many partners of individuals with dementia, because they may worry that they are coercing the partner who cannot truly provide consent. They may also feel turned off by the dementia symptoms or guilty about desires for extramarital affection. Some spouses are upset by disinhibited or uncharacteristic sexual desires or behaviors expressed by their partners with dementia or by repeated requests for sex from partners who cannot remember the last time they had sex (Davies et al. 1992; Hanks 1992; Redinbaugh et al. 1997).

Sexually inappropriate behaviors are seen in 2%–7% of patients with dementia in the community and in up to 25% of those in long-term care facilities (Burns et al. 1990; Hashmi et al. 2000; Kumar et al. 1988; Rabins et al. 1982). These inappropriate behaviors include hypersexual behaviors (e.g., repeated requests for sex, compulsive masturbation), disinhibition (e.g., publicly exposing or sexually stimulating oneself), and sexually aggressive behaviors (e.g., forcibly groping, fondling, or forcing sexual activity on another person). In the assessment, the clinician should look for the following factors that may increase the risk of these behaviors: frontal and temporal lobe pathology, underlying mania or psychosis, medications such as psychostimulants or dopaminergic agents, substance abuse, head trauma, delirium, and lack of sufficient mental or physical stimulation in the environment (Agronin 2005; Bowers et al. 1971; Haddad and Benbow 1993; Hashmi et al. 2000; Raji et al. 2000). The clinician should also keep in mind that most individuals, even in severe states of dementia, still benefit from soothing physical contact of a nonsexual nature. In addition, not all problematic behaviors are sexual in nature.

Case Example 5

A psychiatrist was asked to see a 92-year-old nursing home resident with dementia for reports of sexually inappropriate behaviors. The patient reportedly was disrobing in public and inappropriately touching female staff. Further investigation revealed that the patient often leaves the bathroom with his pants down and genitals exposed because his apraxia prevents him from knowing how to pull up and zip his pants. In addition, he has moderate aphasia and is unable to adequately express his needs. Instead, he often becomes agitated and reaches out physically at staff when he needs help.

In this case, the behaviors under assessment are not sexual in nature, but reflect cognitive impairment and require more attentive caregiving. Unfortunately, many individuals in such settings are incorrectly labeled as sexually aggressive and are in effect punished for their behaviors by physical isolation or chemical restraints. A thorough clinical assessment should prevent such mistakes.

Sometimes the most important thing that a therapist can offer to a couple affected by dementia is reassurance that sexuality can continue to be part of their relationship. As the dementia progresses, however, the clinician should assess the individual's cognitive capacity to make sure that he or she understands the nature of the relationship and is still able to consent to sex. A mental health clinician with training in dementia assessment can help assess this capacity along the lines of the following questions proposed by Lichtenberg and Strzepek (1990): Does the individual know who is initiating sexual contact? Can the individual describe his or her preferred degree of intimacy? Is the sexual activity consistent with the individual's previous beliefs and values? Can he or she say "no" to unwanted activity? Does the individual understand that a sexual relationship with someone other than his or her spouse may be temporary? Can the individual describe how he or she would react if the sexual relationship were to end?

As the partner's ability to answer these questions begins to fade, a shift to simpler forms of physical intimacy, such as hand holding, kissing, and gentle massages and fondling, may be more appropriate for the couple. Actual sexual intercourse and oral sex may be too demanding and potentially upsetting for someone with aphasia, agnosia, and apraxia who is unable to recognize the other person, express his or her needs (e.g., request or refuse physical contact), or physically carry out the behaviors.

Inappropriate sexual behaviors by individuals with dementia can be quite upsetting for partners and for caregivers, and are generally challenging to treat. Such behaviors require verbal limit setting and redirection to more appropriate activities or settings without ever reinforcing them by laughing or joking in response to them. Sometimes one can identify and treat an underlying cause, such as hypersexuality due to mania or psychosis, which may respond to the removal of offending stimulating medications or to the addition of appropriate psychotropic medications. When sexual behaviors appear to reflect unmet needs for intimate contact, available partners can sometimes provide additional physical or even sexual stimulation. This approach is risky, however, and can sometimes backfire.

Case Example 6

Marvin was an 82-year-old divorced man with moderate dementia who had always had a very strong libido and an active sex life. When he was caught forcing himself sexually on another resident in the nursing home, staff informed the son that his father might have to be discharged. The son began bringing in a masseuse to pleasure his father in the privacy of his room on a regular basis. Although Marvin enjoyed this immensely, it only seemed to fuel his libido, and he was again caught forcibly fondling another female resident. He was subsequently discharged from the facility.

In Marvin's case, sexual stimulation worsened the situation. Given the degree of his dementia, a better strategy would have been to try to lessen his libido and impulsivity with one of several medications: an antidepressant, an antipsychotic, or a mood stabilizer. Just as these classes of medications are used to treat agitated behaviors, they sometimes can improve sexually inappropriate behaviors as well (Raji et al. 2000; Segraves 1998). When these fail, hormone therapy with either estrogen (Kyomen et al. 1999) or the antiandrogen medroxyprogesterone (Cooper 1987) can be considered, although these run the risk of problematic side effects such as gynecomastia, glucose intolerance, and liver dysfunction.

Key Points

- Sexuality continues to be an important part of the lives of older individuals, and surveys indicate that a significant percentage of older people remain sexually active and are generally satisfied with their relationships.

- Sexual dysfunction increases with age, with erectile dysfunction most common in older men and low desire most common in older women.

- Assessment of sexual dysfunction in late life must focus on identifying causative factors that can often be treated, such as pain, depression, medication side effects, and chronic medical or psychiatric conditions.

- Sexuality continues to be an important aspect of well-being in long-term care facilities and requires proper staff education and the provision of appropriate accommodations, such as beauty services and adequate privacy.

- Dementia poses a unique challenge to sexuality, because it can cause increased rates of sexual dysfunction and rob individuals of their capacity to engage in and consent to sex. It can also cause sexually inappropriate behaviors.

References

AARP: Sexuality at midlife and beyond: 2004 update of attitudes and behaviors. 2005. Available at: http://assets.aarp.org/rgcenter/general/2004_sexuality.pdf. Accessed March 8, 2009.

Adelman M: Stigma, gay lifestyles, and adjustment to aging: a study of late-life gay men and lesbians. J Homosex 20:7–32, 1991

Agronin ME: Sexual disorders, in Textbook of Geriatric Psychiatry, 3rd Edition. Edited by DG Blazer, DC Steffens, EW Buss. Washington, DC, American Psychiatric Publishing, 2004, pp 303–318

Agronin ME: Geriatric psychiatry: sexuality and aging, in Kaplan and Sadock's Comprehensive Textbook of Psychiatry, 8th Edition. Edited by Sadock BJ, Sadock VA. Philadelphia, PA, Lippincott Williams & Wilkins, 2005, pp 3834–3838

Agronin ME, Westheimer RK: Sexuality and sexual disorders in late life, in Principles and Practice of Geriatric Psychiatry. Edited by Agronin ME, Maletta G. Philadelphia, PA, Lippincott Williams & Wilkins, 2006, pp 523–546

Althof SE, Seftel AD: The evaluation and management of erectile dysfunction. Psychiatr Clin North Am 18:171–192, 1995

Bella AJ, Brant WO, Lue TF, et al: Non-arteritic anterior ischemic optic neuropathy (NAION) and phosphodiesterase type-5 inhibitors. Can J Urol 13:3233–3238, 2006

Bowers MB, Woert MV, Davis L: Sexual behavior during L-dopa treatment for parkinsonism. Am J Psychiatry 127:1691–1693, 1971

Burns A, Jacoby R, Levy R: Psychiatric phenomena in Alzheimer's disease, IV: disorders of behavior. Br J Psychiatry 157:86–94, 1990

Butler RN, Lewis MI: Love and Sex After 40: A Guide for Men and Women for Their Mid and Later Years. New York, Harper & Row, 1986

Centers for Disease Control and Prevention: Cases of HIV infection and AIDS in the United States and dependent areas, 2005. Available at: http://www.cdc.gov/hiv/topics/surveillance/resources/reports/2005report/default.htm. Accessed March 8, 2009.

Centers for Disease Control and Prevention: STD surveillance report 2006. Available at: www.cdc.gov/std/stats/default.htm. Accessed March 8, 2009.

Cooper AJ: Medroxyprogesterone acetate (MPA) treatment of sexual acting out in men suffering from dementia. J Clin Psychiatry 48:368–370, 1987

Crenshaw TL, Goldberg JP: Sexual Pharmacology: Drugs That Affect Sexual Function. New York, WW Norton, 1996

Davies HD, Zeiss A, Tinklenberg JR: 'Til death do us part: intimacy and sexuality in the marriages of Alzheimer's patients. J Psychosoc Nurs Ment Health Serv 30:5–10, 1992

Duffy LM: Sexual behavior and marital intimacy in Alzheimer's couples: a family theory perspective. Sex Disabil 13:239–254, 1995

Dutta TC, Eid JF: Vacuum constriction devices for erectile dysfunction: a long-term, prospective study of patients with mild, moderate, and severe dysfunction. Urology 54:891–893, 1999

Goodwin AJ, Agronin ME: A Woman's Guide to Overcoming Sexual Fear and Pain. Oakland, CA, New Harbinger, 1997

Haddad P, Benbow S: Sexual problems associated with dementia, part 2: aetiology, assessment and treatment. Int J Geriatr Psychiatry 8:631–637, 1993

Hajjar RR, Kamel HK: Sexuality in the nursing home, part 1: attitudes and barriers to sexual expression. J Am Med Dir Assoc 4:152–156, 2003

Hanks N: The effects of Alzheimer's disease on the sexual attitudes and behaviors of married caregivers and their spouses. Sex Disabil 10:137–151, 1992

Hashmi FH, Krady AI, Qayum F, et al: Sexually disinhibited behavior in the cognitively impaired elderly. Clin Geriatr 8:61–68, 2000

Howell S, Shalit S: Testosterone deficiency and replacement. Horm Res 56 (suppl 1):86–92, 2001

Jacoby S: Great sex: what's age got to do with it? Modern Maturity 1999. Available at: http://www.aarpmagazine.org/lifestyle/relationships/great_sex.html. Accessed March 8, 2009.

Kimmel DC: Patterns of aging among gay men. Psychotherapy: Theory, Research and Practice 14:386–393, 1977

Kumar A, Koss E, Metzler D, et al: Behavioral symptomatology in dementia of the Alzheimer type. Alzheimer Dis Assoc Disord 2:363–365, 1988

Kyomen HH, Satlin A, Hennen J, et al: Estrogen therapy and aggressive behavior in elderly patients with moderate-to-severe dementia. Am J Geriatr Psychiatry 7:339–348, 1999

Lichtenberg PA, Strzepek DM: Assessments of institutionalized dementia patients' competencies to participate in intimate relationships. Gerontologist 30:117–120, 1990

Lindau ST, Schumm LP, Laumann EO, et al: A study of sexuality and health among older adults in the United States. N Engl J Med 357:762–774, 2007

Morales A, Buvat J, Gooren LJ, et al: Endocrine aspects of sexual dysfunction in men. J Sex Med 1:69–81, 2004

Morley JE: Testosterone and behavior. Clin Geriatr Med 19:605–616, 2003

Morley JE, Perry HM: Andropause: an old concept in new clothing. Clin Geriatr Med 19:507–528, 2003

Nappi RE, Wawra K, Schmitt S: Hypoactive sexual desire disorder in postmenopausal women. Gynecol Endocrinol 22:318–323, 2006

Pope M, Schulz R: Sexual attitudes and behavior in midlife and aging homosexual males. J Homosex 20:169–177, 1990

Rabins PV, Mace NL, Lucas MJ: The impact of dementia on the family. JAMA 248:333–335, 1982

Raji M, Liu D, Wallace D: Case report: sexual aggressiveness in a patient with dementia: sustained clinical response to citalopram. Annals of Long-Term Care 8:81–83, 2000

Redinbaugh EM, Zeiss AM, Davies HD, et al: Sexual behavior in men with dementing illnesses. Clin Geriatr 5:45–50, 1997

Richardson JP, Lazur A: Sexuality in the nursing home patient. Am Fam Physician 51:121–124, 1995

Segraves RT: Antidepressant-induced sexual dysfunction. J Clin Psychiatry 59 (suppl 4):48–54, 1998

Spector IP, Rosen RC, Leiblum SR: Sexuality, in Psychiatric Care in the Nursing Home. Edited by Reichman WE, Katz PR. New York, Oxford University Press, 1996, pp 133–150

Thomas DR: Medications and sexual function. Clin Geriatr Med 19: 553–562, 2003

Wasow M, Loeb MB: Sexuality in nursing homes. J Am Geriatr Soc 27:73–79, 1979

Westheimer RK, Lopater S: Human Sexuality: A Psychosocial Perspective. Philadelphia, PA, Lippincott Williams & Wilkins, 2002

White CB, Catania JA: Psychoeducational intervention for sexuality with the aged, family members of the aged, and people who work with the aged. Int J Aging Hum Dev 15:121–138, 1982

Wright LK: The impact of Alzheimer's disease on the marital relationship. Gerontologist 31:224–237, 1991

Xu F, Schillinger JA, Aubin MR, et al: Sexually transmitted diseases of older persons in Washington state. Sex Transm Dis 28:287–291, 2001

Zeiss AM, Davies HD, Wood M, et al: The incidence and correlates of erectile problems in patients with Alzheimer's disease. Arch Sex Behav 19:325–332, 1990

Index

Page numbers printed in **boldface** *type refer to tables and figures.*